Food Science and
Nutritional Health

Food Science and Nutritional Health

An Introduction

Theodore P. Labuza

University of Minnesota

John W. Erdman, Jr.

University of Illinois
Urbana-Champaign

West Publishing Company

St. Paul   New York   Los Angeles   San Francisco

Photo Credits

Photographs on pp. 1, 119, 151, 211, 241, 277, 337, 355, 395, and 431 courtesy of the Food and Drug Administration.

Photographs on pp. 37, 293, 309, 375, and 457 courtesy of Land-O-Lakes, Inc.

Photograph on p. 329 courtesy of The Pillsbury Company.

The cover painting *Der Sommer* by Guiseppe Arcimboldo is reproduced with the permission of the Kunsthistorisches Museum, Vienna.

COPYRIGHT © 1984 By WEST PUBLISHING CO.
50 West Kellogg Boulevard
P.O. Box 43526
St. Paul, Minnesota 55164

Library of Congress Cataloging in Publication Data

Labuza, T. P.
  Food science & nutritional health.

  Includes index.
    1. Nutrition. 2. Nutrition disorders. I. Erdman, John.
II. Title. [DNLM: 1. Diet. 2. Food. 3. Nutrition.
QU 145 L127fb]
TX353.L22 1984   641   84–2295
ISBN 0–314–69660–1

In memory of
Dr. Howard Appledorf
who stimulated the ideas
for the first edition
of this book.

Preface

This book represents the cumulative changes that have occurred in the fields of food science and nutrition in the seven years since T.P. Labuza first published *Food and Your Well-Being*. And like *Food and Your Well-Being*, the purpose of this book remains the same: to provide a reliable source of information on the connection between food and health.

This connection is often steeped in controversy and exaggerated claims and, if anything, these controversies and exaggerations have become even more intense since *Food and Your Well-Being* was published. As this book goes to press, EDB is making news as a contaminant and many grain products are being recalled from supermarket shelves. In the recent past, there have been newspaper headlines on the partial banning of saccharin; news articles on sulfite as a cause of instant death; and an alleged connection between the new sweetener, Aspartame®, and brain dysfunction. These controversies will continue and new ones will appear; rarely will these controversies be completely resolved. This places the consumer in an awkward position: whom and what to believe, what to eat and what not to eat, and, above all, how to make the best choices for personal and family health.

These choices can best be made by being informed, by understanding the basic concepts of food science and nutrition. It is our goal to present these basic concepts in a clear and straightforward manner so that the reader can make a better connection between food and food processing, nutrition and health. The hope is that this book will be an invaluable tool in the home as well as in the classroom. Toward this end, and beginning with *Food and Your Well-Being*, John Erdman has extensively revised and expanded the coverage of nutrition in the first half of the book and Ted Labuza has revised and expanded the second half of the book on the technology and preservation of food.

Acknowledgements

No book is written alone, and we owe much to others.

Ted Labuza would like to thank his students for continually asking penetrating questions during and after class, the many consumers who call for help on food problems, the media in the Twin Cities area who call seeking a resource and, collectively, the FDA, the Food Drug Law Institute, and Peter Barton Hutt for instilling the legal sense which helped put the complex food/nutrition issue into a proper perspective. Finally, a large measure of thanks to those who endured the grueling two years of "working on the book," especially Mary Schmidl.

John Erdman would like to recognize the editorial assistance of Edith Erdman and Donald Thompson, the suggestions of Mary Grummer, and the typing of Rita Craighead. A special thanks is due his family and graduate students for their considerable patience during the preparation of this book.

Together, we would like to thank Gary Woodruff and Marge Johnson of West and the reviewers whose comments and suggestions materially helped shape the book into what it now is: Michael E. Mangino, Ohio State University, Clarice Schlickling, Orange Coast College, James Acton, Clemson University, Stan Biede, Louisiana State University. Michael E. Mangino deserves a special mention for his authorship of the accompanying Instructor's Manual.

TPL

JWE

Biographical sketches

Dr. Theodore P. Labuza

Dr. Theodore P. Labuza is a professor of food science and technology in the Department of Food Science and Nutrition at the University of Minnesota. Dr. Labuza is a native of New Jersey. He received a B.S. in Food Science at MIT and a Ph.D. in Food Science and Nutrition at MIT in 1965. After receiving his degree, Dr. Labuza taught at MIT in the Department of Nutrition and Food Science until July of 1971. At that time he joined the University of Minnesota. Dr. Labuza is the author of over 110 scientific articles as well as articles for the popular press concerning food technology and nutrition. He has written three other nutrition books: *Food For Thought* (AVI Publishing Company 1974), *The Nutrition Crisis: A Reader* (West Publishing Company 1975) and *Contemporary Nutrition Controversies* (West Publishing Company 1975). He is a member of many professional organizations. In 1975 he was the National Program Chairman for the Institute of Food Technologists and was responsible for its annual meeting. Dr. Labuza received the IFT award for outstanding research in 1972 and the IFT teaching award in 1978. Besides his regular course in food technology, he also teaches an introductory food processing course and a food law course. Over the last ten years, Dr. Labuza's major research has been in the properties of water in foods as related to nutrient losses and microbiological activity during processing and storage of dehydrated and intermediate moisture foods as well as developing methods for shelf life testing of foods and drugs.

Dr. John W. Erdman, Jr.

Dr. John W. Erdman, Jr., is an associate professor of food science in the Department of Food Science at the University of Illinois. Dr. Erdman received a B.S. degree in food science at Rutgers University. He worked for six months as a flavor chemist for Pepsico and served for two years in the United States Army before returning to Rutgers for graduate school. Dr. Erdman received his Ph.D in 1975. He joined the University of Illinois in 1975. Dr. Erdman is the author of over 50 scientific articles, many dealing with the effects of food processing upon the bioavailability of minerals from foods and others dealing with vitamin A metabolism in man and animals. He has co-authored seven book chapters, and since 1980 has written a monthly column for the magazine *Cereal Foods World.*

Dr. Erdman is a member of many professional organizations including the American Institute of Nutrition, Institute of Food Technologists (IFT), and the Society of Nutrition Education. He is a member of the Subcommittee on the Uses of the RDA, National Research Council, National Academy of Science. He has served on a number of national committees for IFT and is currently chairman-elect of the Nutrition Division of IFT. In 1980 Dr. Erdman received the Samuel Cate Prescott Award for Research from IFT. He has been recognized on numerous occasions by his students at the University of Illinois for his excellence in teaching. In 1983 the University of Illinois presented Dr. Erdman with the Excellence in Off-campus Teaching Award. Dr. Erdman is married and has two children aged three and seven.

Contents

Food Science and Nutritional Health

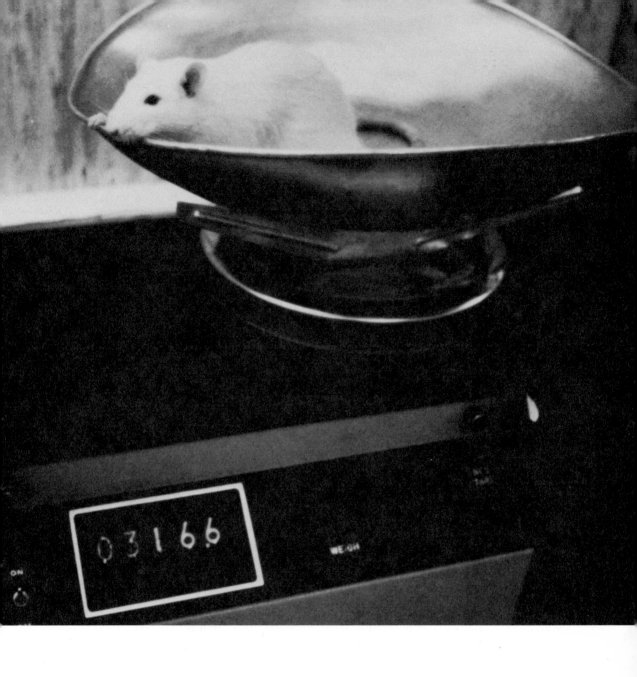

03166

NUTRITIONAL ADEQUACY AND THE STATE OF THE BODY

1

The science of nutrition is a very young science. Prior to 1900 there were few scientific investigators working on nutritional studies. Then the explosion came. New laboratory analytical techniques and a better understanding of biochemical processes resulted in a wide interest in nutritional research. In addition, the ability to synthesize organic compounds increased the study of the effects of various chemicals on health. No vitamins were discovered until 1910. By 1970 there were over 1,300 papers published on vitamin B_{12} alone, and in 1982 just one scientific meeting had almost 1,000 papers presented on various nutrition topics.

Unfortunately, much of this information has not been communicated to the public. This problem is due, in part, to our schools, which require neither an adequate science education nor an integrated food and nutrition education. Moreover, the scientific jargon of nutrition is often too difficult for most people to understand. Consequently, a person's ability to apply findings of nutritional research is limited.

So that we ourselves may begin to better understand how to keep healthy through a good diet, we will first define nutritional adequacy in the most simple terms. We should remember here that nutrition is the sum total of all the processes that occur in the body to break down foods into their various components. The body then uses these substances for growth, repair, and maintenance of all the systems that contribute to health. Food is the input to nutrition. Thus an adequate food intake is a prerequisite to nutritional adequacy, whereas an inadequate food intake can lead to poor health.

CHARACTERISTICS OF NUTRITIONAL ADEQUACY

What are some of the characteristics commonly attributed to nutritional adequacy (or inadequacy)? What state of mind or state of the body makes us feel healthy and gives us vitality? Factors such as body size, weight, longevity, ability to withstand stress, and ability to reproduce can be used as indicators of good health and thus nutritional adequacy. Biochemical and clinical analyses are also extremely helpful in determining nutritional status. Nutrition is not an exact science, however.

Each of us, due to our genetic makeup, differs in our needs for certain nutrients in our diets. Genetically, we all differ in our predisposition to chronic disease. Scientists often speak of the biochemical individuality of people. Just as each of us has different fingerprints, each of us is made up differently. Therefore, we must always think in terms of ranges of nutrient needs or average nutrient needs, not in terms of an absolute need for every person. One person may require 30 milligrams (mg.) of vitamin C daily and his or her neighbor only 15 mg.

Some of the measures we commonly use to define nutritional adequacy are discussed on the following page.

SIZE, WEIGHT AND LONGEVITY

Although body size and weight for a given age is most certainly affected by food intake, many Americans still believe that "the bigger, the better" is true. For example, when a baby is born, the question, "Is it a boy or a girl?" is followed immediately by another question, "How much does it weigh or how big is it?" As the reply to the second question increases in pounds, or length, the opinion that the baby is a healthy one increases accordingly. Certainly very low birth weight is undesirable, but a nine-pound baby is not necessarily healthier than a seven-pound baby.

Grandmothers worry that mother is not feeding the child enough and may try to induce the mother to do so. This attitude is challenged by the facts that show that a correlation may exist between "roly-poly" infants and fat adults. In the United States, over 30% of the population is considered overweight. As we will see in Chapter 12, being overweight may lead to serious health problems. Overweight people have shorter lifespans than the general population has.

The size question is interesting when comparing Japanese who have grown up in the United States with Japanese who were raised in Japan. Comparison between these two groups reveals that the American-raised Japanese are larger in stature than those raised in Japan. This is probably due to a different diet, but is this larger size desirable? Many observers of the Olympic games base the past success of Americans to some extent upon the larger size of the athletes. Yet, in these same Olympic games, the smaller Japanese people have been superior to their larger American counterparts in sports such as gymnastics and volleyball.

The life expectancy of laboratory animals (rats, mice) can be almost doubled by severe underfeeding of balanced diets to the animals from weaning until death. On the other hand, severe underfeeding during the suckling period shortens lifespan for animals. These studies clearly demonstrate the importance of diet in longevity. They suggest that there may be some optimal level of food intake at various periods of life that may extend the lifespan.

The average life expectancy of Americans has risen from 47 years in 1910 to over 73 years by 1983. This amazing increase of 26 years in the average lifespan has, in fact, been steadily growing over the last decade. Much of the increase can be attributed to a decrease in acute and epidemic illnesses, to better health care and awareness, and possibly to a more nutritious diet.

Many areas of the world outside the United States are not as well off as we are. During periods of drought, poor food harvests, or floods, thousands of children may die from malnutrition. Children who have just been weaned from breastfeeding or who are not receiving adequate replacements for breast milk are particularly at risk. The underfed, poorly nourished children of the world have a poor chance of surviving because of poor health care, poor sanitation, and inadequate nutrition. In some places in the world over 50% of children die before they reach the age of seven because they cannot resist various infections, such as measles.

The question of body weight and size does relate to the state of adequacy from a nutrition and health standpoint. Obviously there is a range of optimum sizes and weights for different ages, sexes, and nationalities. The underfed child and the overfed adolescent or adult are beyond these limits and enter into weight ranges that are associated with potential health problems. Medical experts use standard charts of weight and height to determine if a person falls into the normal category. This at least gives some means of measuring health. However, these measures alone do not completely define nutritional adequacy.

Size and weight are often used in animal studies to determine whether a certain diet is nutritionally sound. Rats, for example, may be fed two different experimental diets. One diet that is known to be adequate from previous studies is compared to a new test diet. The weight of young rats on these two diets is then compared over a defined period of time. The rapid weight gain, and thus the larger animal, is a sign of more adequate nutrition. Of course, these studies relate to animals, not humans; translating the results to us is sometimes difficult. Moreover, it may be unethical to test inadequate diets on humans.

ABILITY TO WITHSTAND STRESS

Another criterion for determining nutritional adequacy is the effect of stress on a person. The effects of stress may become noticeable while a person is fighting an infectious disease, doing strenuous work, or suffering from emotional problems. A person who is nutritionally sound usually can better withstand many of these stresses. This is because adequate nutrition helps maintain the body in an optimum state.

REPRODUCTION

A strong correlation exists between the nutritional adequacy of a woman and her reproductive ability and capacity. In those parts of the world where the mother has a nutritionally deficient diet, the number of low birth weight infants, birth defects, stillborn births, miscarriages, and problems during child delivery is very high. These problems can often be alleviated by an adequate diet. In general, nutrients needed to nourish the developing fetus are preferentially supplied to the infant. Therefore, if the mother has poor reserves of nutrients and a poor dietary level of nutrients, the fetus will utilize available nutrients and the mother will suffer. When the mother's nutritional status is very poor, both the mother and the child will suffer from nutrient insufficiency. Frequent pregnancies under these conditions are extremely harmful to both mother and children.

Children who survive periods of severe malnutrition may never develop physically or mentally to their potential. Some studies show that children who were nourished improperly, both in the fetal state through the diet of their mother and during life, had a lower intelligence/testing ability and poorer ability to withstand the stresses of childhood disease. Some studies indicate that the negative effects on learning and behavior caused by improper nutrition are partially correctable.

Unfortunately, in certain areas of the world, some of the poor dietary habits are closely related to the cultures of the people. Education about what constitutes an adequate diet and the subsequent implementation of better diets could help eradicate some of the nutritional deficiencies, but it is difficult to initiate such a program if the poor dietary habits are part of the culture, and there are no money resources to educate and feed. It is hoped that better diets can improve the mental abilities of the children and enhance their chances to live fuller, more productive lives.

Experimental nutritionists can evaluate the adequacy of a specific type of diet by feeding the diet to pregnant rats and determining the effect on the number of offspring and on their health status when they are born. We cannot, however, do this with humans for obvious ethical reasons.

BIOCHEMICAL, CLINICAL, AND DIETARY STATUS

The medical doctor can often spot a serious nutrition or health problem during routine physical exams. The physician can observe the condition of external parts of the body such as eyes, tongue, and skin, and can measure blood pressure, pulse, and heartbeat. In addition, medical laboratories can measure the levels of various important biological chemicals (such as nutrients) in the bloodstream and urine. We do not yet have adequate tests for all nutrients. But one day we may be able to routinely offer a complete nutritional examination. This would probably be the most valuable way to determine whether the diet we are eating is supplying all our needs and providing an adequate basis for good nutrition. For example, if the level of vitamin C in the blood were low, the physician could prescribe a vitamin supplement or, better yet, an addition of orange juice or some other good food source of vitamin C to the diet.

The reader should be wary of clinics that offer complete nutrient analysis of hair, blood, or urine and then prescribe extensive and expensive nutrient supplements based on their results. Nutrient analysis, especially of hair, is an inexact science and the results are difficult to interpret. Problems still exist in assessing the normal values for many nutrients. Moderate to severe deviations from the norm are evidence of nutrition problems, but linking these directly to disease state is often unwarranted.

The doctor can also rely upon information obtained from a dietary history of the patient. A 24-hour or seven-day dietary recall or record for the patient can be analyzed by computer. The results can indicate if the patient is making poor food choices.

Biochemical, chemical, and dietary analyses are valuable tools for indicating nutritional adequacy. However, interpreting results of these tests must be done with caution. Nutrient analysis is still an imprecise science. We must also remember that even the healthiest people become sick; thus, factors other than nutrition do contribute to health and adequacy.

TESTING OF NUTRITIONAL STATUS AND DIETS

A major problem exists in the design and execution of biological tests for nutritional status and measurement of the adequacy of a human diet. Part of the problem relates to the ethical issue of whether we can use humans when the test might cause some possible harmful stress or health problems. Should scientists or clinical nutritionists feed a pregnant mother a new diet to see if it affects the birth of her child? This most certainly could be considered an unethical experiment, but some studies using human subjects may have to be carried out. If the tests involve the use of a drug that may possibly save the mother's life, the decision to use the test is not as difficult. Human studies can be done if the benefit far outweighs the risk, as is the case with some lifesaving drugs. Human studies have been routinely carried out on healthy young men and women to assess, for example, the quality of different proteins. Nutrition tests are usually not dangerous, but if they have a potential to be so, animals must be used instead.

ANIMAL TESTS

If animals are used to study various diets or to determine biochemical data for human nutritional adequacy, a controversy arises. The problem is whether the study of nutrition in animals, such as rats, provides nutrition information applicable to humans. Through long experience, nutritional scientists have found that data collected from tests made on animals can apply to humans under some conditions but may be extremely difficult to apply under other conditions. For example, the growth of an animal on a diet of a certain nutritional value may correlate well with the growth of a child or teenager on a similar diet. A good correlation exists between humans and rats for protein requirements and for the requirement of some vitamins such as vitamins A and D. Diet studies related to reproduction also show similar effects in animals and humans. On the other hand, is it possible to study the effects of diet on the intelligence of animals? Can one state that one animal is more intelligent than another if it can make a choice between two color plaques in a Skinner box to get a food reward or if it can learn to run a maze? This kind of intelligence test with animals may not be a proper criterion for studying nutritional adequacy.

Another problem is that many animal species do not have the same biochemical pathways as humans. Simply, put, this means that some animals do not break down food into its various components and utilize them in the same manner that humans do. A good example of this dissimilarity between animals and humans is found with the dietary requirements of vitamin C.

Humans are unusual animals because they require vitamin C in their diets. Rats and dogs, however, do not need to consume vitamin C because they can manufacture the chemical in their own bodies. Therefore, the effects of a deficiency of vitamin C on the nutritional adequacy of humans could not be studied by using dogs or rats; an animal that requires vitamin C in the diet must be used. Fortunately, the guinea pig is such an animal and is often used when studying the effects of vitamin C deprivation.

Another question that occurs is whether an animal responds to a nutrient or to a diet in the same way that humans do. It is very difficult to use animal studies to calculate the needs of humans. When a special diet is studied we usually express the intake of the test nutrient, drug, or chemical, as in the case of toxicity tests, as the amount of the test substance fed per unit body weight of the animal. This is most often measured in grams (454 g. = 1 lb.) or milligrams (1 mg. = 1/1000 of a gram) per kilogram (1 kg. = 2.2 lb.) of body weight. If an animal is fed one milligram of a nutrient per kilogram of body weight and the animal weighs one kilogram, we could use this number when comparing it to the effects on a 70-kg. (154-lb.) human. We could assume that the same effects that were shown with the rat would occur if the 70-kg. person consumed 70 mg. of the nutrient, that is, the same level as the test animal, namely one miligram per kilogram of body weight. In this way we might be able to establish the minimal requirement of a specific nutrient in the human diet that just prevents any nutritional disease.

We should note that this type of extrapolation (animal to humans or vice versa) may be wrong in certain situations. For example, there were studies done on the effects of LSD (a mind control drug) that used animals as research subjects. In one case, a researcher injected an elephant with a dose of LSD that would effect a "high" in humans based on the number of milligrams per kilogram of body weight. Since the elephant weighs many kilograms, the dose was large. One half hour after the dose was administered, the elephant ran around in circles, trumpeted, defecated, rolled over, and died! A more serious problem would occur if we were testing a drug in an animal that is much less sensitive than man. The human could die or show some ill effects if the same dose were used. In fact, this occurred with thalidomide, an over-the-counter drug that was marketed in Europe. Pregnant mice showed no effects at four grams per kilogram of body weight, yet a single dose of one-half gram taken by a woman during the first months of pregnancy produced horrible birth defects in the fetus.

These are extreme examples of the problems with the scaling up or scaling down of doses in order to relate animal tests to humans. Direct correlation is not always valid and therefore cannot always be used with accuracy. In testing for the safety of food additives scientists regularly use the weight adjustment from animals to humans as described above plus a 100-fold safety factor. Thus, if one microgram per kilogram body weight was the safe level of use of a new food additive determined after extensive testing in rats and monkeys, then 1/100 microgram per kilogram body weight would be used as the upper limit of safe use for humans. This 100-fold safety factor thus protects against variation between species.

In the past, prisoners and people in mental health institutions were extensively used for dietary experiments. A number of cases of unethical research resulted from poor control of human experimentation in these institutions. In one case, normal female patients at a hospital were given without their knowledge, drugs that caused abnormal heartbeats to determine the effect of a second drug to correct this stress condition. In another case, a study of drugs for bronchial asthma was conducted among 130 children in which 91 children received ineffective treatment for up to 14 years so that they could serve as control group in the experiment.

The use of institutionalized persons such as prisoners and the mentally ill for nutrition and drug studies has been questioned by the courts. Fortunately, there are now human research advisory boards at all levels of human research that protect the subjects' rights. It must be pointed out that if human research is discontinued, progress in the field of nutrition will be slow. Human studies, especially those that are federally funded, usually require the filing of numerous forms detailing the experiment, disclosure to the person of the possible effects, and approval by a government agency. This is true even in studies of the characteristics of an artificial flavoring agent that humans must taste.

BIOCHEMICAL ANALYSIS

Another major problem when studying the effects of a diet or a nutrient in animals or humans is tracing the biochemical changes when the chemical is utilized in the body. The needle in the haystack analogy depicts the difficulty of the problem. People usually say it is difficult to find a needle in a haystack. One possible approach greatly reduces the complexity of this problem. By burning the haystack and sifting the ashes, locating the proverbial needle is very much simplified. However, even this has its dangers. The fire could possibly melt the needle or cause the barnyard or barn to burn. Using a magnet would be better (if the needle is made from iron) and would preserve the haystack as well. This second approach is the way the metabolism (the chemical pathways involved in the body) of a nutrient is studied. We don't want to destroy the animal, and certainly not the human, so we design an instrument or biochemical method that can detect what we are looking for.

In cases in which the nutrient is utilized in an unknown way another scientific search technique is used to find the chemical in the body. The chemical or nutrient is labeled by making it slightly radioactive. The chemical can be fed to an animal or, in some highly controlled cases, to humans. Various tissue, blood, or urine samples are taken, digested by acid, heated, or treated in some other way. The radioactive component is separated by this means and identified, much like finding the needle in the hay. This is a useful tool for locating products of the nutrients and drugs in various tissues and organs of the body. Furthermore, it is possible to discover what happens to these chemicals at the various locations in the body and thus to learn their functions. This method has led to many discoveries in the treatment of disease and in the understanding of nutrition.

On the whole, it is evident that some useful information obtained from animal experiments can be extrapolated to establish human needs. In order to better understand human nutritional needs, however, we must also discuss the composition of the human body compared to other living matter.

THE PSYCHOLOGICAL AND PHYSICAL QUALITIES OF THE BODY

The human body may be viewed on two different levels, the psychological and the physical. Certainly, for many of us the most important quality of human life is its spiritual and psychological health. Although psychological health can be considered a mental process, it is important from a nutritional standpoint because a spiritual or psychological state can very much affect physiological or nutritional status. For example, emotional stress can alter eating patterns and intestinal conditions. Digestion can be affected to a great extent in a person who is undergoing an emotional upset. A sound spiritual and emotional state is important for nutritional adequacy, although it is difficult for scientists to measure this. Proper diet is thought to conversely support optimal mental capacity. Therefore, the physical as well as the spiritual aspects of health are interdependent.

THE ENGINE

In order to determine the requirements of the body from a scientific biochemical approach, it is useful to consider the body as an engine. An engine is a machine that performs one or more functions. It requires an input (food) and releases an output (waste products). It also accumulates energy to perform work. In the human body, one type of accumulation is energy. Energy is needed for the work of growth when it occurs, for maintenance of tissues, for movement of muscles, and for basic body functions. Another accumulation is our mental activity and capacity. A primary objective is to make the body operate optimally and to give us a useful and healthy life. An interesting aspect of the human body is that it is a surprisingly efficient engine in that it has the unique characteristic of being able to repair itself, unlike most machines. Of course, not all parts can be replaced. Brain cells, for example, cannot be replaced, but the body has the ability to repair many injured organ tissues. This repair mechanism is important in terms of nutritional requirements, as will be seen in later sections.

In addition to possessing the qualities of an engine, the body can be considered an organic chemical plant. The body is made up of thousands of different biochemicals that are very important in terms of their function and structure. Biochemistry is the study of the metabolic chemistry of living systems. The food we eat is the chemical input needed to repair and maintain the body and to provide the energy needed to carry on the body's life functions. The wastes we excrete are the chemicals the body must remove in the process.

BODY COMPOSITION

Table 1.1 lists the major chemical elements of the body on a weight percentage basis. Four chemical elements account for 96% of the weight of the body. The rest of the body is composed of other

TABLE 1.1 Elemental composition of the body

Element	Percentage by weight
Carbon	18
Hydrogen	10
Oxygen	65
Nitrogen	3
All other elements	4

elements, most of which are the minerals that make up bone tissue. For instance, calcium accounts for almost 2% of body weight. Combining the weights of carbon, hydrogen, oxygen, nitrogen and calcium amounts to 98% of the body weight. Some other elements found in the body are phosphorous (1%), potassium (0.35%), sulfur (0.25%), sodium (0.15%), chlorine (0.15%), and magnesium (0.05%). When added to the others these elements equal over 99.9% of the total body weight.

Table 1.2 lists all the known elements important to the body as well as some of their functions. Twenty-one of the first thirty-four

TABLE 1.2 Nutritional adequacy: chemical elements and nutrition

Element	Nutritional Purpose
Hydrogen	Element in water and all organic compounds
Lithium	Possible use in mental disease
Beryllium	Probably unused; toxic
Boron	Essential in some plants
Carbon	Basic structural backbone of organic compounds
Nitrogen	Part of many organic compounds; basic part of protein
Oxygen	Element in water and all organic compounds
Fluorine	Growth factor in rats; strengthens teeth and bone
Sodium	Principal extracellular ion; involved in nerve impulses, muscular contraction
Magnesium	Required for activity of many enzymes; present in chlorophyll, bone
Silicon	Recently shown to be essential in chicks
Phosphorus	Essential for biochemical synthesis and energy transfer; part of the essential structure of bones
Sulfur	Required for proteins and other biological compounds
Chlorine	Principal cellular and extracellular ion
Potassium	Principal ion in cells; involved in nerve impulses muscular contraction
Calcium	Major component of bone, required for some enzymes, involved in muscular contraction, blood coagulation and nerve transmission
Vanadium	Essential in lower plants, certain marine animals, and rats
Chromium	Essential in higher animals; related to action of insulin
Manganese	Required for activity of many enzymes
Iron	Essential for hemoglobin and many enzymes
Cobalt	Required for activity of several enzymes, part of vitamin B_{12}
Copper	Essential in many enzymes
Zinc	Required for activity of many enzymes
Selenium	Essential for an enzyme system
Molybdenum	Required for activity of several enzymes
Tin	Essential in rats; function unknown
Iodine	Essential constituent of the thyroid hormones

elements of the chemical periodic table are important for the proper biochemistry of the body. This demonstrates the complexity of the human organism.

Zinc is one of the elements needed only in minute amounts in the diet. Because low levels of zinc are found in almost all human diets, no human dietary deficiency for zinc was noted until two decades ago. In the late 1960s zinc deficiency was recognized in certain places in the world as the cause of dwarfism and impairment of sexual development in young males. This nutrient deficiency and others can be recognized by health professionals and corrected by adding foods high in the deficient mineral or nutrient to the diet of the population of the area.

It should be understood that the body is not a random combination of these various elements. In a healthy individual the complex biochemistry of the body is well organized and efficient.

Some knowledge of the composition and chemistry of the organs and tissues of the body is important to understand how nutrition affects body function. Blood, which can be considered a fluid tissue, makes up about 8% of the total weight of the body, skin 7%, liver 2.5%, and the brain 2.5%. The amount of fat tissues can vary greatly.

The condition of the liver, muscle tissue, and fat tissue are extremely important when studying the nutritional adequacy of a diet. For instance, if one consumes an excess of alcohol and has a poor diet, the liver grows in size (hyperplasia) and the cells become infiltrated with fat. Scientists studying the effect of certain diets on an animal dissect the animal, remove and weigh the liver, and other tissues, and make a compositional comparison to normal tissue. Any significant change from normal tissue composition would indicate a dietary and/or health problem.

The amount of muscle tissue and fat tissue in a human may also be examined as a function of diet. The amount of fat tissue in humans can vary from as low as 13% to as high as 70%. If a person has a body composed of 50% or more fat, it is usually evident from the external appearance that a form of nutritional disease exists. It has been estimated that 30% of the population of the United States is overweight. This form of malnourishment occurs not because of lack of proper nutrients, but because of the excessive number of calories in a diet. Having a large percentage of the body weight composed of fat can, as previously mentioned, reduce life expectancy.

The other tissue that can vary to some extent from one person to another is muscle tissue. The range can be from 25% to 45% of body weight. A weightlifter may possess a large percentage of muscle tissue compared to body weight, whereas an average person does not have such a high percentage of muscle tissue. Despite a commonly held notion, excess consumption of protein has little to no effect on the amount of muscle tissue a person has. Only exercise can affect this amount.

As we get older there is a general increase in body fat and decrease in muscle tissue. Both these processes can be slowed by better control of food intake and continued exercise.

The composition of the body is about 60% water (see Table 1.3). The percentage of water varies among the different types of tissues. For example, muscle tissue, is about 75% water, about 20% protein, and about 3% fat. Bones, on the other hand, are about 20% water, 30% protein, very little fat, and 45% minerals. These measurements have been determined by analysis of cadavers and of organs removed by surgery. The bodies, tissues, and organs are ground up into a finely comminuted product. To measure water content, a portion of this product is put into a heated vacuum chamber where the water is extracted by drying. The weight of the remaining material is then measured; the weight lost is the water content. The protein and fat content can also be determined. Protein is measured by determining the nitrogen content of the tissue, while the fat content is measured by extraction with ether or some other organic solvent. Measurements of the minerals that are left are obtained by putting a portion of the dried tissue into a very hot oven (600° F) that burns off all the organic matter. The material left is a gray-white ash, the minerals. For this reason total minerals are referred to as ash in food analysis tables. Carbohydrates make up the remaining part of the sample. This same type of analysis is used to determine the proximate (gross) composition of foods.

Table 1.4 lists the proximate composition of some foods and living organisms. Compared to human tissue, cabbage, for example, has more water, ten times less protein, a higher carbohydrate content, 85 times less fat, and about 5 times fewer minerals. Obviously, studying the effects of nutrients on the growth and development of a

TABLE 1.3 Composition (%) of various tissues and organs

Organ or Tissue	Water	Solids	Protein	Fat	Carbo-hydrate	Minerals
Muscle	72–78	22–28	18–20	3.0	0.6	1.0
Blood	79	21	19	1	0.1	0.9
Liver	68–80	20–40	15	3–20	1–15	1
Brain	78	22	8	12–15	0.1	1.0
Skin	66	34	25	7	trace	0.6
Bones	20–25	75–80	30	trace	trace	45.0
Overall Body Composition						
	59–62	38–41	16–18	13–18	1	4–7

Adapted from FS201, University of Florida, Dr. H. Appledorf.

TABLE 1.4 (% By weight) composition of various organisms in comparison to various foods

Organism		H₂O	Protein	Carbo-hydrate	Fat	Minerals (Ash)
Microorganisms	E. coli	78	18.0	1.0	1.0	2.0
	Yeast	72	12.0	13.0	1.0	2.0
Invertebrates	Fly	73	20.0	3.0	3.0	1.0
	Scallop	80	15.0	3.4	0.1	1.4
Bird	Hen's egg	74	13.0	0.7	11.0	1.1
	Hen	56	21.0	trace	19.0	3.2
Mammals	Pig	58	15.0	trace	24.0	2.8
	Horse	60	17.0	trace	17.0	4.5
	Rat	60	30.0	trace	7.0	3.0
	Human	61	18.0	trace	17.0	4.0
Vegetables	Cabbage	92	1.4	6.3	0.2	0.8
	Onion	87	1.0	11.0	0.2	0.6
	Spinach	93	2.3	3.8	0.3	0.6
Meat (cooked)	Hamburger	57–70	16.0	trace	15.0–30.0	2.0
	Steak	49	15.0	trace	36.0	0.7
Milk—Cow's		87	3.5	4.9	3.7	0.7

Adapted from FS201, University of Florida, Dr. H. Appledorf.

cabbage would not give much information about the nutritional need for humans because the two are very different in composition, especially in the amount of vitamins, minerals, and proteins they contain.

Because the metabolism and composition of a human is close to that of a pig, the pig has been used in some nutritional studies. A major problem, however, is that pigs are too large to allow studying many of them at the same time, and they cost too much to feed and maintain. However, a miniature pig (about 200 lbs. fully grown) has been bred for nutrition and drug studies. Unfortunately, it is sometimes difficult to handle and at 200 lbs., the pig is still too big and requires a lot of food. The rat is the most common experimental animal used for nutritional studies, despite problems outlined earlier in this chapter. As seen in Table 1.4, the rat has much more protein than humans and less than 50% of the fat.

SUMMARY

In this chapter we have examined the concept of nutritional adequacy. Many factors can be used to assess the nutritional status of a human and the adequacy of a diet, including body size and weight, longevity, ability to withstand stress, reproduction, intelligence (to some degree), and biochemical tests. We have also noted that animal studies are most commonly used to determine the needs of the human to achieve optimum nutritional status. The relationship between humans and animals is not always clear, but if we carefully analyze the information, we can obtain meaningful results that may be useful in our study of nutrition. The composition of the human body is different from that of other animals and very different from that of most foods.

Multiple Choice Study Questions

1. Which item is probably the least precise measure of nutritional adequacy?
   A. condition of eyes, tongue, skin
   B. intelligence
   C. blood chemistry
   D. body size and weight

2. The most frequently utilized animal of those below in nutrition research is the
   A. rabbit
   B. rat
   C. mouse
   D. pig
   E. hamster

3. The major element in the body is
   A. carbon
   B. hydrogen
   C. oxygen
   D. nitrogen
   E. sulfur

4. Which component makes up the largest percentage of the average human body?
   A. fat
   B. carbohydrate
   C. water
   D. protein

5. Which component makes up the smallest percentage of the average human body?
   A. fat
   B. carbohydrate
   C. water
   D. protein

6. Which is not measured by proximate analysis?

A. fat
B. water
C. protein
D. fiber
E. vitamin C

Essay Study Questions

1. List the important criteria for establishment of nutritional adequacy. Discuss how they are used and determined.

2. Define and discuss the problems involved in the use of animals for nutritional studies of humans.

3. How is the proximate composition of a food determined?

4. Point out some positive and negative aspects of body size and weight with respect to health.

5. Does diet have any effect on intelligence?

6. What problems exist in ascertaining the measurement of the adequacy of a particular diet?

7. What are the pros and cons of the use of animals in studying human nutritional needs?

Things to Do

1. Keep a record of food intake for seven days. Using U.S. Department of Agriculture Handbook No. 456 or Appendix I calculate the nutrient composition and caloric value of each meal and average out the seven days. Discuss the difficulties in estimating serving sizes and in recordkeeping.

2. Try to relate eating habits to periods of good and poor health.

Chapter 1. Answers to Multiple-Choice Study Questions: 1, B; 2, B; 3, C; 4, C; 5, B; 6, E.

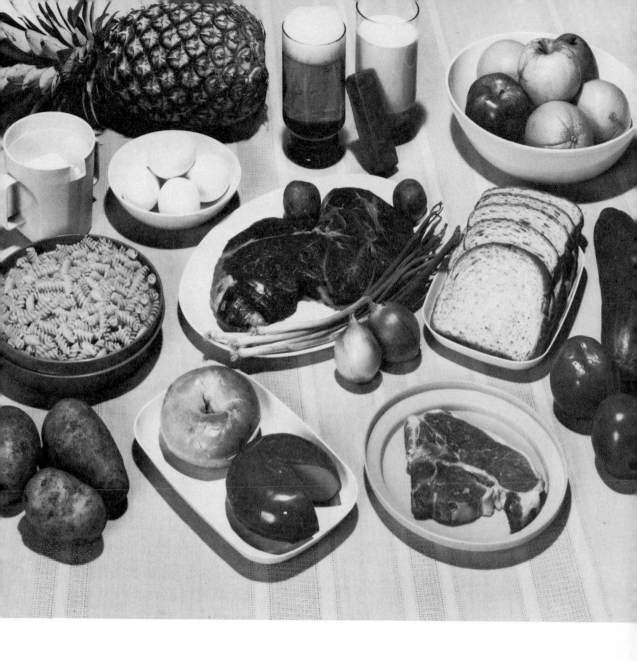

NUTRIENT REQUIREMENTS AND ENERGY NEEDS OF THE BODY

2

DISCOVERY OF NUTRITIONAL REQUIREMENTS

Epidemiology is the branch of health sciences that studies population groups to interrelate the effects of genetic history and environmental factors (including diet) affecting the group with the amount and type of diseases contracted by that group.

Epidemiologists have found that many of the deaths occurring from the time of primitive peoples through the Dark Ages were due to food poisonings and nutritional deficiencies. Many other deaths were due to the lack of medical care for minor injuries and wounds, which may have eventually become infected and resulted in death. The average lifespan during the thirteenth through the seventeenth century was about 30 years, mainly because so many young children died. Today, it is over 73 years of age.

It is probable that discoveries by early explorers would have been made sooner had there been a greater awareness of nutritional requirements. For example, as a result of nutritional disorders caused by diet deficiencies Vasco da Gama lost 60 out of 110 members of his ship's crew before he rounded the Cape of Good Hope. Historians tell us that the discovery of the New World and India and expeditions to other places such as the Arctic Circle, would have taken place sooner if the nutritional requirements of the body were known in order to prevent the loss of crews to illness.

In Vasco da Gama's expedition, scurvy was responsible for the high percentage of fatalities. Scurvy, a condition produced by the lack of vitamin C in the diet, caused stress on the body and lowered the body's resistance to disease. Death probably did not result directly from the lack of vitamin C but from the contraction of pneumonia or some other infectious malady that the body could not fight off.

Beriberi, a paralytic disease (polyneuritis) caused by the lack of thiamin (vitamin B_1), was also common in the past because of the consumption of polished rice in many parts of the world. As early as 2600 B.C. rice was polished. During polishing the hulls and the bran are removed and the rice is surface ground to make it white. This also makes it last longer, cook more easily, and taste better. Unfortunately, the people who polished rice did not know that the polishing process also removed essential B-complex vitamins, including thiamin. In the 1800s, Japan lost thousands of sailors yearly due to the prevalence of beriberi on board ships. The basic diet of these sailors consisted of white rice stripped of its B-complex vitamins by polishing.

Nutritional deficiency diseases have occurred frequently throughout history. For example, the work of Louis Pasteur in the 1860s revealed that milk carried two bacteria that caused deadly disease, brucellosis and tuberculosis. His discoveries showed that subjecting milk to a heat treatment killed these organisms and made it safe to drink. This was a great public health benefit; however, within one year after pasteurization was initiated on a large scale, scurvy became prevalent in children, especially among those living in large cities. The pasteurization process destroyed most of the vitamin C in milk. Even though milk contains very low levels of vitamin C, it contains enough to prevent scurvy. The milk was the main source of vitamin C for children in large cities at that time and the nutrient was destroyed by making the milk safe for consumption.

It has only been during the last 60 years that the basic causes of disease resulting from outright nutrient deficiencies have been thoroughly researched and understood. Many of the major discoveries concerning vitamins occurred between 1920 and 1950. Since that time it has become possible to prevent direct nutrient deficiencies by choosing the proper foods, using foods fortified with vitamins, or using vitamin supplements.

HUMAN NUTRITIONAL REQUIREMENTS

What are the specific requirements for individual nutrients for humans? What amounts will insure adequate nutritional status, not just prevent direct nutrient deficiency diseases? Nutritional requirements depend upon the nutrient in question, what stage of life cycle the person is in, his/her own biochemical individuality, and sometimes other factors such as body weight or caloric intake. Biochemical individuality refers to the fact that like fingerprints each of us has a unique biochemical makeup and a specific set of nutrient requirements.

The stage of the life cycle is extremely important. An infant or a growing child requires nutrients for growth of new tissues, whereas most adults are not growing and need nutrients primarily for maintenance and repair of tissues. Pregnant or lactating women have higher nutrient requirements to support growth of their fetus or infant child.

Availability of all essential nutrients during growth of infants and children is critical for optimal development of the child. In general the nutrient requirements for a two-year-old are higher, when expressed per kilogram of body weight, than they are at any other period of the life cycle.

A mature adult cannot ignore nutritional requirements just because he or she is no longer growing. Approximately one billion cells per minute are under constant repair and replacement in the human body. In order to grow and repair cells, the intake of nutrients such as protein is essential. The process is sustained by the energy supplied from the intake of fats and carbohydrates. Vitamins and minerals are also essential for carrying out the various steps in the process.

Based on studies with both humans and animals, and examinations of people who have inadequate diets, the requirements for each of the nutrients in the growth or maintenance periods of life can be estimated. For example, during the treatment of young children who have developed kwashiorkor much has been learned about protein requirements. Kwashiorkor is a disease resulting from lack of protein during early life (see Chapter 6).

Early studies in nutrition focused upon the search for the level of an essential nutrient that was necessary to prevent a serious disease. Information based on the history of diseases, as well as information from animal and biochemical studies was collected. A value called the MDR or *minimum daily requirement* was established for each nutrient. The MDR was useful in assessing the adequacy of a diet and was used extensively in dietary surveys throughout the 1960s. However, it did not completely serve the purpose of assessing the nutritional status of a large population and is no longer used by most nutritionists. One problem was that in most cases no adjustment in the requirement was made for age, sex, or other factors such as stress.

Nutritional scientists recognized that the MDR was established as a minimum for the population as a whole and did not account for the effects mentioned above. In addition, they realized that because each person has a biochemical individuality, the requirement of a nutrient varied somewhat from person to person. The scientists also recognized the fact that some people were misusing the MDR; they thought that if a given level of a nutrient was the minimum, consuming twice that level was twice as good, three times the level was three times better, and so on.

In 1943 the Food and Nutrition Board of the National Academy of Sciences–National Research Council (NAS/NRC) published the first Recommended Dietary Allowances (RDA) to "provide standards serving as a goal for good nutrition." The RDAs are not considered permanent and are revised based on the best scientific evidence available. The NAS/NRC, at approximately five-year intervals, publishes revised RDAs. The ninth revised edition was published in 1980 (see Tables 2.1 and 2.2).

The Recommended Dietary Allowances are the levels of intake of essential nutrients thought to be adequate to meet known nutritional needs of *practically* all healthy persons in the USA. You will note in Table 2.1 that RDAs are listed for different ages and sexes. This reflects the different needs of nutrients throughout the life cycle.

The specific RDAs are, in general, developed using a statistical approach. The RDA is established at a level above the average requirement level. This RDA level is carefully assigned after consideration of the variation of people's actual nutrient needs. Often the range of needs of a population for a nutrient forms a bell-shaped curve similar to the left-hand curve of Figure 2.1. The actual shape of the population curve is calculated from a statistical formula that includes information based on deviations from the average requirement. For example, if the mean value of the requirement for a

TABLE 2.1 Food and nutrition board, national academy of sciences–national research council recommended daily dietary allowances,[a] Revised 1980 (Designed for the maintenance of good nutrition of practically all healthy people in the U.S.A.)

	Age (years)	Weight (kg)	Weight (lb)	Height (cm)	Height (in)	Protein (g)	Fat-soluble vitamins			Water-soluble vitamins							Minerals					
							Vitamin A (μg RE)[b]	Vitamin D (μg)[c]	Vitamin E (mg α-TE)[d]	Vitamin C (mg)	Thiamin (mg)	Riboflavin (mg)	Niacin (mg NE)[e]	Vitamin B6 (mg)	Folacin[f] (μg)	Vitamin B12 (μg)	Calcium (mg)	Phosphorus (mg)	Magnesium (mg)	Iron (mg)	Zinc (mg)	Iodine (μg)
Infants	0.0–0.5	6	13	60	24	kg × 2.2	420	10	3	35	0.3	0.4	6	0.3	30	0.5[g]	360	240	50	10	3	40
	0.5–1.0	9	20	71	28	kg × 2.0	400	10	4	35	0.5	0.6	8	0.6	45	1.5	540	360	70	15	5	50
Children	1–3	13	29	90	35	23	400	10	5	45	0.7	0.8	9	0.9	100	2.0	800	800	150	15	10	70
	4–6	20	44	112	44	30	500	10	6	45	0.9	1.0	11	1.3	200	2.5	800	800	200	10	10	90
	7–10	28	62	132	52	34	700	10	7	45	1.2	1.4	16	1.6	300	3.0	800	800	250	10	10	120
Males	11–14	45	99	157	62	45	1000	10	8	50	1.4	1.6	18	1.8	400	3.0	1200	1200	350	18	15	150
	15–18	66	145	176	69	56	1000	10	10	60	1.4	1.7	18	2.0	400	3.0	1200	1200	400	18	15	150
	19–22	70	154	177	70	56	1000	7.5	10	60	1.5	1.7	19	2.2	400	3.0	800	800	350	10	15	150
	23–50	70	154	178	70	56	1000	5	10	60	1.4	1.6	18	2.2	400	3.0	800	800	350	10	15	150
	51 +	70	154	178	70	56	1000	5	10	60	1.2	1.4	16	2.2	400	3.0	800	800	350	10	15	150
Females	11–14	46	101	157	62	46	800	10	8	50	1.1	1.3	15	1.8	400	3.0	1200	1200	300	18	15	150
	15–18	55	120	163	64	46	800	10	8	60	1.1	1.3	14	2.0	400	3.0	1200	1200	300	18	15	150
	19–22	55	120	163	64	44	800	7.5	8	60	1.1	1.3	14	2.0	400	3.0	800	800	300	18	15	150
	23–50	55	120	163	64	44	800	5	8	60	1.0	1.2	13	2.0	400	3.0	800	800	300	18	15	150
	51 +	55	120	163	64	44	800	5	8	60	1.0	1.2	13	2.0	400	3.0	800	800	300	10	15	150
Pregnant						+30	+200	+5	+2	+20	+0.4	+0.3	+2	+0.6	+400	+1.0	+400	+400	+150	h	+5	+25
Lactating						+20	+400	+5	+3	+40	+0.5	+0.5	+5	+0.5	+100	+1.0	+400	+400	+150	h	+10	+50

a The allowances are intended to provide for individual variations among most normal persons as they live in the United States under usual environmental stresses. Diets should be based on a variety of common foods in order to provide other nutrients for which human requirements have been less well defined.

b Retinol equivalents. 1 retinol equivalent = 1 μg retinol or 6 μg β-carotene.

c As cholecalciferol. 10 μg cholecalciferol = 400 IU of vitamin D.

d α-tocopherol equivalents. 1 mg d-α tocopherol = 1α-TE.

e 1 NE (niacin equivalent) is equal to 1 mg of niacin or 60 mg of dietary tryptophan.

f The folacin allowances refer to dietary sources as determined by Lactobacillus casei assay after treatment with enzymes (conjugases) to make polyglutamyl forms of the vitamin available to the test organism.

g The recommended dietary allowance for vitamin B12 in infants is based on average concentration of the vitamin in human milk. The allowances after weaning are based on energy intake (as recommended by the American Academy of Pediatrics) and consideration of other factors, such as intestinal absorption.

h The increased requirement during pregnancy cannot be met by the iron content of habitual American diets nor by the existing iron stores of many women; therefore the use of 30–60 mg of supplemental iron is recommended. Iron needs during lactation are not substantially different from those of nonpregnant women, but continued supplementation of the mother for 2–3 months after parturition is advisable in order to replenish stores depleted by pregnancy.

TABLE 2.2 Mean heights and weights and recommended energy intake [a]

Category	Age (years)	Weight (kg)	(lb)	Height (cm)	(in.)	Energy needs (with range) (kcal)		(MJ)
Infants	0.0–0.5	6	13	60	24	kg × 115	(95–145)	kg × 0.48
	0.5–1.0	9	20	71	28	kg × 105	(80–135)	kg × 0.44
Children	1–3	13	29	90	35	1300	(900–1800)	5.5
	4–6	20	44	112	44	1700	(1300–2300)	7.1
	7–10	28	62	132	52	2400	(1650–3300)	10.1
Males	11–14	45	99	157	62	2700	(2000–3700)	11.3
	15–18	66	145	176	69	2800	(2100–3900)	11.8
	19–22	70	154	177	70	2900	(2500–3300)	12.2
	23–50	70	154	178	70	2700	(2300–3100)	11.3
	51–75	70	154	178	70	2400	(2000–2800)	10.1
	76 +	70	154	178	70	2050	(1650–2450)	8.6
Females	11–14	46	101	157	62	2200	(1500–3000)	9.2
	15–18	55	120	163	64	2100	(1200–3000)	8.8
	19–22	55	120	163	64	2100	(1700–2500)	8.8
	23–50	55	120	163	64	2000	(1600–2400)	8.4
	51–75	55	120	163	64	1800	(1400–2200)	7.6
	76 +	55	120	163	64	1600	(1200–2000)	6.7
Pregnant						+ 300		
Lactating						+ 500		

[a] The data in this table have been assembled from the observed median heights and weights of children shown in Table 2.1, together with desirable weights for the mean heights of men (70 in.) and women (64 in.) between the ages of 18 and 34 years as surveyed in the U.S. population (HEW/NCHS data).

The energy allowances for the young adults are for men and women doing light work. The allowances for the two older age groups represent mean energy needs over these age spans, allowing for a 2–percent decrease in basal (resting) metabolic rate per decade and a reduction in activity of 200 kcal/day for men and women between 51 and 75 years, 500 kcal for men over 75 years, and 400 kcal for women over 75 years. The customary range of daily energy output is shown in parentheses for adults and is based on a variation in energy needs of ± 400 kcal at any one age, emphasizing the wide range of energy intakes appropriate for any group of people.

Energy allowances for children through age 18 are based on median energy intakes of children of these ages followed in longitudinal growth studies. The values in parentheses are 10th and 90th percentiles of energy intake, to indicate the range of energy consumption among children of these ages.

nutrient is 14 mg. and the standard deviation (a statistical term denoting variation) is plus or minus 2 mg. as measured by surveys (i.e., the requirement is 14 ± 2), then about 68% of the population requires 12 to 16 mg. If the RDA is set based on two standard deviations above the mean for a nutrient, 18 mg. would be the RDA for this nutrient and this level should be adequate for a total of 97.5% of the total healthy population (if the original data were adequate).

The curve at the right of Figure 2.1 is an example of the average nutrient intake pattern of the population as a whole for a particular nutrient. How far it is displaced to the right or left would depend on the nutrient. For example, the curve for iron intake for women may in fact be displaced to the left side of the requirement curve. In the example shown in Figure 2.1, one can see that most of the population ingests much more of the nutrient than the RDA, with only a small percentage falling below the RDA. Over a certain period of time, those who have a high requirement and a low intake will be in a state of marginal nutritional status for that nutrient. It would be impossible, however, to determine precisely the number of people in this category without making biochemical tests.

The RDA should be applied to population groups rather than to individuals. Many schools, universities, and private companies now have computer programs that rapidly determine the quantities of nutrients in diets based on the food intake data supplied. There also are calculators on the market that do this. It should be remembered that this information can only be an estimate of nutrient status because it is based on estimates of food intake, and on average food composition data. Furthermore, the length of time over which the food intake is estimated influences the accuracy of the estimate. Some investigators only evaluate a 24-hour recall period, which is a poor representation of an overall diet. A seven-day evaluation gives much better results and is useful in assessing nutritional status of groups.

It is a misuse of the RDA to evaluate a 24-hour recall for an individual and make dietary recommendations for an individual based on that data and the RDA. As pointed out in the ninth edition

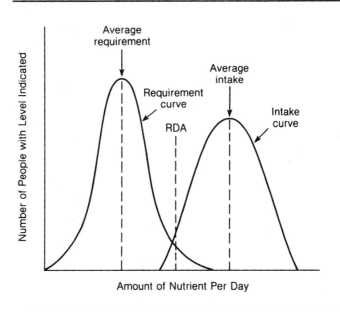

FIGURE 2.1 Nutrient intake and requirements

of the *Recommended Dietary Allowances,* "even if a specific individual habitually consumes less than the recommended amounts for some nutrients, his diet is not necessarily inadequate for those nutrients. However, since the requirements of each individual are not known (i.e., we don't know exactly where an individual lies in the bell-shaped curve in Figure 2.1), it is clear that the more (an individual's) intake falls below the RDA and the longer the low intake continues, the greater is the risk of deficiency."

Certain ranges of nutrient intake are often used to assess the level of nutritional adequacy. If the intake of a nutrient falls within 80% to 100% of the RDA, the diet is usually considered adequate; at 60% to 80% there is some cause for concern; below 60% the population may have a nutrient intake problem and some general population nutritional intervention may be necessary. Chronic intake of 60% of the RDA for a nutrient places the population in marginal nutritional status for that nutrient. Outright nutritional deficiency disease usually occurs only at extremely low intake levels.

Consuming nutrients at levels over the RDA will not make a person healthier and, in fact, may cause health problems as will be discussed later (Chapters 7 and 8) with respect to the vitamins and minerals. It should also be noted that RDAs for energy (calories) are not recommendations but are based on average energy expenditures for each age and sex group. Thus about half the population would be expected to consume less than the RDA for calories and the other half more.

The reader should be reminded that the values in Table 2.1 were established for healthy people in the United States. Other countries have established similar guidelines, but the values may differ, based on their interpretations of the scientific literature. For example, for women the NAS/NRC RDA for iron is 18 mg. while in Canada it is 12 mg. This does not mean that a woman consuming 12 mg. is nutritionally inadequate in the United States and is healthy in Canada. These are guidelines and should be used as such.

For the first time in the 1980 edition of RDAs, safe and adequate daily dietary intakes of selected vitamins and minerals were published (Table 2.3). These suggested intakes are based upon less complete scientific data and therefore must be regarded as more tentative than the RDAs. Due to potential toxicity problems, upper levels of intakes listed in Table 2.3, especially for trace elements, should not be habitually exceeded.

The RDAs have been used by the United States government as a basis in nutritional labeling of food products. Basically the USRDAs on a food label (see chapter 24) are the highest levels for a nutrient listed in Table 2.1. The consumer can compare nutritive value of food products by utilizing USRDA figures and serving size (see Chapter 24).

TABLE 2.3 Estimated safe and adequate daily dietary intakes of selected vitamins and minerals

	Age (years)	Vitamins		
		Vitamin K (μg.)	Biotin (μg.)	Pantothenic Acid (mg.)
Infants	0–0.5	12	35	2
	0.5–1	10–20	50	3
Children and Adolescents	1–3	15–30	65	3
	4–6	20–40	85	3–4
	7–10	30–60	120	4–5
	11 +	50–100	100–200	4–7
Adults		70–140	100–200	4–7

	Age (years)	Trace Elements					
		Copper (mg.)	Manganese (mg.)	Fluoride (mg.)	Chromium (mg.)	Selenium (mg.)	Molybdenum (mg.)
Infants	0–0.5	0.5–0.7	0.5–0.7	0.1–0.5	0.01–0.04	0.01–0.04	0.03–0.06
	0.5–1	0.7–1.0	0.7–1.0	0.2–1.0	0.02–0.06	0.02–0.06	0.04–0.08
Children and Adolescents	1–3	1.0–1.5	1.0–1.5	0.5–1.5	0.02–0.08	0.02–0.08	0.05–0.1
	4–6	1.5–2.0	1.5–2.0	1.0–2.5	0.03–0.12	0.03–0.12	0.06–0.15
	7–10	2.0–2.5	2.0–3.0	1.5–2.5	0.05–0.2	0.05–0.2	0.10–0.3
	11 +	2.0–3.0	2.5–5.0	1.5–2.5	0.05–0.2	0.05–0.2	0.15–0.5
Adults		2.0–3.0	2.5–5.0	1.5–4.0	0.05–0.2	0.05–0.2	0.15–0.5

	Age (years)	Electrolytes		
		Sodium (mg.)	Potassium (mg.)	Chloride (mg.)
Infants	0–0.5	115–350	350–925	275–700
	0.5–1	250–750	425–1275	400–1200
Children and Adolescents	1–3	325–975	550–1650	500–1500
	4–6	450–1350	775–2325	700–2100
	7–10	600–1800	1000–3000	925–2775
	11 +	900–2700	1525–4575	1400–4200
Adults		1100–3300	1875–5625	1700–5100

CALORIES DO COUNT: A DEFINITION

The recommendations for caloric (energy) intakes are listed in Table 2.2. Calories are a measure of energy. A certain amount of energy is necessary for maintenance and growth of the body. A calorie (cal) is the amount of energy required to raise the temperature of one gram of water by one degree centigrade. The Calorie (capitalized) used when referring to food energy is actually a kilocalorie (Kcal or Cal), which is 1000 times as large as a calorie, or the amount of energy required to raise one kilogram (approximately 2.2 lbs.) of water by one degree centigrade. To illustrate how much energy the Calorie is, it takes about four Kcal to melt three one-inch ice cubes in a drink of soda pop. This is the same amount of energy obtained by the body in burning (metabolizing) about one gram (1/28 oz.) of sugar in the body.

The exact number of Calories necessary for an individual varies. For the adult the amount usually ranges from 1,500 to 3,000 Calories (or more) per day. The higher value is needed by a person under more stress or with a higher degree of physical activity. The lower number might be required by a person of small body size whose physical activity is minimal, for example, someone with a desk job. Over the years, daily life in the United States has been simplified by an increase in mechanization, and caloric requirements have decreased proportionately. For example, chopping wood was at one time a part of the daily routine of many early Americans, but this type of physical exertion became unnecessary. Men and women also have different caloric requirements. Women usually need fewer calories than men due to their smaller body size and, in some cases, less strenuous work activities. Also, men generally have more lean body tissue (i.e., less body fat). Lean body tissue requires more calories for maintenance than does fat tissue. As stated previously, the caloric values in Table 2.2 are averages and not recommendations; close to 50% of the population for each category will consume fewer calories than listed.

Calories are supplied by the components of food. Protein supplies about four Calories per gram. The National Research Council recommends 44 to 56 grams of protein per day for adults. This is about the amount of protein present in 10 oz. of meat. Adult Americans usually consume 80 to 120 grams of protein per day, which amounts to 320 to 480 Calories. Thus, about 12% to 15% of the total calories in our diet comes from protein. Protein functions and requirements other than caloric value will be discussed in greater detail in a later chapter.

Carbohydrates also supply about four Calories per gram and make up from 35% to 45% of our caloric intake. As seen in Table 2.1, there is no recommended RDA value for carbohydrates. However, in order to meet energy needs, a minimum of about 300 grams of carbohydrates should be consumed per day. Many nutritionists stress that this should not be in the form of simple sugars alone, but that more complex carbohydrates in the form of starches should be included (see Chapter 4). Today, in the U.S., the various types of simple sugars account for about one-third of the total carbohydrate intake with starches supplying the other two-thirds.

Fats, another source of energy, account for the remaining 30% to 50% of our caloric intake. As with carbohydrates, there is no RDA for fat. In the U.S., approximately 100 to 150 grams of fat are consumed daily, averaging about 42% of the calories. One should note that there is a great difference between the caloric value of fat and carbohydrates. Even though a lesser amount of fat is consumed in the diet, more energy from fat is supplied to the body. This is due to the difference between the way the body metabolizes fats and carbohydrates. Carbohydrates and protein supply four Calories per gram while fats supply nine Calories per gram. Diets prescribed for purposes of weight reduction often advocate the intake of lesser amounts of fats because of their higher caloric content. The high intake of fats is also of concern because of the possible relation that has been shown between fat intake and heart disease. Many nutritionists feel that fat intake should be reduced to 30% to 35% of the calories or lower, and that the type of fat consumed should be changed. This issue will be discussed in depth in Chapter 11.

It should be noted that alcohol often supplies a significant percent of the calories in some people's diet. One gram of alcohol is estimated to supply about seven Calories.

Overall, the values of energy supplied by food components are:

> nine Calories per gram from fat,
> four Calories per gram from carbohydrates,
> four Calories per gram from protein, and
> seven Calories per gram from alcohol.

These values can be used to calculate the caloric value of foods, if the composition is known. For example, referring to Table 1.4 we see that a cooked steak has 49% water, 15% protein, 0% carbohydrate, 36% fat, and 0.7% minerals. Thus, for a 3.5-oz. (about 100 gram) piece of meat we have:

water:	49 grams × 0 Calories =	0
protein:	15 grams × 4 Calories =	60
carbohydrate:	0 grams × 4 Calories =	0
fat:	36 grams × 9 Calories =	324
minerals:	0.7 grams × 0 Calories =	0
	Total =	384 Calories

This is the way the caloric values of most foods are calculated.

The body needs other nutrients in much smaller amounts. In some cases microgram levels (one microgram = 1 μg. = 1/1,000,000 of a gram) or milligram levels (one milligram = 1 mg. = 1/1,000 of a gram) are required. For example, although calcium makes up almost 2% of the body, the RDA recommendation is only about one gram per day. Three glasses of milk (8 oz. each) will provide the needed calcium. The metabolic function of the other nutrients, vitamins, and minerals are discussed in Chapters 7 and 8.

CHOOSING AN ADEQUATE DIET

The RDAs are not very helpful for an individual in designing his or her own diet. The major problem is that people are accustomed to choosing and eating foods rather than adding up percentages of RDAs. It is our hope that this book may teach people that it is important to choose a variety of foods to insure nutritional adequacy and meet these needs.

A number of food group plans have been suggested to aid the consumer in selecting a balanced diet. Several decades ago the United States Department of Agriculture (USDA) suggested use of the Basic Four food groups. In 1980, the USDA added another group (called the miscellaneous group) that includes foods high in fats, sweets, and alcoholic beverages. This last group thus contains foods high in calories, but low in nutrients such as protein, vitamins, and minerals. Consumption of foods from this group should be reduced or eliminated when a person is overweight. Table 2.4 lists the Basic Four food group plan. It is useful in planning daily menus.

For those who want to determine specific nutrient content of foods, a detailed list of the amounts of nutrients present in foods can be found in the "Nutrient Value of American Foods In Common Units" Agricultural Handbook No. 456, published by the United States Government Printing Office. An excerpt of some of this data is in Appendix I.

DETERMINATION OF ENERGY NEEDS

Food energy values can be measured by burning food in a bomb calorimeter—an enclosed device containing oxygen. The heat energy so generated is then measured. Food energy value can also be calculated, as we have seen, from the composition of the food.

Human energy requirements and the energy produced in the body when we eat a food can be determined by placing a person in a chamber equipped with thermocouples (sensitive electronic devices for measuring temperature). The inward flow of oxygen and the outward flow of carbon dioxide are measured. To get energy values the heat gain inside the chamber is calculated, which is the heat output of the person enclosed. The amount of oxygen consumed and carbon dioxide released can also be used to estimate energy use. By this process the body's caloric requirements can be determined during rest or during some physical activity.

The Basal Metabolic Rate (BMR) is an important factor in overall energy requirements of an individual. The BMR is the minimum amount of energy in Calories (Kilocalories) per hour required to maintain the body while awake but at rest so that one is not undergoing any voluntary physical actions. To assure reliability and reproducibility, the BMR should be measured 14 hours after eating and directly following eight hours of sleep. This amount of energy

TABLE 2.4 Servings in the four food group plan

Food group	Recommended number of servings (adult)	Serving size
Meat and meat substitutes	2	2–3 oz. cooked meat, fish, or chicken; 1 cup cooked legumes
Milk and milk products	2[a]	1 cup (8 oz.) milk, 1–2 oz. cheese
Fruit and vegetables	4[b]	½ cup fruit, vegetable, or juice
Grains (bread and cereal products)	4[c]	1 slice bread, ½ cup cooked cereal; 1 cup ready-to-eat cereal
Miscellaneous category: Fats, sweets, and alcohol	variable [d]	

[a] For children up to 9, 2–3 servings; for children 9 to 12, 3 servings; for teenage and pregnant women, 4 servings
[b] One should be rich in vitamin C; at least one every other day should be rich in vitamin A
[c] Enriched or whole-grain products only
[d] Depends upon energy needs; moderation recommended

is the minimum needed for the involuntary body functions, including blood flow, breathing, normal muscle contraction, and the electrical and chemical functions of the brain. It has been found that the BMR varies with age, size, and sex. From birth to about 20 years of age, the basal metabolic caloric requirement increases due to the body's growth process, but above age 20 basal requirements begin to decrease. Older people may have weight problems partially because at age 40 a person may have the same eating habits used at age 15, while the BMR has decreased. This, however, is not the only reason for becoming overweight.

Men usually have higher BMRs than women, due to their larger body size. The basal metabolic rate has been estimated to be 1,200 to 1,500 Calories per day for women and about 1,600 to 1,800 per day for men. Diets that have a caloric intake of less than 1,200 Calories per day for women and 1,600 Calories per day for men may cause stress to the body by failing to supply enough energy to maintain normal body functions. Because of this, the body would have to burn stored energy sources, such as fat, to supply the energy requirements. Of course, these diets result in loss of weight and are the basis for dieting plans.

Any activity that exceeds basal metabolic functions requires more calories. Table 2.5 lists some of the caloric values of various activities for an adult in terms of total calories spent. This table includes the BMR in the values listed, but does not account for different body size.

TABLE 2.5 Estimated adult caloric expenditures of various activities

Activity	Calories per minute
Baseball	3.4–4.0
Basketball	8.6
Bowling	4.0–5.0
Canoe rowing	
slow (2–3 mph)	2.0–3.0
moderate (4 mph)	5.0–7.0
rapid (5–6 mph)	7.0–8.0
Classwork	1.0–2.0
Climbing	10.7–13.2
Cycling	
5 mph	4.5
9 mph	7.0
13 mph	11.1
Dancing	
slow	3.0
fast	4.0–7.0
Domestic work	
bed making	3.5
dusting	2.5
ironing	1.7
meal preparation	2.5
cleaning floors	3.5
standing	2.6
typing	1.6
washing	2.6
Dressing	1.5–2.0
Driving a car	2.0
Driving a motorcycle	2.8–3.5
Eating	2.5
Farm chores	2.0–3.0
Football	
touch	8.9
tackle	12.0
Golf	5.0
Gymnastics	
balancing	2.5
abdominal	3.0
trunk bending	3.5
hopping	6.5
Handball	10.0–13.3
Hockey	12.0–15.0
Jogging—slow	10.0–15.0
Reclining (watching TV)	1.5–1.6
Running	
7 mph	10.0
9 mph	11.0
12 mph	14.5
Shivering	5.0–6.7
Skating	11.1
Skiing	
moderate speed	10.0–16.0
maximum speed	15.0–19.0
Sleeping	1.0–1.2

TABLE 2.5 Estimated adult caloric expenditures of various activities *(Continued)*

Activity	Calories per minute
Squash	10.0–11.0
Swimming	
breaststroke	11.0
backstroke	11.5
crawl	14
Talking	1.0–1.2
Tennis	7.1
Walking	
2 mph	2.5
3 mph	3.5
5 mph	5.5
up stairs	10.0–12.0
Wrestling	7.0–9.0

Table 2.5 may be used to calculate a person's caloric expenditure. To do this you must make up the following list:

Activity	Minutes Spent		Value From Table 2.5		Calories Expended
_____	_____	×	_____	=	_____
_____	_____	×	_____	=	_____

One would keep the list for all activities in the day. The last value, Calories Expended, is equal to minutes spent times the value from Table 2.5. As a very simple example, Table 2.6 shows the calculations for an active young male based on average values from Table 2.5. This person is very active since the caloric expenditure was over 3,200 Calories for a 24-hour period.

If we were to examine how many Calories were consumed that day for the same student, it would probably range from 2,500 to 3,500. Studies with people show that on a day-to-day basis caloric

TABLE 2.6 Energy expenditure for an active young male

Activity	Time spent	Table 2.5 value Cal./min.	Total
Sleeping	8½ hr. = 510 min.	1.0	510 Cal.
Reclining (TV)	4 hr. = 240 min.	1.5	360 Cal.
Classroom	4 hr. = 240 min.	1.5	360 Cal.
Eating	2 hr. = 120 min.	2.5	300 Cal.
Handball	1 hr. = 60 min.	13.0	780 Cal.
Walking	2 hr. = 120 min.	3.0	360 Cal.
Dancing	1½ hr. = 90 min.	6.0	540 Cal.
Talking	1 hr. = 60 min.	1.0	60 Cal.
Total	24 hours	Total	3,270 Cal.

intake and expenditure are rarely equal. However, over several days' time, input of calories is often close to expenditure of calories. If weight remains constant over a long period of time, obviously the person is eating just the right amount to meet expenditures.

A person sleeping ten hours, eating three hours, and perhaps watching television the rest of the time would require only about 2,000 Calories. Unfortunately, many people do live such a sedentary existence, yet they eat over 2,500 Calories per day. Since one pound of body fat tissue is equivalent to about 3,500 Calories, a person consuming an excess of 500 Calories per day could gain one pound every week. This is because the body does not excrete the excess calories but stores them as fat tissue for future use. Calories from excess carbohydrates and proteins are also converted to fat. An excess of just 50 Calories per day would lead to a five-pound weight gain in one year or 50 pounds in ten years. Fifty Calories is less than one slice of toast or one-half glass of beer. This small daily excess is one important way in which people can gain weight. The weight gain is usually not rapid but instead is very slow and occurs without one knowing it. Increased exercise of any kind, even spaced over the whole day, would make up for this slight excessive intake. Fifteen to thirty minutes of walking or bicycle-riding would be more than sufficient to burn this extra 50-Calorie intake. Of course, this is difficult for many people to do, so they gain weight. A simple approach is to reduce food intake and do a moderate amount of simple exercise, even 10 to 15 minutes per day. We will cover obesity and overweight in greater detail in Chapter 12.

SUMMARY

We have seen that there is a series of different nutrient requirements needed to attain nutritional adequacy. The requirements for essential nutrients are met by eating a variety of foods from the four basic food groups: protein foods, dairy products, cereal products, and fruits and vegetables. In order for nutritionists to assess the quality of a population's diet, we can compare the nutrient content of the population's diet to that of the recommended dietary allowances (RDA). These are standards that have been set for different population groups and are revised periodically.

One basic nutrient requirement is the need to supply energy for the various processes that occur in the body. This is met by ingestion of carbohydrates, fats, and proteins. The caloric value of food can be calculated from the composition of these components in that food. The total calories we eat are important since an excess will yield an undesirable increase in body weight in the form of fat tissue. The important thing is to find the weight at which you function best and eat enough food to supply that caloric need as well as to supply the other desired nutrients. It is important to exercise and reduce food intake to lose weight. The caloric need can be calculated from energy expenditures for various activities.

Multiple Choice Study Questions

1. Biochemical individuality refers to
   A. the over 200,000 different chemical reactions that occur in the body
   B. the fact that only certain biochemical enzymes can help a reaction to occur
   C. the fact that each vitamin has a different function
   D. the fact that each individual may have a specific set of nutrient requirements that differ from the average
   E. none of the above

2. The RDA is
   A. the maximum amount of an essential nutrient necessary for health
   B. the statistical best estimate of the requirements for non-essential nutrients
   C. the recommendations for intake of fat and carbohydrate
   D. greater than the MDR

3. The RDAs were formed to establish
   A. the amounts of nutrients required by all individuals
   B. absolute nutritional standards
   C. recommendations for an ideal diet
   D. goals to aim for in providing nutrition to meet the physiological needs of groups of people
   E. none of the above

4. The RDA for calories has been established so that ___ percent of a given population group will be expected to consume less than the recommended amount.
   A. 2.5
   B. 5
   C. 20
   D. 50
   E. 60

5. The RDA for most vitamins is established to meet the needs of ___ percent of the population.
   A. 50
   B. 66.6
   C. 85.5
   D. 95
   E. 97.5

6. Nutritional risk could occur if the diet drops below ___ percent of the RDA.

   A. 100
   B. 90
   C. 80
   D. 70
   E. 60

7. Soy products like textured soy best fit into which food group of the Basic Four?

   A. meats
   B. cereals
   C. fruits and vegetables
   D. milk
   E. sugars

8. A Calorie is a measure of

   A. the amount of heat needed to synthesize a protein
   B. the heat derived from burning a food
   C. nutrition status
   D. the carbon content of a food

9. A Calorie is the amount of heat needed to raise

   A. 1 g. water 1°F
   B. 1 g. water 1°C
   C. 1 kg. water 1°F
   D. 1 kg. water 1°C
   E. 1 lb. water 1°C

10. Physical requirements over and above the BMR account for about ___ percent of calorie requirements.

   A. 0
   B. 10
   C. 20
   D. 50
   E. 100

11. The smallest percentage of total calories in the diet on the average is supplied by

   A. fats
   B. protein
   C. carbohydrate
   D. lipid

12. The most Calories per unit of weight (per gram) is supplied by

    A. starch

    B. alcohol

    C. olive oil

    D. steak

13. How many Calories are in a 100-gram hamburger that is 65% water, 15% protein, 1% carbohydrate, 18% fat and 1% minerals?

    A. 126

    B. 212

    C. 226

    D. 262

    E. 312

14. Calculate the approximate body weight gain (in pounds of fat) over a 10-year period for daily consumption of 1,980 calories, assuming an average daily expenditure of 1,900 calories, and no change in lean body mass.

    A. 16 lbs.

    B. 83 lbs.

    C. 8 lbs.

    D. 35 lbs.

    E. none of the above

15. Handball playing will consume 14 Cal./min. How many *hours* of handball playing will be required to reduce from 250 pounds down to 240 pounds body weight (assuming lean-body mass and water content did not change)?

    A. 2,500

    B. 25

    C. 42

    D. 4

    E. none of the above

*Essay Study
Questions*

1. What are the specific major nutrient requirements for humans?

2. Discuss the methods by which the RDA is established for an essential nutrient.

3. What is the difference between the RDA and the MDR of a nutrient?

4. How can the RDA be used to assess nutritional status?

5. What dietary problems might be caused by relying solely on the Basic Four food guide?

6. Define a Calorie and indicate how the body obtains it.

7. How are caloric requirements measured?

8. What is the BMR?

Things to Do

1. Calculate the percentage of RDAs for each of the vitamins and minerals from your seven-day diet survey.
   A. Are there any serious deficiencies?
   B. How can this be corrected?

2. Using food composition tables, calculate the caloric content of various canned fruits and vegetables. How does this compare to the value on the can label?

3. Using the Basic Four food guide determine which days met the recommendations and which days did not. How can it be corrected?

4. Make a 48-hour record of all activities and calculate the caloric expenditure from values in Table 2.5. How does this compare to the caloric intake average?

Chapter 2. Answers to Multiple-Choice Study Questions: 1, D; 2, D; 3, D; 4, D; 5, E; 6, E; 7, A; 8, B; 9, D; 10, D; 11, B; 12, C; 13, C; 14, B; 15, C.

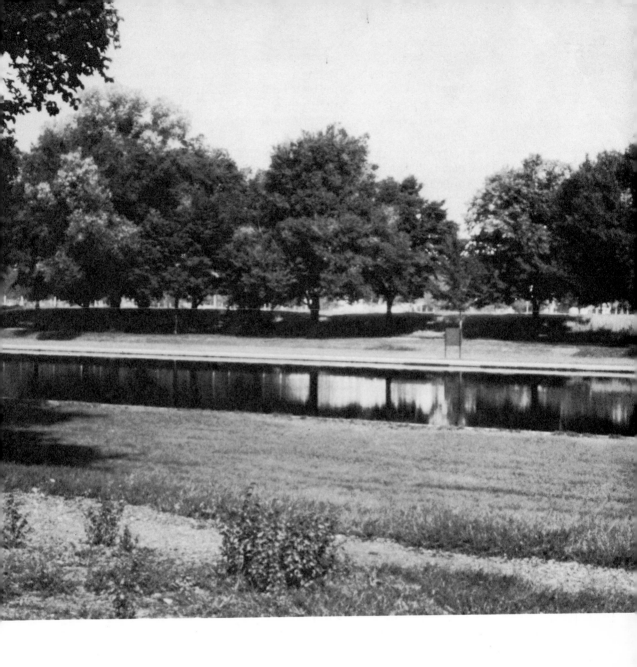

WATER AND OXYGEN: TWO ESSENTIAL SUBSTANCES

3

OXYGEN

Oxygen is probably the most critical substance for human metabolism. However, most of us do not recognize it as such because it is not eaten, but involuntarily consumed in the process of breathing. If the oxygen supply were eliminated, we would die in a few minutes.

Oxygen is consumed in the body in the respiration-reaction (catabolism) to form ATP, when fats, carbohydrates, and proteins are broken down. ATP or adenosine triphosphate is the compound made by the body that acts as an energy storage form and is the major energy source for most of our physical and metabolic functions. Thus without oxygen, we could not use our calorie sources, could not form ATP efficiently, and could not survive.

Ironically, human beings have an inefficient mechanism for utilizing the oxygen taken into the lungs. Close to 3,300 gallons of air (which is 21% oxygen) are breathed in each day. However less than 10% of the total oxygen in this air is utilized by the body for energy production. The rest is exhaled along with the carbon dioxide.

Carbon dioxide is a breakdown product from the catabolism (breakdown) of the calorie-supplying nutrients in the diet. As shown in Figure 3.1, carbohydrates, fats, and certain portions of the protein we eat (see Chapter 6) undergo respiration to yield energy, carbon dioxide, and water. Water from respiration may be exhaled from the lungs, perspired through the skin, or excreted in the urine or feces.

WATER

Water makes up about 60% of the human body. A human can survive only about four days without water. Water is consumed in several ways. Most of it is obtained by drinking approximately three pints of liquids (1,650 cc) per day in the form of water, tea, coffee, soft drinks, milk, etc. The water in the solid foods we eat contributes about 750 cc and the metabolic water (water that forms when sugar, fat, and proteins are metabolized to produce energy) amounts to another 350 cc. Output of water by the lungs is about 400 cc per day; perspiration through the skin amounts to about 500 to 800 cc;

$$\left.\begin{array}{r} \text{Carbohydrate} \\ \text{Fat} \\ \text{Protein} \end{array}\right\} \quad \begin{array}{l} + \text{ Oxygen} \longrightarrow \text{Energy } + \begin{array}{l}\text{Carbon}\\\text{dioxide}\end{array} + \text{ Water} \\[2mm] + \quad O_2 \quad \longrightarrow \quad \text{ATP } + \quad CO_2 \quad + \quad H_2O \end{array}$$

FIGURE 3.1 Catabolism of nutrients

by excretion in the urine about 1,700 cc; and excretion in the feces 150 cc per day.

Water Balance
The intake of water should equal the output of water. During the progress of some diseases, a condition called edema occurs in which water is retained by the tissues in the body. This is usually seen first as a swelling of the limbs. This condition is extremely dangerous if prolonged, since it usually indicates a salt imbalance as well as a protein imbalance in some cases. Drugs can be used to decrease edema, but the causative disease should be treated as well. Protein deficiency in the diet (see Chapter 6) can cause edema. In some cases the severity of protein malnutrition (kwashiorkor) may be masked by the accompanying edema, which reduces measured weight loss. Thus, mothers of children with kwashiorkor usually do not seek help until irreversible biological damage has occurred. Body weight is not always a good indicator of physical condition.

Uses of Water in the Body
Water has several functions in the body. It is a medium in which chemical reactions take place. It also serves as the means of controlling excess body heat through evaporation. Evaporation of one gram of water removes about six Calories of heat from the body. This is equivalent to raising the temperature of eight ounces of water from 68°F up to 83°F. Water serves a transport function. As the main constituent of blood, it carries the various nutrients to the tissues and carries away the metabolic toxic substances to the kidneys where they can be removed from the body. Water is a lubricant, functioning as the main component of tears, saliva, and mucus.

Water and Exercise
Frequent water consumption during prolonged exercise is essential for maintenance of water balance. Loss of body heat occurs by evaporative cooling in two ways: evaporation of perspiration and evaporation in the lungs. As a result, considerable water must be replaced during and after heavy exercise.

For a nonconditioned person, serious water balance problems (heatstroke) can occur if there is loss of 3% of body weight during an exercise session. Conditioned athletes can still perform with 4% to 5% body weight loss but this water loss must still be replenished.

Water should be replaced frequently during heavy exercise. Salt tablets are rarely necessary and can be dangerous, if not consumed with abundant water. Salts can be easily replaced by means of foods or by light salting of foods. Commercially available drinks that contain salts and simple sugars may be consumed. However, with major water loss some plain water should be consumed along with those drinks.

Water and Dieting

Extra water consumption is very important for people who go on high-protein or high-fat diets. In a high-protein diet that involves the consumption of large amounts of meat and eggs, there is an inherent simultaneous decrease in carbohydrate intake. Utilizing fat for energy produces acids and ketones in the blood. Without a high water intake, which increases urination and consequently flushes the toxic substances of metabolic origin out of the bloodstream, one could reach the state of excessive ketosis (see Chapter 5). Similarly, using protein solely for energy can result in uremia (see Chapter 6). Both these conditions result from a higher-than-normal level of metabolic products in the blood. High-protein or high-fat diets are thus not recommended because of the possible adverse health effects.

A person should normally consume at least one and one-half quarts of liquid a day. Diets that recommend the intake of lesser amounts of water are dangerous to the kidneys because the concentration of metabolic end products increases in the bloodstream with the potential to cause severe reactions. In addition, consumption of smaller amounts of water over a period of time may contribute to the formation of kidney stones.

SUMMARY

Oxygen and water are two of the most critical chemical molecules required by the body. Oxygen is used in the process of producing energy from our calorie sources. Water serves as the major tissue component and as a reaction medium. It is also involved in the process of controlling body heat through perspiration.

1. Oxygen is primarily used by the body to produce

    A. ATP
    B. RNA
    C. DNA
    D. protein
    E. fat

2. The water content of the human body is ___ percent.

    A. 20
    B. 40
    C. 50
    D. 60
    E. 94

3. How much liquid should an average person consume in the diet daily?

    A. 1 pint
    B. 1 quart
    C. 1½ quarts
    D. 2 quarts
    E. 1 gallon

4. Restricted consumption of water during heavy exercise leads to

    A. the requirement of higher salt intakes
    B. early fatigue
    C. improved performance
    D. fewer muscle cramps during exercise
    E. none of the above

5. What substance if we were deprived of it, would most quickly lead to adverse health effects?

    A. water
    B. oxygen
    C. vitamin B_1
    D. lysine
    E. protein

1. What functions does water perform in the body?

2. Discuss the needs of water for a person undergoing strenuous work.

3. What is water balance? (How is water consumed and excreted?)

4. Why is oxygen essential for humans?

*Things
to Do*

1. Using the dietary survey, determine the amount of water from each food.

2. Keep a record of liquid intake and urine excretion for several days. Using an estimate for fecal excretion and perspiration, determine your water balance.

3. Determine the viewpoint of athletic coaches and athletes on water consumption, and discuss these in class.

Chapter 3. Answers to Multiple-Choice Study Questions: 1, A; 2, D; 3, C; 4, B; 5, B.

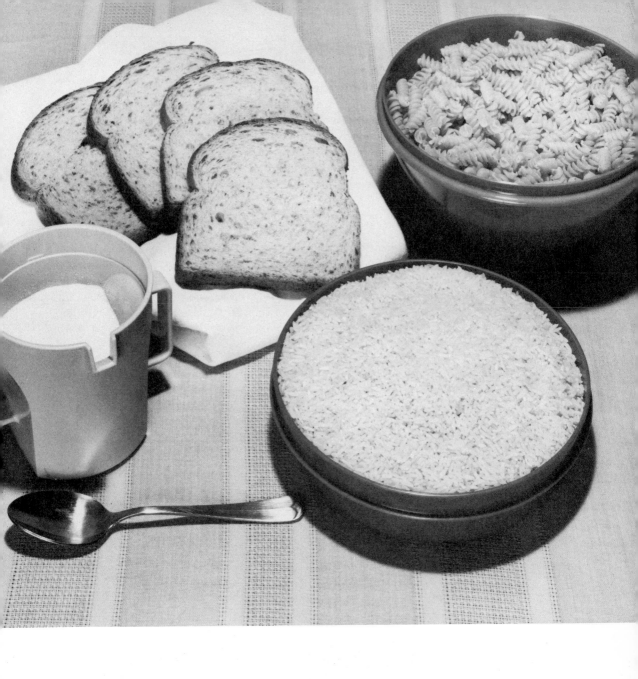

CARBOHYDRATES AND THEIR EFFECT ON HEALTH

4

THE DIFFERENT FORMS OF CARBO-HYDRATES

Simple Carbohydrates

Carbohydrates (sugars and starches) supply from 35% to 45% of the calories consumed in the average American diet. Carbohydrates are present in many different foods and in many different forms. These forms are illustrated in Figure 4.1.

Simple sugars are basic building blocks of all carbohydrates and are called monosaccharides. The majority of simple sugars in foods are made up of six atoms of carbon, twelve atoms of hydrogen, and six atoms of oxygen, as seen in the detailed structure. Glucose and fructose are the major types of simple sugars. They have exactly the same chemical content in terms of carbon, hydrogen, and oxygen but the atoms are arranged slightly differently. Most carbohydrates digested by the body are converted into glucose; glucose is the major carbohydrate that cells use to produce energy. Fructose, for example, may be readily converted into glucose in the body. Honey, as well as some corn syrups, have a high concentration of both glucose and fructose.

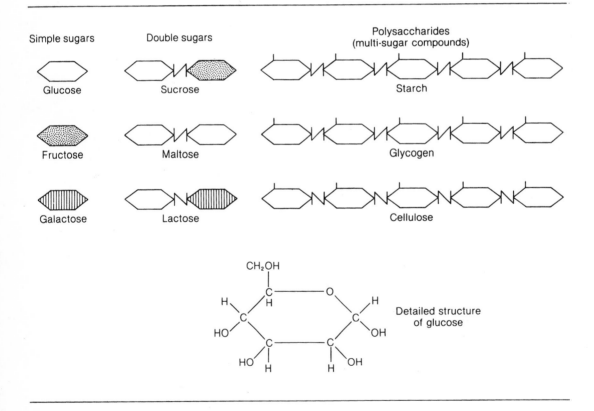

FIGURE 4.1 Carbohydrates

Another type of simple sugar is ribose, which has only five carbons. Ribose is important in the structure of the chemicals that make up the genetic materials of cells, RNA and DNA. Ribose is usually present in very low quantities in the diet and is not therefore considered a major energy source.

Disaccharides are made up of two simple sugars chemically combined. Sucrose, known as table sugar, is the most common example of a disaccharide. It is extracted from sugar cane or sugar beets. Sucrose is composed of one molecule of glucose connected to a molecule of fructose. It also has a very high level of sweetness and is used in many formulated foods. The body breaks down this sugar into glucose and fructose during digestion in the intestine. The fructose may then be converted into glucose, which can be used by the body for production of energy-rich components such as ATP. Glucose can also be used as a basic building block for synthesis of other chemicals.

There has been much concern about how much sugar, as sucrose, we eat. The average person is said to consume 90–100 pounds of sucrose per year or about 112 grams per day based on the total amount of sucrose used in this country. This disappearance figure has essentially remained the same for the last 50 years. Disappearance figures are based on the total production of a food item plus imports minus exports divided by the total population. Obviously, this figure can only be an estimate of an individual's intake, which can range from only a fraction to four to five times higher than disappearance. Sucrose is an important food because it is the most efficient food calorie source from an agricultural standpoint. For example, sugar cane or beets provide three times the caloric yield per acre that rice does and twice that of potatoes. Thus, it should not be discounted since it is an economical food that can supply considerable energy.

Total consumption of nutritive sweeteners averages about 130 pounds per person per year. As mentioned, sucrose accounts for 90–100 pounds, while the rest is made up largely from syrups, such as corn syrups, and high fructose sweeteners derived from corn. Intake of these corn-derived sweeteners has increased rapidly in the last few decades. Currently, high fructose corn syrups are replacing sucrose in soft drinks, salad dressings, jam, jellies, and other products at a rapid rate because they can create the same sweetness at a lower level of addition. Therefore, Americans are beginning to increase consumption of fructose and decrease consumption of sucrose.

Lactose is another disaccharide common to the diet. Lactose, milk sugar, is the natural carbohydrate found in both cow's and mother's milk. Lactose is made up of one molecule of glucose and one molecule of galactose, a six-carbon sugar compound, which has a structure very similar to glucose. Lactose is unusual because its occurrence is limited to mammalian secretions biologically intended for the very young. Most adult North Americans of European descent and most Western Europeans retain the ability to digest lactose throughout their lives. However, in many parts of the world, including the Middle East, the Orient, and the African nations, many people beyond childhood have difficulty digesting this sugar. The problem is created by the relative absence of lactase enzyme activity in the digestive tract. Lactase is necessary to break down lactose (see Chapter 9). As a result, the sugar passes into the intestine where bacteria begin to ferment it. Gas, diarrhea, and other problem conditions can result. Fortunately, the children are capable of digesting lactose because they have the enzyme during early life. Therefore, by consuming milk they are able to obtain the proper nutrient intake during the early stages of growth and development. It is only later in life that they lose this digestive ability. The same is true of many animal species such as cats and dogs. Today special packets containing the needed enzyme can be purchased and added to a quart of milk. Milk is held in the refrigerator for about 24 hours and the lactose (about 70% to 80% of it) is broken down into the simple sugars that the body can absorb.

Complex Carbohydrates

More complex sugars take the form of polymers. These molecules are made up of simple sugars that join together to form very long chains, much like the links in a long necklace made of beads as shown in Figure 3.1. In addition, these chains can form branches and thus produce a very complex structure. They are produced by both plants and animals to serve as storage carbohydrates as well as to impart structure.

In plants this polymer form of storage carbohydrate is known as starch. Potato starch and corn starch have molecules of glucose bound together in long branched chains. These are formed and stored in the plant to be used as the need arises. In humans the polymer form of storage carbohydrate is called glycogen and is one form of storage energy in the body. The main location for storage of glycogen is in the liver and muscle tissue. A total of about 300 to 350 grams of gycogen can be stored in these places. This accounts for almost 1,200 to 1,400 Calories, which can be made available for quick energy needs in muscular movement. This is also just about enough to meet the basal metabolic needs for one day. Under starvation or extended exercise the glycogen is used up rapidly. A false sense of weight loss occurs because the glycogen is structurally associated (bound) with a considerable quantity, three to four pounds, of water. When the glycogen is metabolized, the water is released and is passed into the bloodstream. To maintain balance, the water is eventually excreted in the urine. People who therefore deplete their glycogen stores through exercise or starvation will rapidly lose three to four pounds, but most of it is just water. As soon as food is eaten again, the glycogen along with water is redeposited and the weight is regained.

Fiber

The various types of celluloses, hemi-celluloses, and other complex carbohydrates as well as the noncarbohydrate lignin are poorly digested in the human digestive tract. These compounds are largely found as components of the cell walls of grass, wood, cereal grains, fruits, and vegetables and are known as fiber. Some of these chemical compounds are composed of long chains of sugars containing branches similar to some starches. They also may contain other chemical structures attached to the simple sugars at various positions. Interestingly, cellulose, like starch, is a polymer of glucose but the linkages between the glucose molecules in the cellulose chains are constructed in such a way that human enzymes cannot break down the connection. Therefore, we cannot digest cellulose and utilize it for energy. Hemi-celluloses and gum fibers, such as pectin, are only partially digestible and degraded by humans whereas lignin is almost completely indigestible. Hemi-celluloses, lignins, and gums have a sugar different than glucose in the chains.

Ruminant animals, such as cows, have a modified digestive tract for dealing with these fiber materials. When the cow chews grass and swallows it, it is deposited in the "rumen" or first stomach. The rumen is a "digestive vat" filled with bacteria that excrete enzymes to break the polymers down into simple compounds that can be used to supply energy. Humans do not have these enzymes in their digestive tract. The partially digested substance (the cud) is then regurgitated into the cow's mouth, rechewed, swallowed, and sent into the remaining portion of the digestive tract where the compounds from the digested fiber can be absorbed and used by the cow.

The relationship between the microorganisms in the cow's body that assist in the digestive process and the animal's digestive process is known as symbiosis. The same relationship is found with the termite. The termite cannot digest wood, but the bacteria in its mouth can, thus supplying food for the growth and maintenance of the insect.

Although the different types of food fiber sources supply little or no calories for a human, they are still very important in our diet. Fiber, like glycogen, can bind large quantities of water. Since it is poorly digested, it passes into the large intestine where it absorbs water from the body to become a large, but well-formed soft stool containing the other waste matter. Stools from diets high in fiber pass easily. An increase in dietary fiber increases the frequency and volume of defecation, thus acting as a natural laxative. In addition, the greater defecation frequency reduces the pressure in the large intestine, possibly preventing diverticulosis. Diverticulosis is a problem in many elderly people. Because of pressure exerted to pass hard stools, the large intestine may balloon out at various points where infections can subsequently develop. This problem, along with hemorrhoids, is said to be frequent among low fiber consuming populations, such as those found in the United States. Diverticulosis could possibly be prevented by increasing dietary fiber, but no direct evidence for fiber as a preventive factor in diverticulosis or hemorrhoids has yet been shown.

Based on epidemiological evidence, some toxicologists feel that fiber also helps prevent cancer of the colon. (Epidemiology is the study of the relationship between population statistics—such as incidence of heart disease, food habits—and health status.) In some parts of Africa, certain groups of people eat large amounts of fiber. They defecate three to five times daily and have a low incidence of diverticulosis and colon cancer. The theory is that the fiber helps to pass any toxic chemicals through the colon quickly. Thus, some nutritional scientists feel that dietary fiber is beneficial in reducing certain health risks.

Another factor attributed to dietary fiber is a reduction in the risk of coronary heart disease (CHD). This theory is also based on epidemiological studies rather than on direct scientific evidence. The reasoning given is that some types of fiber bind to cholesterol and bile salts in the digestive tract, preventing them from being absorbed into the bloodstream. Cholesterol in the intestine comes from the diet as well as from the bile excreted by the liver during digestion. Bile salts are synthesized from cholesterol (see Chapter 9). Pectin is one fiber that will act to remove cholesterol and bile salts from the body. More discussion on diet and heart disease can be found in Chapter 11.

There is very little information on the amount of dietary fiber a person should consume. The African's daily fiber consumption ranges from 25 to 30 grams, whereas in the United States it is only 4 to 6 grams per day. The many different definitions of fiber complicate this problem even further. Crude fiber, as measured by food chemists, is that organic material that is left after digestion by alcohol, acid, and alkali. However, this process digests more of the fibrous compounds than can be digested by the body. True dietary fiber values for food are anywhere from two to three times higher. Dietary fiber is that food fiber that we do not digest.

Table 4.1 lists crude fiber content in selected foods. A prudent suggestion for individuals consuming the usual low-fiber American diet is to increase the dietary level by about 3 grams of crude fiber per day. In a typical daily diet, this could be met by eating a large apple and one serving of popcorn or peanuts as a snack. Of course, this also increases the caloric intake, unless the high-fiber food replaces a low-fiber food. The reader should be warned that sudden increases in fiber consumption with fiber supplements, such as wheat bran, are not recommended. Not only may gas and discomfort follow, but very high levels of fiber may decrease mineral absorption.

As seen in Table 4.2 we have significantly decreased our consumption of complex carbohydrates compared to 1910 while total simple sugars have increased by 50% since 1910. Some reversal of this trend would probably be beneficial to our health. One problem, however, is that in areas where dietary fiber consumption is high, the incidence of stomach cancer is also high. Thus, massive changes in dietary patterns may decrease one problem and increase another.

TABLE 4.1 Crude fiber content of foods

Item	Portion	Crude fiber content in grams
Asparagus	6 spears	0.7
Beans, snap green	1 cup	1.0
Broccoli, flower & stalk	1 large uncut stalk	1.5
Carrots, raw	1 large	1.0
Lettuce, Romaine	3½ oz.	0.7
Lettuce, iceberg	3½ oz.	0.5
Lettuce, leaf	3½ oz.	0.5
Mushrooms, raw	10 small	0.8
Green onions	5 pieces, 5" long	1.0
Peppers, raw green	1 large	1.4
Apple, raw whole	1 medium	1.5
Apple, raw whole	1 large	2.3
Dried fruit	½ cup	2.0
Watermelon	1 slice	1.8
Cucumber	½ medium	0.3
Radish	10 small, 1" diameter	0.7
Celery	1 outer stalk	0.3
Tomato	1 medium	0.8
Bran, whole wheat, unrefined	2 tsp. (20 grams)	1.0–2.0
Bread, white	1 slice	0.1
Peanuts	3 oz. roasted	2.0
Popcorn	3 oz.	2.0

Adapted from Handbook No. 8 USDA 1975.

TABLE 4.2 Changing pattern of carbohydrate consumption; percentage of amount consumed compared to 1910. (1910 = 100%)

Carbohydrate	1920	1930	1940	1950	1960	1970	1980
Sucrose	113	145	127	133	129	135	111
Total simple sugars	116	143	125	131	127	135	140
Potatoes	76	67	63	53	51	55	54
Flours & cereals	80	75	66	55	47	45	47
Total complex carbohydrates	78	71	65	54	49	25	50
Total carbohydrates	84	82	74	66	61	63	64

THE USE OF CARBO-HYDRATES IN THE BODY

Carbohydrates are a source of energy, supplying the body with four Calories per gram. Energy derived from these carbohydrates is used in many different processes in the body. Muscle movement is an important use of energy derived from the utilization of glucose. In general, glucose and fat supply energy for muscle movement. Glucose is the major source of energy for red blood cells and other body cells. In addition, the burning of glucose for muscle movement creates heat that is useful in maintaining body temperature. The energy is produced from carbohydrates via a complex series of reactions. These reactions require oxygen for optimal energy yield and produce carbon dioxide and water as waste products. The carbon dioxide and some water is exhaled while the rest of the water is passed out of the body via urination and perspiration.

The Biochemistry of Carbohydrate Breakdown

The process of metabolizing carbohydrates is a complex series of chemical reactions that are represented in a simplified form in Figure 4.2. After sugars and starches are digested into monosaccharides, they are transported to the liver where they are converted to glucose. The glucose then enters the bloodstream where it can be transported to the cells where it is needed. The liver also converts some of the glucose to the storage form—glycogen. Excess carbohydrates are converted to fats and stored in fat tissues. Some glucose that passes into the muscle tissues is also converted to glycogen for storage there.

Within the liver some of the simple sugars are converted to body starch (glycogen) and stored until needed. When the body cells require more energy than is available from the free glucose in the blood, glycogen is broken down into glucose. The steps by which this occurs are very complex and are controlled by hormones. For example, when we become excited or increase physical activity, the adrenal glands release the hormone adrenalin. Adrenalin is a chemical compound that induces the enzymes of the liver and muscles to

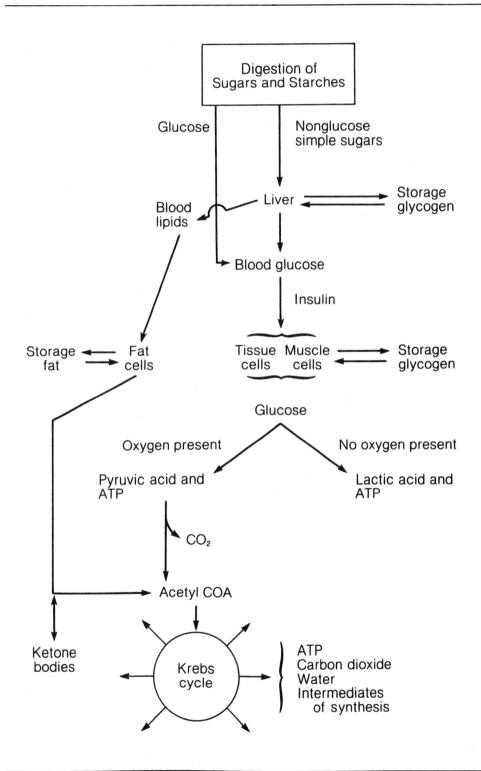

FIGURE 4.2 Metabolic pathway for energy production

cause the breakdown of glycogen. The glucose level in the blood then increases and glucose is distributed among the various tissues of the body. The glucose cannot enter the tissues, however, until another reaction occurs. A certain portion of the pancreas, stimulated by the increase in glucose levels in the bloodstream, secretes insulin (another hormone) into the bloodstream. This hormone enables the glucose to enter the cells (as yet, this is not a completely understood process). Once inside, the glucose can be metabolized to provide the energy for the necessary functions of the cells.

When glucose enters a cell it can be utilized in one of two different pathways depending on the availability of oxygen in the cell. Oxygen is necessary for the complete breakdown or metabolism of the sugar. Normally, an adequate supply of oxygen is available for this process. Under these conditions, glucose is broken down into two molecules of pyruvic acid, and two molecules of a high-energy compound called ATP are formed from two molecules of ADP. ATP (*Adenosine Triphosphate*) is a large molecule containing three phosphate (PO_4) groups. The addition of the third phosphate group onto ADP (*Adenosine Diphosphate*) to form ATP is a means of storing energy. The bonds between the phosphate groups are of "high energy." The energy stored in a molecule of ATP can be released for a specific purpose (for example, muscle contraction) when needed by simply cleaving off one or two phosphate groups. This energy-trapping mechanism allows us to store energy released from catabolism (breakdown) of components of our foods. ATP is the major high-energy compound for mammals.

Complete catabolism of the two molecules of pyruvic acid in a complex set of reactions called the Krebs Cycle, which was named after Dr. Hans Krebs, produces an additional 36 molecules of ATP from ADP as well as 6 molecules of carbon dioxide and water. Thus a complex set of reactions is necessary to completely catabolize glucose. Most of the reactions take place in the mitochondria within cells and require the presence of numerous enzymes and coenzymes. Mitochondria are small bodies within a cell that act as the metabolic factory site where the enzymes and coenzymes are packaged. Enzymes and coenzymes are necessary because a chemical barrier has to be overcome in order to initiate the reaction. The chemical state of the body at the normal temperature does not permit initiation of these reactions. However, the enzymes (which are largely protein molecules), sometimes associated with coenzymes (which are often forms of vitamins) and trace metals, act as catalysts to push the reaction along while the body maintains normal temperature. These reactions can therefore take place at a temperature at which they would not normally occur. This is one example of the subtlety of living organisms.

By studying these reactions, the functions of some of the vitamins we require have become evident. The reaction that initially breaks down pyruvic acid to acetyl COA (prior to the Krebs Cycle) requires three different enzymes and five different coenzymes organized into a multienzyme complex. Vitamin B_1 (thiamin) is one of the five vitamins in the complex. Niacin, riboflavin, and pantothenic acid are other vitamins involved as coenzymes in this set of reactions. Similarly, other reactions occurring within the Krebs Cycle require the presence of other B vitamins, some of which serve many different functions in producing the ATP through a process known as oxidative phosphorylation. If these vitamins are absent from the diet for extended periods, these reactions will not proceed and deficiency symptoms and diseases will occur (see Chapter 7).

Many acids are produced in the Krebs Cycle. Some of these, produced industrially by either fermentation or synthetically, are also utilized in food processing. For example, citric acid, one of the chemicals produced during metabolism of pyruvic acid, is used industrially to increase the acid level in foods. (Acidity is usually defined as pH where the pH is a measure of the hydrogen ion (H^+) content. A pH of 7 is defined as neutrality, a lower value means a more acid solution, a higher value is more alkaline. In the body the CO_2 produced from the Krebs Cycle helps keep the pH of the blood around 7.2, which is just slightly alkaline.) Addition of citric acids to foods is done for flavoring purposes as well as to prevent deterioration of the food by microorganisms. Microbiological deterioration will be discussed later. Succinic acid, fumaric acid, and oxaloacetic acid, which are other Krebs Cycle acids, are also used in food processing. When they are used as food ingredients, they must be indicated on the label of the food product as an additive. Some of them can be seen listed as part of the ingredient list on cake mixes and carbonated beverages. In normal metabolism these acids are present as neutral salts because the blood buffers them.

The Krebs Cycle is also important as it is the point of origin for many of the other chemical pathways that occur in the synthesis of the chemicals required for many of the body's functions, such as the production of building blocks for the synthesis of new protein tissues and hormones.

As indicated before, high oxygen levels in the blood and tissues are necessary for the complete breakdown of glucose. There are instances, however, when an adequate supply of oxygen does not reach the cells. For example, strenuous exercise can deplete the muscles of oxygen, i.e., the oxygen delivery from the lungs to blood to tissues cannot keep up with the demand. In this situation glucose does not break down into pyruvic acid; lactic acid is formed instead, along with two ATPs. Lactic acid causes the pH in the muscles to drop, i.e., it becomes more acid. Not only is this process inefficient (since lactic acid cannot be further broken down to yield more ATP or energy), but cramps may result when the muscles are overstressed in the absence of an adequate supply of oxygen. Fat stores in muscle may also be called upon to provide energy for muscle contraction, but this process also requires oxygen. Fat utilization will be discussed in the next chapter, but the pathway is illustrated in Figure 4.2.

CARBOHYDRATE INTAKE AND HEALTH

Obesity

Many people associate consumption of foods high in carbohydrates with calories and with fatness. Dieters often eliminate bread, potatoes, and other carbohydrate-rich foods from their diets. Sometimes these foods are replaced with foods higher in fat, and caloric intake is increased instead of decreased. For a balanced perspective on weight control see Chapter 12.

Diabetes Mellitus

Diabetes mellitus is a condition resulting from the failure of the pancreas to provide an adequate supply of insulin or from a failure of the tissues to adequately react to insulin. In this condition, a person can have high levels of glucose in the bloodstream after a meal, but the cells cannot take in the glucose to produce the needed energy. There are two major types of diabetes mellitus: early onset and adult onset. In the former type, there is a decrease in insulin production while in adult-onset diabetes, insulin production is normal, but insulin no longer facilitates cell uptake of glucose from the blood.

Under extreme conditions, a diabetic can go into a coma and shock unless there is a readily available alternative source of energy. Body fat can serve partially as this alternative source. A problem may occur when fat is solely utilized as the energy source. Under these conditions the Krebs Cycle may not provide enough ATP for the body. In addition, the central nervous system needs glucose as an energy source. Without glucose, nerve functions may begin to deteriorate and a coma can result. The ketone bodies and acids, which are produced during incomplete burning of fat, can be harmful to the body. One of these chemicals is acetone, which can be smelled on the person's breath. Persons with severe diabetes can develop brain damage caused by these chemicals as well as by the lack of glucose uptake by the brain cells. At low levels, the ketone bodies can also cause hallucinations. Some people with diabetes need insulin injections so that their cells can take in the needed glucose. Others must modify their diets to restrict foods high in simple sugars. Frequent feedings (five or six times a day) rather than three meals per day are preferred.

Obesity is highly correlated to the incidence of adult-onset diabetes. Statistics show that obese persons have a two or three times greater chance of developing diabetes of this type than are persons of normal weight. Obese persons who begin to show signs of diabetes (i.e., sugar in the urine) can often control the problem by weight loss and control of diet.

Hypoglycemia

In the last decade it was popular to blame a wide variety of symptoms on the "disease" hypoglycemia. Hypoglycemia, or abnormally low blood sugar, is neither a disease nor a diagnosis. It is a symptom of one of several rare conditions. Hypoglycemia is so rare that at the Mayo Clinic, where one-quarter million people come yearly with rare diseases, fewer than 100 have a bona fide hypoglycemia disorder. In the United States, people are spending millions on books and remedies to treat this "undisease." We are told that if we are irritable, impatient, depressed, or lack concentration we have hypoglycemia.

Hypoglycemia can be caused by several different factors, all of which are rare. As a result of genetic disorders, the intestine might not be able to digest the starches or sugars so carbohydrates cannot enter the body. This can result in a low blood-sugar level as well as in severe intestinal distress. However, the body compensates by utilizing fats or protein to raise the blood glucose.

In a second type of hypoglycemia, insulin is produced at too high a level so that glucose is too rapidly removed from the bloodstream. Low blood glucose results in insufficient glucose being supplied to the brain and can result in shock and coma. Low blood glucose also results if a diabetic person injects too much insulin. Some tumors that form in the body can produce an insulin-like compound that causes glucose to be rapidly removed from the bloodstream. This has the same effect as an oversupply of insulin. Contrary to popular belief, overeating sugar or sweets has not been shown to cause hypoglycemia. Neither has overconsumption of simple sugars been shown to cause diabetes. However, if caloric expenditures are less than the intake of calories, sweets can contribute to obesity and this can lead to diabetes in some persons.

Sugars and Dental Caries

Consumption of simple sugars, including sucrose, can result in dental caries. However, this does not mean that sugars and sugary foods should be eliminated entirely from the diet. Moderation of sugar consumption and proper care of the teeth are important to control dental decay. Research results with both humans and animals show that the amount of dental caries is a function of the amount and type of sugar consumed and the frequency of consumption. Recent work suggests that repeated eating of sugars over the day produces more caries than if the same amount is consumed in only two or three meals.

Caries result because certain bacteria in the mouth use the starches and simple carbohydrates for energy. As a result, they produce lactic acid. This acid can eat away at the enamel of the teeth. These bacteria stick to the teeth by forming a complex sticky matrix, especially at the gum line. Removing plaque material helps keep the teeth healthy. This is done by proper brushing, flossing daily, and periodic cleaning by a dental hygienist.

If sugars are consumed, the mouth should be rinsed with water soon afterwards or a liquid should be consumed along with the food to wash the sugar out of the mouth. The Tufts University Forsythe Dental Clinic has shown that the sugared breakfast cereals children consume with milk do not increase the number of caries. Some mothers have eliminated sugared cereals from breakfast for their children, replacing them with the unsugared types despite these scientific facts. Both sugared and unsugared cereals are a good source of energy and protein. Since children frequently consume milk and fruit along with the cereal they end up with a balanced meal. Most experts agree that it is continuous snacking on sugary foods, especially sticky ones (such as some candy or raisins), without proper rinsing or tooth care, that is the leading cause of caries. Thus, moderate use of sugar should produce no health problem, as was concluded by a report by the National Academy of Science in early 1976. More recent work has also shown that some foods, such as chocolate and cheddar cheese, may actually have an anticaries effect.

Alcohol

Alcohol is not a true carbohydrate, but it is best classified with this nutrient group. Alcohol produces seven Calories per gram and is absorbed very rapidly from the intestinal tract. See Table 4.3 for the caloric value of some common drinks. Alcohol consumption, even for the "social drinker," can result in a challenge to proper nutrition and health. Social drinkers consuming only three to four drinks per day, may consume up to 10% to 20% of their calories as alcohol. These persons must pay particular attention to the non-alcohol portion of their diet to insure that the remaining 80% to 90% of calories come from foods of high nutrient density (see Chapter 2). Often, however, social drinkers neglect fruits, vegetables and whole-grain cereal items and eat low nutrient density snack items. This practice may lead to poorly balanced nutrient intake.

TABLE 4.3 Alcohol beverages: Caloric values and alcoholic content of portions commonly used

Liquor	Measure (Approx.)	Weight (g.)	Cal	Carbohy-drates (g.)	Alco-hol (g.)
Distilled liquors					
Liqueurs					
Anisette	1 cordial glass	20	75	7.0	7.0
Apricot brandy	1 cordial glass	20	65	6.0	6.0
Benedictine	1 cordial glass	20	70	6.6	6.6
Creme de menthe	1 cordial glass	20	67	6.0	7.0
Curacao	1 cordial glass	20	55	6.0	6.0
Brandy	1 brandy glass	30	73		10.5
Gin, dry	1 jigger, 1½ oz.	45	105		15.1
Rum	1 jigger, 1½ oz.	45	105		15.1
Whiskey, rye	1 jigger, 1½ oz.	45	119		17.2
Whiskey, scotch	1 jigger, 1½ oz.	45	105		15.1
Wines					
California, red	1 wine glass	100	85		10.0
California, sauterne	1 wine glass	100	85	4.0	10.5
Champagne, domestic	1 wine glass	120	85	3.0	11.0
Madeira	1 wine glass	100	105	1.0	15.0
Muscatel or port	1 wine glass	100	158	14.0	15.0
Sherry, dry, domestic	1 wine glass	60	85	4.8	9.0
Vermouth, dry	1 wine glass	100	105	1.0	15.0
Vermouth, sweet	1 wine glass	100	167	12.0	18.0
Malt liquors (American)					
Ale, mild	8 oz.	230	100	8.0	8.9
Ale, mild	1 bottle, 12 oz.	345	148	12.0	13.1
Beer	8 oz.	240	114	10.6	8.9
Beer	1 bottle, 12 oz.	360	175	15.8	13.3
Beer (lite)	1 can, 12 oz.	360	96	2.8	12.1
Cocktails					
Daiquiri	1 cocktail glass	100	125	5.2	15.1
Eggnog (Christmas)	4 oz. punch cup	123	335	18.0	15.0
Gin rickey	1 glass, 8 oz.	120	150	1.3	21.0
Highball	1 glass, 8 oz.	240	165		24.0
Manhattan	1 cocktail glass	100	165	7.9	19.2
Martini	1 cocktail glass	100	140	0.3	18.5
Mint julep	1 glass, 10 oz.	300	212	2.7	29.2
Old Fashioned	1 glass, 4 oz.	100	180	3.5	24.0
Planter's Punch	1 glass, 4 oz.	100	175	7.9	21.5
Rum Sour	1 glass, 4 oz.	100	165		21.5
Tom Collins	1 glass, 10 oz.	300	180	9.0	21.5

Adapted from FSN 201, University of Florida, Dr. H. Appledorf, and Handbook No. 456 USDA.

Far more harm comes with chronic alcohol consumption. After years of alcohol abuse, the liver becomes infiltrated with fat and gradually loses its capacity to function. Toxic substances build up in the blood and other organs are affected. As a result of both poor nutrient intake and poor absorption, storage, and utilization of many trace nutrients by the alcohol, nutritional deficiency diseases are common in alcohol wards in hospitals. Symptoms of folic acid, thiamin, vitamin A, zinc, and other deficiency diseases are common in alcoholics.

ATHLETES AND THE USE OF CARBO-HYDRATES

Quick-Energy Food

Quick-energy foods have been reported to be useful for athletes. A few years ago, several liquid and solid products were put on the market and advertised as good sources of quick energy. However, it may take an hour or more for solid foods to be transported from the stomach into the small intestine where they can be absorbed by the body. Therefore, high solid content quick-energy foods such as candy bars, cookies, and so on do not provide immediate energy. Some nutritionists believe that the high energy "spurt" that some people report for certain quick-energy foods is actually psychological.

Quick-energy liquid drinks on the market are composed of sugars in the form of glucose, sucrose, and sometimes fructose. The remaining ingredients in the drink are salts that are similar to those found in the bloodstream. This liquid, if it is very dilute and contains no fat, can pass quite quickly to the intestine, where the glucose would be rapidly absorbed through the lining of the digestive tract. These drinks would thus begin to produce the needed quick energy within one half-hour of consumption.

High solid content food consumption during exercise can be dangerous if the athlete is sweating profusely and thus losing a lot of water from the body. When the product is consumed there is further loss of internal blood water and tissue water because the solids in the digestive tract must be diluted by large quantities of water. Water loss is prevented by the liquid products that are designed to have a solids concentration similar to that of the blood. However, they still should not be used in unlimited quantities because stomach cramps can occur (see Chapter 3).

Glycogen Loading

Glucose released from glycogen stores in muscle is an important fuel for muscles (except for heart muscle), especially during the first minute or two of exercise. After a minute or so, however, fat in muscle tissue begins to be broken down (see Chapter 5) and provides the major source of energy for the remaining period of activity. After a dramatic fall in muscle glycogen in the initial minutes of exercise, glycogen loss is slow. Total loss of muscle glycogen seems to occur simultaneously with fatigue of that muscle.

Weightlifting which requires short bursts of muscle activity, may rely only upon glycogen while endurance events such as long-distance running or cross-country skiing draws largely upon fat for energy.

Some athletes involved in endurance events use a technique known as carbohydrate or glycogen loading to increase their muscle glycogen stores. The athlete will consume a high fat and high protein (low carbohydrate) diet and vigorously exercise from about seven to three days prior to an event. This period depletes muscles of glycogen stores. Then, for the day or two just prior to the event, the diet is modified to a very high carbohydrate content and training is vastly reduced. This last day or two is the glycogen loading period. Well-conditioned athletes may increase their glycogen stores two- or three-fold with this diet-exercise modification plan. In addition, more glycogen is retained in muscle after long periods of intensive exercise and this is said to provide a competitive edge for the final part of the competition.

Problems associated with glycogen loading have been reported. The early low carbohydrate diet period often leaves the athlete fatigued, while the glycogen loading period gives the athlete a feeling of heaviness and stiffness. These latter symptoms are associated with large increases in water content in muscles. This water is bound to the newly deposited glycogen. There have also been reports of cardiac pain and abnormal electrocardiograms after glycogen loading.

Based upon the possible harm to heart function, glycogen loading cannot be recommended for athletes unless supervised by a competent physician. Furthermore, even the best-trained and supervised world-class athlete should not undergo this diet plan more than two or three times a year. The college or high school competitor is likely to lose more from fatigue and/or heaviness and stiffness during training than he or she will gain at the end of an event.

Wrestlers who starve themselves before an event also create an endurance problem for themselves. They usually reduce food consumption drastically so they can compete in a lower weight class. Others may even try to sweat off more weight by using a hot sauna. What happens is that they deplete their glycogen stores (along with three to four pounds of water) and sweat off a lot of water. With no energy stores, fats must be used for energy during the competition, which cannot yield the needed energy as quickly. The water loss is also detrimental in competition.

SUMMARY

Carbohydrates are a major source of energy in the body. They can be found in most foods in both simple and complex forms. The simple carbohydrates are the sugars such as glucose, fructose, and sucrose; the complex ones are polymers made up of long chains of simple sugars. In metabolism, most sugars are converted into glucose, which serves as the major energy source for cellular processes. When utilized, the glucose forms water, carbon dioxide, heat, and ATP. The latter is the major energy storage molecule used in all reactions in the body.

Much controversy exists about carbohydrate nutrition. Of recent interest is dietary fiber, an undigestable form of carbohydrate. Some nutritionists suggest increasing fiber consumption to decrease risk of diverticulosis, coronary heart disease, and colon cancer. It has also been suggested that reduction of sucrose intake would reduce dental caries significantly. Although all these corrections have not been borne out scientifically, some modification of the diet to increase dietary fiber and decrease simple sugar intake of the population would be prudent.

Multiple Choice Study Questions

1. Sucrose is made up of
   A. glucose and galactose
   B. glucose and ribose
   C. glucose and fructose
   D. ribose and lactose
   E. lactose and galactose

2. Which of the following is not a disaccharide?
   A. maltose
   B. fructose
   C. sucrose
   D. lactose

3. Glucose supplies four Calories per gram. The same amount would also be supplied by
   A. dry potato starch
   B. linoleic acid
   C. alcohol
   D. fluid whole milk

4. Which of the following is the storage starch of man?
   A. cellulose
   B. amylose
   C. lactose
   D. glycogen

5. Lactose is the major carbohydrate found in
   A. bread
   B. meat
   C. milk
   D. blood
   E. beer

6. Honey contains mainly

    A. sucrose and xylose

    B. raffinose and stachiose

    C. ribose and marmose

    D. glucose and fructose

    E. maltose and lactose

7. Besides carbon dioxide, what is formed when one molecule of glucose is totally burned?

    A. one molecule of water

    B. two ATPs

    C. three molecules of water

    D. eight ATPs

    E. six molecules of water

8. Excess sugar in the diet is mainly converted to

    A. adrenalin

    B. protein

    C. fat

    D. insulin

    E. cellulose

9. Sugar is stored in the body as

    A. cellulose

    B. cellophane

    C. glucagon

    D. glycogen

    E. insulin

10. Diabetes can be the result of

    A. excess glycogen production

    B. low glycogen levels in the blood

    C. excess bile salts

    D. excess insulin production

    E. too little insulin production

11. True hypoglycemia is the result of

    A. excess glycogen production

    B. low glycogen levels in the blood

    C. excess bile salts

    D. excess insulin production

    E. too little insulin

12. Dietary fiber

    A. is not the same as crude fiber

    B. increases the fecal excretion of bile salts, fats, and sterols

    C. is not digestible by the human system

    D. all of the above

    E. none of the above

13. Which of the following average servings provides the lowest dietary fiber content?

A. 3 oz. meat
B. 3 oz. popcorn
C. 1 medium apple
D. 1 slice watermelon
E. 1 cup green beans

14. Dietary fiber consumption is probably not related to

A. diverticulosis
B. stool size
C. diabetes
D. coronary heart disease (CHD)
E. colon cancer

15. A recommended daily intake of crude fiber by the adult in the U.S. diet is

A. 2–3 grams
B. 4–6 grams
C. 10–12 grams
D. 15–20 grams
E. 25 grams

*Essay Study
Questions*

1. What differentiates simple carbohydrates from complex carbohydrates?

2. What is lactose intolerance?

3. What is dietary fiber and what are the potential benefits of increased consumption of it?

4. What is the difference between plant starch and glycogen?

5. What is epidemiology?

6. Discuss the metabolism of carbohydrates to form ATP.

7. What is diabetes?

8. Explain the concept of glycogen loading used by athletes for long-distance events.

9. Discuss the evidence connecting dental caries with the consumption of carbohydrates.

10. What is hypoglycemia?

*Things
to Do*

1. Obtain food labels. Determine the types of added carbohydrates and the fiber content.

2. Obtain a pH meter or pH paper. Using a blender, make slurries of various foods and measure their pH. Prepare a pH chart with the various foods marked on it.

3. Obtain a test kit for ketone bodies from a pharmacy. Check for the presence of ketones in the urine of normal people and people on various diets.

4. Design two diets, one with less than 20% carbohydrates and one with about 50% carbohydrates.

Chapter 4. Answers to Multiple-Choice Study Questions: 1, C; 2, B; 3, A; 4, D; 5, C; 6, D; 7, E; 8, C; 9, D; 10, E; 11, D; 12, D; 13, A; 14, C; 15, C.

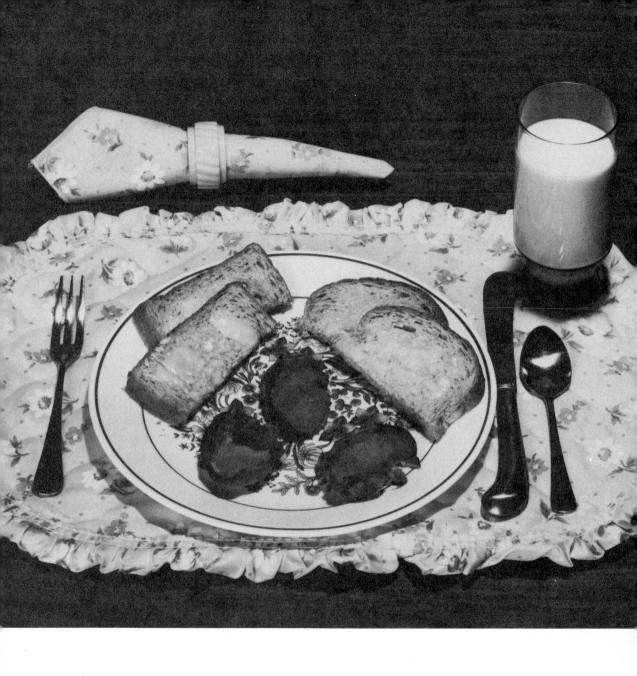

FATS, FATTY ACIDS, AND CHOLESTEROL

5

COMPOSITION OF FATS

About 30% to 50% of the calories in the diets of Americans is derived from the various types of fats. Fats are complicated molecules containing less oxygen per unit of carbon and hydrogen than is found in carbohydrates. Because there is proportionately less oxygen, the complete metabolism of fats demands more oxygen and thus fats produce more energy, approximately nine Calories per gram compared to four Calories per gram from carbohydrates.

TRIGLYCERIDES

Figure 5.1 shows the structural appearance of a triglyceride, which is the most prevalent fat molecule found in most foods and body tissues. The molecule is composed of three fatty acids connected to a glycerol molecule. Triglycerides serve as the major storehouse of fats in the human body as well as in animal and some plant tissues.

The backbone of the triglyceride fat molecule is a molecule of glycerol. Glycerol is an intermediate product in the metabolic pathway where glucose is converted to pyruvic acid. To the backbone of glycerol are attached fatty acids. Fatty acids are long-chained polymers of carbon atoms (see Figure 5.2).

Figure 5.1 also shows two other kinds of fat molecules found in much lower levels in foods and in the body. A monoglyceride has only one fatty acid connected to the glycerol; a diglyceride has two fatty acids on the glycerol molecule. Labels of many foods such as salad dressings and breads show that they contain monoglycerides and diglycerides as food additives (see Chapter 21). These chemicals are used because the molecules, due to their structures, possess the unusual property of being able to stabilize foams and emulsions. They concentrate at the water/oil interface and keep oil or water drops in suspension. Although these food additives are usually made synthetically, they closely resemble their natural counterparts.

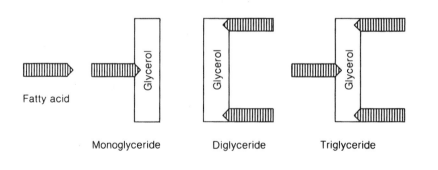

Fatty acid

Monoglyceride   Diglyceride   Triglyceride

FIGURE 5.1 Monoglycerides, diglycerides, and triglycerides

FATTY ACIDS

The fatty acids that are important in the functioning of the human body are separated into two types: saturated and unsaturated. A triglyceride, which contains mostly saturated fatty acids, is usually a solid at room temperature. The fat found in beef is an example of triglycerides made up of mostly saturated fatty acids. They do not melt from the tissue unless they are heated. One saturated fatty acid found commonly in animal tissue is stearic acid. It has 18 carbons connected in a long chain (see Figure 5.2.).

Triglycerides contain many different saturated fatty acids. For example, Figure 5.2 shows the structure of the 16-carbon palmitic acid, which is found in high concentrations in palm kernel oil. Palm oil is becoming one of the more important fats in making salad dressings and margarine. Also shown is butyric acid. This fatty acid is found in butter fat and has only four carbons. One form of

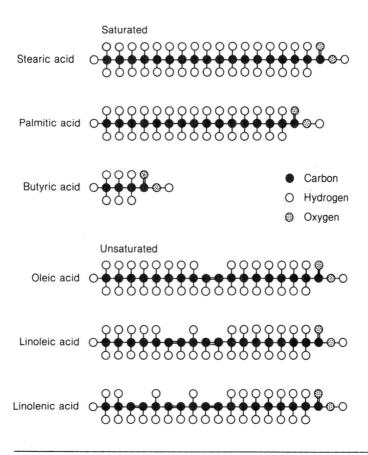

FIGURE 5.2 Chemical structure of fatty acids

rancidity in foods occurs when butyric acid is broken off from the triglyceride of butter fat. In the free form, butyric acid produces a foul odor, which makes the butter unacceptable. The result of cleaving off fatty acids from triglycerides is known as hydrolytic rancidity.

Chemically, unsaturated fatty acids differ from saturated fats because of the presence of one or more double bonds in the structure. At each double bond in the molecule, a hydrogen is missing on two adjacent carbons. These double bonds make the fat more susceptible to oxidative breakdown, an undesirable chemical reaction with oxygen. When unsaturated fatty acids predominate in triglycerides, the fat is usually liquid at room temperature. Most of the fatty acids of vegetable oils are unsaturated, thus accounting for the liquidity of salad oils at room temperature.

Differences among the unsaturated fatty acids are based on the number of double bonds present, the placement of the bonds, and the length of the carbon chains. Those having only one double bond are known as monounsaturated fats. Oleic acid is a monounsaturated fatty acid commonly found in olive oil (see Figure 5.2 for structure). It differs from stearic acid only by the double bond. Oleic acid is not required by the body because the body is able to synthesize it from the breakdown products of sugars, amino acids, and other fats. The polyunsaturates are those fatty acids containing two or more double bonds. Polyunsaturated fats (PUFA) are most susceptible to breakdown in the presence of oxygen. This chemical reaction causes the rancidity that occurs in potato chips and peanuts.

Liquid salad oils, such as corn oil, cottonseed, and soybean oil, contain a high amount of polyunsaturated fatty acids. Butter is a relatively saturated fat containing stearic acid and is solid at room temperature. The production of solid vegetable shortenings or margarine requires the hydrogenation of liquid oils. This process adds hydrogen to double bonds, decreases unsaturation, and leads to greater saturation. Through manipulation of this process, various textures of margarine may be achieved and a more stable fat with the proper plastic texture may be formed.

Linoleic acid, also shown in Figure 5.2, is an example of a polyunsaturated fat with two double bonds. Linoleic acid is found in high concentrations in some vegetable oils and to a far smaller extent in meats. Linoleic acid cannot be synthesized by humans and is therefore one of the essential nutrients required in the diet. Some fish have fatty acids that have many more double bonds (like linolenic acid in Figure 5.2), and thus are very unstable.

A deficiency of linoleic acid has never been found in humans eating a balanced diet. Deficiency symptoms have occurred, however, in infants and people who were in hospitals on certain improperly designed elemental diets or intravenous feeding solutions. The signs of essential fatty acid deficiency are dermatitis (a skin disorder) and metabolic disorders of cholesterol and fat transport. Animal studies have also shown impairment of reproduction, a key sign of nutritional inadequacy. The amount of linoleic acid required in a normal diet is about 2% of the total calories or from five to six grams per day. Soybean oil, the major oil used in this country, is over 50% linoleic acid so that a couple of teaspoons (1 tsp. = 5 g.) would supply the needed amount. Corn oil and cottonseed oil are also very high in linoleic acid, whereas olive oil has only about 10% linoleic acid. Thus, 10 times more olive oil would be needed in the diet, if this were the only fat source. Most meats supply only a small part of the required linoleic acid. Table 5.1 lists the percentages of saturated, monounsaturated, and polyunsaturated fats in some common foods. Some nutritionists feel that mixing fats to achieve a ratio of 1/1/1 of saturated to monounsaturated to polyunsaturated fats (S/M/P) is the best dietary pattern to achieve nutritional adequacy. As can be seen in Table 5.1, to achieve this one should mix the diet with both animal and vegetable fats.

For many years, nutritionists have recommended that people increase their intake of polyunsaturated fatty acids (PUFA) because saturated fats, in contrast to PUFA, may cause an increase of blood cholesterol in experimental animals (see Chapter 11). Over the last half decade Americans have increased consumption of PUFA, but have not substantially reduced intake of saturated fats. As a result, our total fat intake has increased about 25% in the last 60 years.

TABLE 5.1 Fatty acid distribution in some foods

| | Percentage of Fatty Acid | | | S/M/P * Ratio |
Food	Saturated	Oleic (mono)	Linoleic (polyunsaturated)	
Corn oil	10	28	53	1/2.8/5.3
Safflower oil	8	15	72	1/1.9/9.0
Peanut butter	9	25	14	1/2.8/1.6
Soybean oil	17	30	50	1/1.8/2.9
Butter	46	27	2	1/0.6/0.4
Margarine	22	58	17	1/2.6/0.8
Beef	18	16	1	1/0.9/0.06
Pork	36	37	8	1/1.0/0.2
Chicken	5	6	3	1/1.2/0.6
Cheddar cheese	18	11	1	1/0.6/0.06
Eggs	4	5	1	1/1.25/0.25
Milk	54	27	0.1	1/0.5/0.002

Derived from USDA Handbook No. 456.
* Saturated/Monounsaturated/Polyunsaturated

Consumption of diets containing over 40% of calories as fat have been associated with high rates of obesity in our population, may well increase the incidence of coronary heart disease, and have been recently related to higher incidence of colon and breast cancer. Therefore, it has been recommended by several health groups that Americans reduce their fat intake to 35% of calories or lower.

PHOSPHOLIPIDS   Other fats that are very important in the metabolism of the body are the phospholipids. They are similar to the diglycerides in structure. Where the third fatty acid would attach they instead contain phosphate (hence the name) attached to an alcohol or nitrogen containing group (Figure 5.3). The composition of the two fatty acids in a phospholipid can vary greatly.

Lecithin is one of the phospholipids that is manufactured by the body. It is shown in Figure 5.3. Lecithin and other phospholipids are major structural components of cell membranes and blood lipoproteins. In addition, they take part in many metabolic processes. Lecithin occurs in high concentrations in eggs and soybeans. It is extracted from soybeans for use in salad dressing and cake mixes because it helps give stability to the emulsion. The presence of lecithin is one reason eggs can be beaten into foam. Lecithin functions even better than monoglycerides or diglycerides as an emulsifier. When absorbed on the surface of an oil droplet, lecithin adds a charge that repels other droplets. This slows down breakdown of an emulsion much better than the uncharged monoglycerides or diglycerides because if two droplets combine they can rise to the liquid surface much faster than a smaller droplet.

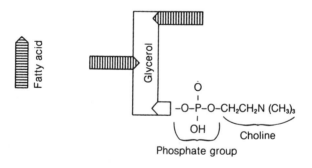

FIGURE 5.3 Structure of the phospholipid lecithin

CHOLESTEROL   The last major form of fats in the diet are the sterols. Cholesterol is the major sterol found in animal tissue. Much controversy has surrounded the role of cholesterol in heart disease. This will be discussed further in Chapter 11. The sterols are part of the structure of the membranes of cells, are the basic building block of steroid hormones, and help transport fats in the bloodstream. Cholesterol is found in every cell of the body and it is the precursor of vitamin D.

The cholesterol level in the average American diet is roughly 400 to 700 milligrams per day. Common sources of cholesterol are shown in Table 5.2. Cholesterol is not found in foods of plant origin. Advertising claims that a salad oil, a margarine, or a peanut butter contain no cholesterol should not be surprising as only foods of animal origin contain cholesterol.

TABLE 5.2 Cholesterol content of some foods

	Amount of cholesterol in:	
Item	100 grams,* edible portion	Edible portion of 1 pound as purchased
	Milligrams	Milligrams
Beef raw:		
With bone	70	270
Without bone	70	320
Brains, raw	>2,000	>9,000
Butter	250	1,135
Caviar or fish roe	>300	>1,300
Cheese:		
Cheddar	100	455
Cottage, creamed	15	70
Cream	120	545
Other (25% to 30% fat)	85	385
Cheese spread	65	295
Chicken, flesh only, raw	60	—
Crab:		
In shell	125	270
Meat only	125	565
Egg, whole	550	2,200
Egg white	0	0
Egg yolk:		
Fresh	1,500	6,800
Frozen	1,280	5,800
Dried	2,950	13,380
Fish:		
Steak	70	265
Fillet	70	320
Heart, raw	150	680
Ice cream	45	205
Kidney, raw	375	1,700

TABLE 5.2 Cholesterol content of some foods *(Continued)*

Item	Amount of cholesterol in:	
	100 grams,* edible portion	Edible portion of 1 pound as purchased
	Milligrams	Milligrams
Lamb, raw:		
With bone	70	265
Without bone	70	320
Lard and other animal fat	95	430
Liver, raw	300	1,360
Lobster:		
Whole	200	235
Meat only	200	900
Margarine:		
All vegetable fat	0	0
Two-thirds animal fat,		
One-third vegetable fat	65	295
Milk:		
Fluid, whole	11	50
Dried, whole	85	385
Fluid, skim	3	15
Mutton:		
With bone	65	250
Without bone	65	295
Oysters:		
In shell	>200	>90
Meat only	>200	>900
Pork:		
With bone	70	260
Without bone	70	320
Shrimp:		
In shell	125	390
Flesh only	125	565
Sweetbreads (thymus)	250	1,135
Veal:		
With bone	90	320
Without bone	90	410

Adapted from USDA Handbook No. 456.

*About 3½ ounces

As seen in Table 5.2, pork, beef, and veal supply about the same amount, approximately 70 mg. in a three and one-half ounce (100-gram) serving. One egg, which is about 50 grams, supplies 250 mg. of cholesterol. Shellfish have a much higher cholesterol content. It is important to note that the amount of cholesterol in the diet (exogenous cholesterol) is usually much less than that made by the body every day. The endogenous cholesterol is produced in the liver and other tissues for various functions such as the formation of hormones. Some is also converted into bile salts. When we eat, the gall bladder releases the bile salts into the small intestine where they help emulsify and digest the fats in the foods.

Most of the bile salts are reabsorbed from the intestine and recycle through the bloodstream to the liver for reuse. For most people, consumption of low cholesterol diets will result in increased synthesis of endogenous cholesterol, primarily in the liver. In the same regard, the body adjusts for the consumption of high quantities of cholesterol by reducing synthesis of cholesterol. Thus for most of us reducing the amount of cholesterol in the diet will only have a small effect on the total cholesterol levels found in the blood despite claims made by many people. However, some people have defects in the control of cholesterol metabolism that result in elevated blood and tissue levels of cholesterol. These persons must modify their diet under medical supervision.

FAT METABOLISM

When fats are metabolized to provide energy in the body, they follow a pathway that enters into the Krebs Cycle (see Figure 4.2). As with carbohydrates, complete oxidation of fatty acids yields water, carbon dioxide, and energy. Because of their lower oxygen content compared to carbohydrates, fats supply more energy per gram (nine Calories per gram).

An undesirable condition exists if fats become the major source of calories, that is, when carbohydrates drop below 100 Calories per day (5% of total calories). In this case, there are not enough intermediates in the Krebs Cycle to draw in the fat metabolites and break them down. Thus, certain chemicals build up in the bloodstream. These chemicals are acids and ketones. The three major ones are acetone, acetoacetic acid, and β-hydrobutyric acid. If the acid and ketone levels get too high, they can affect the brain. As a result, a person may have hallucinations and may eventually go into a coma. This has occurred with people during starvation; consumption of severely low calorie diets has produced the same effect. Consumption of certain "fad" diets without medical supervision can be harmful (see Chapter 12). It should also be remembered that the brain and central nervous system require glucose almost exclusively for energy metabolism. Thus, as carbohydrates drop in the diet and glycogen stores are used up, the central nervous system may not function optimally.

DEPOSITION OF FAT TISSUE

In Chapter 12 we will discuss obesity, but we should point out how the buildup of fat tissues (adipose tissue) occurs. If we consume more calories, either as protein, carbohydrates, or fat, than we expend, the remaining protein, carbohydrate, or fat molecules will be converted into storage triglycerides for deposition in fat tissues. In adults the storage of fat occurs by a process called hypertrophy; the fat cells grow larger as they are stuffed further and further and are stretched out. In infants and children some research shows that hyperplasia—increase in cell numbers—may also occur when excess calories are consumed. It is, therefore, possible that overfeeding infants causes hyperplasia, which gives overfed infants a greater chance to become obese by hypertrophy when they become adults, especially if their eating habits do not change.

SUMMARY

Fats supply a major part of the calories in the diet of Americans. They provide more energy than carbohydrates, yielding nine Calories per gram. The major food and body fats are composed of complex molecules called triglycerides, which are fatty acids attached to a glycerol base. Fatty acids may either be saturated or unsaturated. The latter are important since they can react with oxygen and break down, and one of them, linoleic acid, is essential for body growth. In addition to the triglycerides, fats are also present as sterols, predominately cholesterol, and phospholipids. The liver also produces cholesterol so that diet modification to reduce cholesterol may only have a small effect on blood cholesterol levels. Body fats are also important from the standpoint of obesity. The excess calories consumed in a diet are deposited as fat tissues. When a person goes on a reducing diet to decrease fat tissue, some adverse effects may occur if not enough carbohydrates are consumed.

Multiple
Choice
Study
Questions

1. A diglyceride is composed of

    A. glucose and two fatty acids
    B. glycose and two amino acids
    C. glycerol and two fatty acids
    D. glycerol and three fatty acids
    E. cholesterol and two fatty acids

2. Triglycerides are made up of

    A. glycogen and amino acids
    B. glycogen and citric acids
    C. glucose and fatty acids
    D. glycerol and fatty acids
    E. glycerol and phospholipids

3. Which of the following is a phospholipid?

    A. butyric acid
    B. cholesterol
    C. retinol
    D. choline
    E. lecithin

4. Diglycerides are used in food processing

    A. to increase transport of blood lipids

    B. to prevent microbial growth

    C. to prevent rancidity

    D. to stabilize emulsions

5. Which fatty acid is uniquely found in milk fat and can cause off-odors?

    A. butyric

    B. stearic

    C. oleic

    D. palmitic

    E. none of these

6. Which of the following foods has the highest amount of unsaturated fat?

    A. pork

    B. beef

    C. butter

    D. margarine

    E. corn oil

7. Which food has the highest polyunsaturated to saturated fat ratio?

    A. peanut butter

    B. coconut oil

    C. safflower oil

    D. butter

    E. milk

8. What is the best ratio to achieve for the Saturated/Monounsaturated/Polyunsaturated Fatty Acid ratio in the diet?

    A. 1:1:1

    B. 1:1:2

    C. 2:1:1

    D. 1:2:1

    E. 0.5:1:1

9. The most essential fatty acid for humans is

    A. oleic acid

    B. linoleic acid

    C. linolenic acid

    D. pyruvic acid

    E. stearic acid

10. When fat is used as a primary energy source in the body

    A. high blood sugar levels (glucose) occur

    B. urea is formed, which overtaxes the kidney

    C. more water should be drunk because high concentrations of metabolites (ketones) are formed

    D. a person will become diabetic quickly

    E. more energy is available for short bursts of strength

11. The minimum amount of carbohydrate required daily is

    A. 10 grams

    B. 50 grams

    C. 100 grams

    D. 200 grams

    E. 500 grams

12. Cholesterol is a sterol that

    A. comes only from the diet

    B. is produced in the liver as a precursor to hormones

    C. is the major cause of heart disease

    D. combines with fatty acids to form triglycerides

    E. causes cancer of the liver

13. Endogenous cholesterol comes from

    A. the diet

    B. eating liver

    C. corn oil

    D. eggs

    E. the liver

Essay Study Questions

1. Discuss the types of fats found in foods.

2. Relate the similarities and differences between fat and carbohydrate metabolism to produce energy.

3. Describe the difference between saturated and unsaturated fats.

4. What fatty acid is essential for humans and what happens if a deficiency exists?

5. What is a phospholipid and what is its function?

6. What is exogenous cholesterol and what foods are major sources of it in the diet? How does this compare to endogenous cholesterol?

7. What complications could arise if one were to go on a starvation diet or on a very low carbohydrate diet?

*Things
to Do*

1. Using the diet survey, determine what foods were major sources of fats in the diet.

2. Look for foods that have fat-type labeling. Do they meet the 1:1:1 S/M/P ratio and are they low in cholesterol?

3. What is the average cholesterol consumption found in the seven-day survey? Which foods are responsible for high cholesterol intake?

4. Find someone who is dieting and test their urine for ketone bodies.

Chapter 5. Answers to Multiple-Choice Study Questions: **1,** C; **2,** D; **3,** E; **4,** D; **5,** A; **6,** E; **7,** C **8,** A; **9,** B; **10,** C; **11,** C; **12,** B; **13,** E.

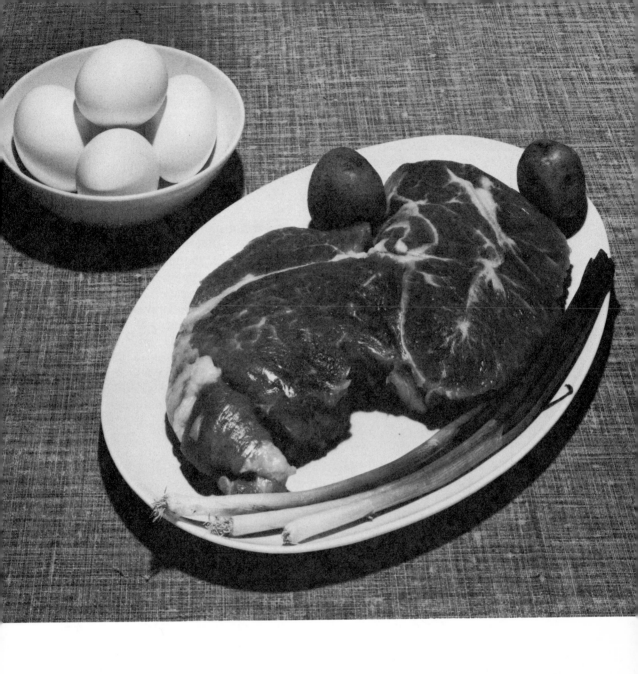

**PROTEIN:
HOW MUCH DO
WE NEED?**

6

**PROTEIN
AND NUTRITION
IDEAS**

One of the most misunderstood aspects of nutrition concerns the need for dietary protein by humans. A popular misconception is that the proteins from meat cause one to become aggressive. This misconception can be traced back to an experiment conducted at the London Zoo in the early 1800s. The London Zoo was having problems with some overly noisy, aggressive bears. An experiment was set up to see if a change in diet would quiet the bears down. They had been fed raw meat as the major part of their usual diet. In order to establish the effects of the meat on animals, bread was substituted for the meat. As a result, the bears became extremely docile and lethargic. As we will see, they became docile because they did not get a balanced diet and were too malnourished to have enough energy to be active. This experiment was regarded as definitive proof that meat protein caused aggression. The study was eventually published in a scientific journal! It was regarded by many as an established fact for quite some time.

Today athletes and their coaches carry a similar misconception to an extreme. Most athletes feel they have to consume enormous amounts of protein to build muscles and perform well. In actuality, consuming an average American diet to meet their caloric needs is all that is necessary. Some athletes consume three pounds of steak and five or six eggs a day. Others spend large amounts of money for powdered or liquid protein supplements.

The body will increase muscle mass if the right exercises are performed and the athlete consumes a well-rounded diet. Americans, on the average, already consume twice the amount of protein that is necessary for adequate health. Even athletes undergoing the most vigorous training require little additional protein although they certainly need more calories. It has been estimated that for an increase in one pound of muscle per week, only 13 grams of protein above our basal requirement are needed daily. Most of us already consume 40 or more grams above our basal daily needs. Therefore, it is a waste of money to buy protein supplements or high protein animal foods to supplement normal training meals. It may even be harmful, in some cases, to consume large amounts of supplemental protein.

**COMPOSITION
OF PROTEINS**

Proteins, like carbohydrates, are made up of molecules linked together in long chains to form polymers with hundreds of units. The individual units are called amino acids and they are the building blocks of protein connected together by what is called the peptide bond. The amino acids are basically composed of nitrogen, carbon, oxygen, and hydrogen, although three of them also contain sulfur.

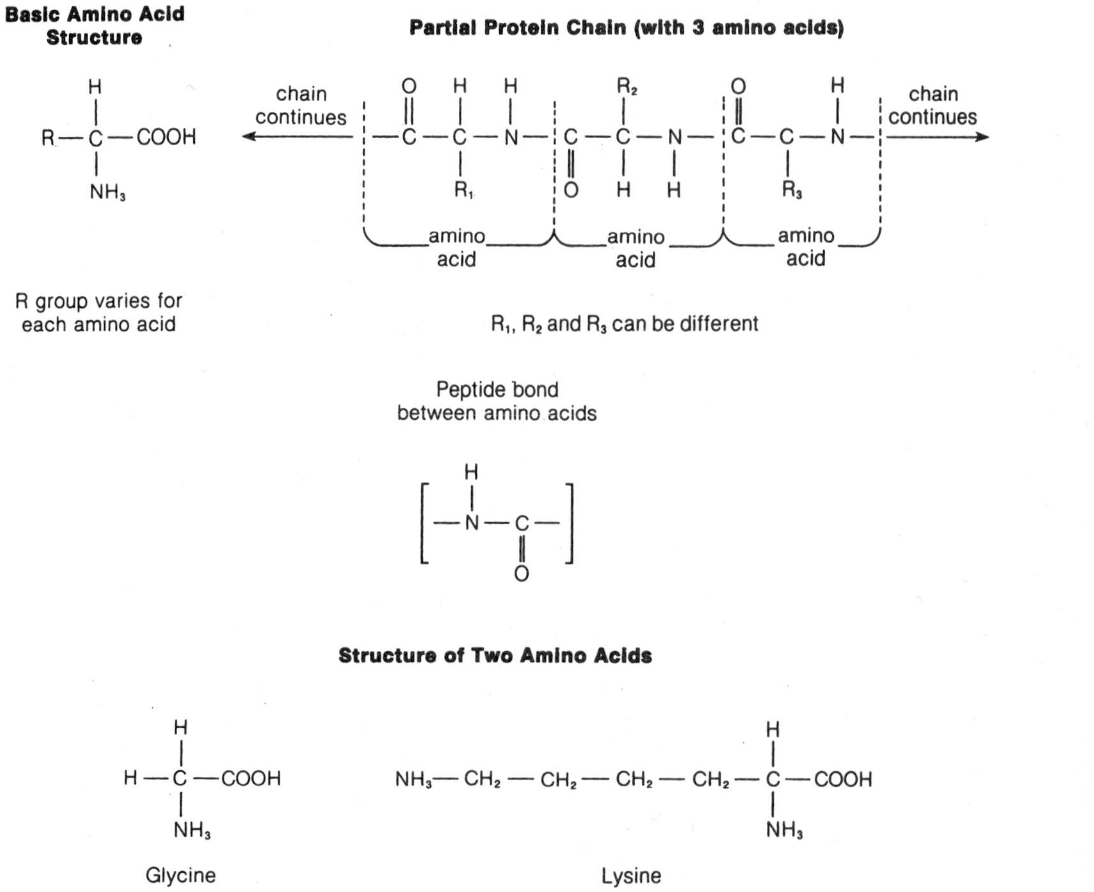

Basic Amino Acid Structure

Partial Protein Chain (with 3 amino acids)

R group varies for each amino acid

R_1, R_2 and R_3 can be different

Peptide bond between amino acids

Structure of Two Amino Acids

Glycine

Lysine

FIGURE 6.1 Basic structure of amino acids and proteins

The basic structure of an amino acid and of a protein chain is shown in Figure 6.1. Amino acids differ in their R group, which is the location on the backbone where different molecular structures are attached. For example, glycine has a simple hydrogen (H) for the R group while lysine has a $-CH_2-CH_2-CH_2-CH_2-NH_2$ group attached. Different R group attachments result in over 20 different kinds of amino acids that can also be combined in different sequences. The possibilities for producing different proteins are almost limitless with this many different amino acids, different sequences, and the many polymer lengths. The amino acids occur in different sequences for each protein. The sequence determines the shape and function of the individual protein. For example, myosin, a muscle protein, has a linear chain; hemoglobin, the molecule that carries oxygen in the blood, has a globular appearance; and casein, a milk protein, has different-sized chains held together by the mineral calcium in a very complex arrangement. Many other proteins are composed of several chains wound around each other in helices. Some of these helices have extremely complicated structures. In addition, protein chains can have cross-linkages between them to impart a rigid structure. Such is the case with collagen, a major protein in cartilage and bone. Another is gluten, which helps form the texture of bread.

ESSENTIAL AMINO ACIDS

Of the known amino acids, only eight have been identified as being absolutely essential to the adult human body. These are listed in Table 6.1 and are called essential because the body cannot synthesize them in high enough rates to meet body needs. They must come from the diet.

Recent evidence has shown that arginine, another amino acid, may be an essential amino acid for humans. Histidine is required only for infants. Adults can make enough histidine to meet needs. The remaining amino acids can be manufactured in the body, but are also supplied in almost all foods containing protein. If the nonessential amino acids are not in the diet they can be built from other components in the diet. Protein in the diet serves as the major source of nitrogen in the body. This nitrogen is necessary for the production of the other nonessential amino acids, because the carbohydrates and fats in the diet cannot supply the nitrogen for amino acid synthesis.

Protein found in foods is of varied quality. If a protein has all the essential amino acids in the right balance, it is a high quality protein. A poorer quality protein may be low in one or more of the

TABLE 6.1 Essential amino acids required for humans

Isoleucine	Phenylalanine
Leucine	Threonine
Lysine	Tryptophan
Methionine	Valine

Arginine (presently under investigation)
Histidine (infants only)

essential amino acids. Proteins from plant sources are generally of lower quality than are proteins from animal sources. Gluten, the protein in wheat flour, for example, is low in the essential amino acid lysine and thus it has lower protein quality than milk or eggs. However, when wheat bread is consumed with sufficient other protein that is adequate or high in lysine, such as the protein in milk, the body can use the wheat protein more efficiently. Because the bread used for the experiment with the bears in the London Zoo was probably not supplemented with other protein, the animals had an inadequate diet. They were probably missing other needed nutrients as well. Dr. Norman Borlaug (a Nobel Prize winner) and others have been working on a genetic strain of wheat that has a higher lysine content and thus a better protein quality.

Tryptophan, another essential amino acid, is significant on a worldwide nutritional scale because corn is low in tryptophan. Corn, also known as maize, serves as a major part of the diet in many countries. Because corn is also low in lysine, it is a fairly poor quality protein source. The areas of the world that use corn as the basic protein source in the diet have suffered major malnutrition problems. Through genetic manipulation researchers at Purdue University have developed a strain of corn, Opaque-2, that is high in lysine and tryptophan. It might have been the answer to the problems of malnutrition in South America and Mexico where corn is used as a major part of the diet. Unfortunately, due to growing conditions that are unsuitable for Opaque-2 in hot climates, the high requirement for fertilizer in its growth, the corn's poor resistance to pests and disease, and the negative response of the people in these areas to the yellow corn instead of the old white corn, Opaque-2 has not enjoyed as much success as originally anticipated. Subsequent work on other genetic varieties of corn has solved some of these problems.

Soy protein is quite high in lysine, but is low in methionine. Substitution of soy flour for 12% of wheat flour in bread can greatly increase growth when fed to experimental animals. The mixing of two poorer quality proteins to balance protein qualities is known as complementation.

Because vegetable sources of protein are of poorer quality, vegetarians must be careful to complement protein sources to obtain optimal protein quality. This is particularly true for strict vegetarians who consume no fish, egg, or milk products.

Egg-white protein is considered one of the best-balanced proteins. Often the amino acid make-up of other proteins are compared to egg. In Table 6.2, the amino acid profiles of some plant and animal proteins are listed. The profile for egg-white protein is listed at the top of the table for comparison.

TABLE 6.2 Essential amino acid composition of some plant and animal foods based on USDA Composition Data (Grams of amino acid per 100 grams of food)

Food	Histi-dine	Isoleu-cine	Leucine	Lysine	Meth-ionine	Phenyla-lanine	Threo-nine	Tryp-tophan	Valine	% Protein
EGGS	.312	.863	1.144	.832	.408	.751	.647	.214	.965	13.0
Bananas				.055	.011[†]			.018		1.2
Barley	.004	.008	.013	.006	.003[†]	.010	.006	.002	.009	0.2
Beans (dried)	.627	1.250	1.890	1.633	.222[†]	1.214	.954	.204	1.334	22.0
Bread (white enriched)	.180	.330	.351	.207[†]	.206	.448	.258	.085	.331	8.7
Broccoli	.059	.119	.153	.138	.047[†]	.112	.115	.035	.160	3.1
Buckwheat flour	.256	.440	.683	.687	.206[†]	.442	.461	.165	.607	11.7
Cabbage	.027	.043	.061	.071	.014[†]	.033	.042	.012	.046	1.5
Carrots	.014	.038	.054	.043	.009[†]	.035	.036	.008	.047	1.0
Cauliflower	.050	.108	.168	.140	.049[†]	.078	.106	.035	.150	2.5
Chickpeas (dried)	.551	1.178	1.515	1.414	.272[†]	.997	.728	.167	1.010	20.5
Coconut meat (fresh)	.060	.157	.235	.133	.062	.152	.113	.029[†]	.185	3.5
Corn, cornmeal, & grits (dry)	.180	.402	1.128	.251	.161	.395	.347	.053[†]	.444	8.7
Cottonseed flour	1.278	1.816	2.840	2.063	.662[†]	2.517	1.701	.570	2.370	48.1
Cowpeas (immature)	.297	.445	.625	.590	.125[†]	.501	.338	.095	.491	9.0
Cowpeas (dried)	.690	1.105	1.707	1.485	.350[†]	1.193	.897	.219	1.288	22.8
Cucumbers (whole)	.013	.028	.038	.039	.009[†]	.021	.024	.007	.031	0.9
Eggplant (cooked)	.017	.051	.061	.027	.005[†]	.043	.034	.009	.059	1.0
Filberts	.242	.718	.790	.351	.117[†]	.452	.349	.177	.786	12.6
Fish (cooked)	.574	1.429	2.091	1.982	.704	1.003[†]	1.035	.282	1.320	22.0
Gluten flour	.828	1.835	6.472	.742[†]	1.166	2.312	1.424	.245	2.120	41.4
Lentils (dried)	.541	1.300	1.739	1.510	.178[†]	1.091	.885	.213	1.344	24.7
Lima beans (dried)	.659	1.182	1.700	1.358	.326[†]	1.204	.966	.193	1.280	20.4
Lima beans (immature)	.277	.515	.677	.531	.090[†]	.435	.379	.109	.543	8.4
Meat (beef, cooked)	1.005	1.586[†]	2.381	2.625	.825	1.191	1.342	.415	1.557	30.5
Milk (whole, cow)	.077	.235	.423	.259	.098	.193	.161	.049[†]	.249	3.5
Mung beans (sprouted)	.085	.210	.343	.260	.041[†]	.182	.119	.028	.225	3.8
Oats, oatmeal (cooked)	.034	.010	.140	.069	.028[†]	.100	.062	.024	.111	2.0
Okra	.033	.077	.112	.085	.025[†]	.072	.073	.021	.101	2.0
Peanut butter	.676	1.143	1.690	.992	.245[†]	1.406	.747	.307	1.383	27.8
Peas (cooked)	.088	.248	.337	.255	.043[†]	.207	.198	.449	.221	5.4
Peas (dried)	.659	1.357	1.994	1.766	.289[†]	1.215	.929	.255	1.350	24.1
Peppers (raw, green)	.014	.046	.046	.051	.016[†]	.055	.050	.009	.033	1.2
Potatoes (cooked)	.037	.114	.129	.139	.032[†]	.115	.102	.028	.139	2.6
Rice (cooked)	.040	.112	.205	.094	.043[†]	.120	.093	.026	.166	2.5
Sesame seeds (dry)	.360	.777	1.372	.476[†]	.521	1.190	.577	.271	.276	18.6
Snap beans (cooked)	.030	.072	.093	.084	.023	.038[†]	.060	.022	.077	1.6
Sorghum	.211	.598	1.760	.299[†]	.190	.547	.394	.123	.628	11.0
Soybeans (textured)	1.550	3.494	5.013	4.108	.874[†]	3.214	2.558	.894	3.411	65.0
Soybean milk (fluid)	.110	.214	.279	.246	.049[†]	.178	.161	.046	.170	3.4
Spinach (raw)	.068	.149	.245	.198	.054[†]	.138	.141	.052	.176	3.2
Sunflower seeds	.518	1.129	1.536	.768[†]	.392	1.117	.806	.303	1.198	24.0
Sweet potatoes (cooked)	.040	.096	.115	.094	.037[†]	.111	.094	.035	.150	2.0
Tapioca	.009	.017	.025	.025	.004[†]	.017	.017	.008	.018	0.6
Tomatoes	.017	.032	.045	.046	.007[†]	.031	.036	.010	.031	1.1
Turnip greens (cooked)	.032	.066	.129	.080	.033[†]	.090	.078	.028	.092	1.8
Wheat, white flour	.192	.440	.738	.218[†]	.126	.526	.276	.118	.413	10.5
Wheat, whole grain flour	.267	.567	.876	.358[†]	.199	.645	.376	.161	.605	14.0
Yeast, baker's (dry)	.325	.604	1.061	.842	.228	.560	.604	.112[†]	.774	12.1
Yeast, brewer's	1.049	2.011	2.707	2.769	.702[†]	1.596	1.974	.596	2.285	38.8

[†] Indicates limiting amino acid.

FUNCTIONS AND METABOLISM OF PROTEIN

Protein is needed both to synthesize new body tissues and to repair or maintain those already present. Tissues are constantly undergoing repair, and dietary protein is constantly needed to provide the amino acid building blocks for new synthesis or for replacement of components excreted in the feces or urine.

Proteins, such as collagen, elastin, and contractile muscle fibers, provide structure for tissues. Other proteins include major components of enzymes, hormones (such as insulin), blood transport vehicles for other nutrients, and antibodies.

When dietary protein consumption exceeds protein needs for synthesis or repair of tissues, amino acids are not stored in the body. The excess amino acids pass through the bloodstream to the liver, where the nitrogen component of the amino acids (i.e., the amino group) is cleaved off as ammonia and is converted to urea. The urea then passes through the blood to the kidney where it is excreted in the urine. The remaining carbon backbone of an amino acid can either be converted to fat, or if ATP energy is needed, it can enter the Krebs Cycle to produce ATP, CO_2, and H_2O. In the case of very low carbohydrate consumption, carbon backbones from certain amino acids can be converted to glucose. In all cases, therefore, the excess protein consumed is eventually used for energy or finds its way to fat cells to be deposited as fat.

EVALUATION OF PROTEIN QUALITY

When we consider the nutritional adequacy of protein in our diet, we must ask two questions. First, we must ask about the total quantity of dietary protein. Then we must be concerned with the quality of the protein—the amino acid makeup or balance of that protein. The total quantity of protein in a food is easily determined by analysis of total nitrogen in the food. Since most nitrogen in food is from protein, we can convert grams of nitrogen to the approximate grams of protein by a simple equation (grams of nitrogen $\times$ 6.25 = grams of protein). The quality of protein is more difficult to ascertain. Nutritionists can use chemical, animal, human, or microbiological assay techniques to estimate protein quality.

Chemical Methods

Direct analysis of amino acid composition of a protein is a rapid technique of estimating protein quality. The food proteins are hydrolyzed (usually with strong acid) to break the peptide bond between individual amino acids. Then the individual amino acids are separated and quantified using column chromatography. The amount of each essential amino acid in a certain quantity of protein is determined and compared to a good quality protein such as egg-white protein.

In Table 6.3, we see how one can determine protein quality by a method called chemical score. For clarity, only four essential amino acids have been listed. The amount of amino acid is expressed as per 100 grams of nitrogen.

In Table 6.3 the content of each amino acid is compared to that in egg; for example, for corn the lysine content of 18 grams per 100 grams nitrogen is divided by 40 grams lysine per 100 grams nitrogen in egg, which gives 45%. The lowest ratio obtained by dividing each amino acid content by the corresponding one in egg determines the most limiting amino acid. In this case, for corn the limiting amino acid, tryptophan, is equivalent to 40% of that in egg. This limiting amino acid then determines the chemical score, which is 40. The soy protein also shows a chemical score of 40, but in this case the limiting amino acid is methionine. Of course, chemical methods do not account for any differences in digestibility of the protein (see Chapter 9).

To improve the protein quality, several things can be done. One of the most interesting from the world food standpoint is to achieve a higher score by genetic manipulation, that is, by finding a strain that has a naturally higher limiting amino acid content. Secondly, one can supplement the poor-quality protein with the limiting amino acid. For example, some cereals are supplemented with lysine to achieve a higher score. Of course, this now means some other amino acid then becomes limiting. Corn supplemented with tryptophan and lysine would then become limiting in methionine, but in a diet with meat this would be no problem since meat is high in methionine. Lastly, one can complement the poor quality protein with other foods containing the missing amino acids to increase its quality.

From Table 6.2 we can see that most foods of plant origin are low in total protein on a percentage of weight basis. The limiting amino acid is indicated with a dagger in Table 6.2. Plant proteins are often limiting in methionine or lysine.

TABLE 6.3 Determination of the quality of a protein by chemical score (Amino acid content g. / 100 g. Nitrogen)

Protein	Lysine	Methio-nine	Phenyl-alanine	Tryp-tophan	Chemical score	Limiting amino acid
Eggs	40	20	36	10	100	
Corn (% of egg)	18 (45%)	12 (60%)	28 (78%)	4 (40%)	40	tryptophan
Soy (% of egg)	40 (100%)	8 (40%)	31 (86%)	9 (90%)	40	methionine

Table 6.4 summarizes the average chemical scores for a number of foods. As shown, gelatin is one of the poorest of proteins if eaten alone. It contains no tryptophan, thus the chemical score is zero. It also has a low lysine content. Contrary to popular belief, eating gelatin probably does not contribute much to nail growth unless one has a very low protein level in the diet. In fact, the protein in nails is keratin, which is entirely different from the protein in gelatin. Keratin contains a lot of methionine, which gelatin lacks. Only balanced nutrition (such as by mixing gelatin with meat), nail care, and a little luck will help. Gelatin capsules consumed alone for helping nails is not satisfactory.

Rice, a major food source in the world, is, according to Table 6.4, a medium-quality protein since it has a chemical score of only 72. Mixing it with vegetables helps to upgrade the overall protein quality. It must be emphasized that to achieve proper protein complementation, the two (or more) protein sources must be eaten at the same meal. Otherwise the body cannot efficiently utilize the amino acids of the foods for growth or maintenance of tissues.

Animal Methods

PER Protein quality as measured by the Protein Efficiency Ratio (PER) is a better test of protein quality than chemical analysis since it involves use of a biological test system with animals. Protein

TABLE 6.4 Protein quality values as determined by different methods

Food	Chemical score [a]	Biological value	
		Growing rat	Adult human [b]
Egg	100	87	94, 97
Milk (cow's)	85	90	62, 79, 100
Casein	80	69	70
Beef	83	76	67, 80, 84, 75
Fish	80	75	94
Oats	79	66	89
Rice	72	—	67
Corn meal	42	54	24
White flour	47	52	42, 40, 45, 67, 70
Wheat germ	61	75	89
Soy flour	73	75	65, 71, 81
Potato	56	71	80, 71, 81
Peas	58	48	56, 90
Gelatin	0	20	—
Cassava	22	—	—

[a] Based on a comparison to eggs
[b] Values are from different studies

digestibility and body utilization can be accounted for. The PER test uses rats that have just been weaned. They are fed for 28 days on a test diet containing 10% of the protein being studied. Weight gain versus protein intake is measured and is compared to growth of rats on a similar diet in which casein, the major protein from milk, is used as the protein source. Weight gain over the period divided by the amount of protein fed yields the PER. The PER for the control diet (casein) is then adjusted to a value of 2.5 and the test protein is compared to this number. Since weight gain can also be affected by the other components in the diet and not just by the intake of protein, many interpretation problems exist with this type of measurement. However, PER is commonly used because it is the only method currently approved by the Food and Drug Administration for nutritional labeling of the protein quality in foods (discussed in Chapter 24). Interestingly, the PER value can be rather closely correlated with the chemical score, so the latter is not a bad estimate of quality. It should be noted here that a protein with a corrected PER equal to or greater than 2.5 is considered to be of high quality, while one with a lower PER is considered to be of lower to poor quality.

Biological value and other methods Another method used to estimate protein quality is called Biological Value (BV). This test can be used on either humans or rats. BV measures the percent of absorbed nitrogen that is retained for growth and maintenance of tissues. The amount of nitrogen absorbed is simply total intake of nitrogen minus fecal losses. The quantity of nitrogen retained is determined by subtracting fecal and urinary losses of nitrogen from the total ingested nitrogen. BV is determined by dividing nitrogen retained by nitrogen absorbed and multiplying this figure by 100. This test is usually performed on growing animals (rats) or on adult humans.

Table 6.4 lists the biological values for various proteins. As can be seen, the number varies for the same protein when several human tests are compared. This is an inherent biological problem when comparing human studies done at different places and with different people. However, for most cases in Table 6.4, all three protein quality indices are similar.

There are a number of other rat test procedures used by different research groups to evaluate protein quality. These include nitrogen balance, net protein ratio, net protein retention, and slope ratio. Nitrogen balance is of special note because it, like BV, can also be used with human subjects.

Protein quality test procedures with animals are often used even though the results cannot be applied to humans with consistency.

Human tests are very expensive and difficult to perform. Moreover, there would be moral and medical considerations in subjecting a growing child, a pregnant woman, or an aged person to a low-quality protein diet for any length of time. Therefore, tests such as PER are relied upon to estimate protein quality.

Microbiological and Enzymatic Tests

A considerable amount of effort has gone into development of microbial or enzymatic tests to predict protein quality. The protozoan *Tetrahymena pyriformis* has an essential amino acid requirement similar to that of humans, and under proper conditions the growth rate of this protozoan can be correlated quite well to PER or BV. Gas production by the anaerobic bacteria *Clostridium perfringens* grown on substrate containing test proteins has also been used to measure protein quality of various proteins. These microbiological test procedures require further refinement. However, they only require a few days to perform and are inexpensive.

In vitro digestion of food proteins by digestive enzymes (see Chapter 9 for discussion of digestive enzymes) such as pepsin and trypsin, with subsequent chemical analysis, is a promising method for the future. The enzymatic tests are rapid and relatively inexpensive to perform.

PROTEIN REQUIREMENTS

Based on PER, biological value, nitrogen balance studies, and other biochemical studies, protein recommendations for humans have been established. The RDA (Recommended Dietary Allowance) set by the National Research Council is approximately 44 to 56 grams of protein for adults who consume a mixed diet. Table 6.2 lists protein contents of many foods. Proper complementation of these various protein sources serve to provide the body with all essential amino acids. In terms of grams per kilogram of body weight, infants and children require much more protein than adults do (see below).

Infants	2.0–2.4 g./kg./day
Six months to 15 years	1.5 g./kg./day
Adults (men and women)	0.8 g./kg./day

A pregnant woman should add 30 grams of protein daily to her requirement to provide for fetal growth. During lactation, the mother should add 20 grams of protein to the requirement. Recent studies suggest that persons over 70 years of age may have an increased need for protein above the adult level of 0.8 g./kg./day possibly due to very poor efficiency of utilization.

The RDAs have been set to account for the efficiency of utilization and the fact that people eat a mixed diet. Studies indicate that it is possible for healthy adults to live on only 20 to 30 grams of high-quality protein per day. Therefore, there is a substantial safety factor included in the RDA figures. No extra protein is required for extra activity or stress; only extra energy need be supplied.

PROTEIN CONSUMPTION PROBLEMS

Protein supplies vary throughout the world. In the Orient, where the major portion of the diet consists of rice, 20 to 30 grams of moderate-quality protein are consumed in an average day. Since cooked rice is only 2% or 2.5% protein, about five pounds of rice would have to be consumed in a day to meet an RDA of 50 grams. Actually, many Orientals do consume over two pounds of rice per day; however, this protein is of moderate quality and must be complemented with vegetables, beans, and nuts. Many do not do this and thus live on the borderline of protein malnutrition.

In areas of Africa, Asia, and Central America severe protein shortages occur during certain periods of the year and can be particularly severe during water shortages or flooding. The disease of protein deficiency is known as kwashiorkor, named after the Ghanaian word for "the evil spirit that infects the first child when the second child is born." When the first child is removed from breastfeeding because the second child has taken its place, the first child must be provided with a high-quality diet. Often, in these poor areas, the child is given a thin cereal gruel or a mashed fruit paste. Consumption of these low-protein weaning foods leads to poor growth, discolorization of skin and hair, edema, bloated stomachs, open, unhealing sores, anemia, and death if untreated. Death usually comes from a common malady like measles or viral infection. The child with kwashiorkor is unable to produce antibodies to fend off familiar illnesses. Availability of adequate weaning foods, improvement of sanitation, and better food education would help diminish the incidence of this disease.

Problems also exist with consuming too much protein. In the United States the average adult may consume over 100 grams per day, with a range from 80 grams to 150 grams. Of this, a large percentage comes from animal protein. Males eat more protein because they associate this with increased strength and vigor. For a person with normal kidney and liver function this is no problem. Persons with either kidney or liver disease must limit their intake of protein to levels near their actual requirement. Excess protein must be broken down in the liver to yield carbon skeletons and ammonia. Normally the liver converts ammonia to urea, which flows through the blood to the kidney where it is excreted in the urine. In liver disease, urea is not efficiently produced and ammonia levels increase. Ammonia is extremely toxic. In kidney disease, the urea is not efficiently excreted in the urine and blood urea levels rise. In either of these diseases, high protein intake produces nausea, vomiting, and, in extreme cases, shock. With kidney failure, routine blood dialysis is necessary to remove toxic substances from the blood.

We again remind athletes who may want to consume several hundred grams of protein daily that this is useless and perhaps dangerous. Protein consumed in excess of the RDA is just used for energy or for production of fat stores. Protein consumption is a very expensive way to produce energy or fat.

PROTEIN INTOLERANCE

An intolerance for certain sugars such as lactose, which was discussed in Chapter 4, can result in intestinal discomfort. Likewise, intolerance for certain proteins can also cause allergy. One type of intolerance is celiac disease or, as it is also known, non-tropical sprue. This is an intolerance for one specific protein subfraction of gluten, the protein found in wheat and other cereals such as rye and barley. It does not show up until babies begin eating bread or certain cereals. The infants then begin to lose weight instead of gaining. Diarrhea, fatty stools, and weight loss are the first symptoms. Celiac disease affects about one in every 2,000 infants to some degree, but the cause was not discovered until the 1950s. If gluten is eaten, the food in the intestine cannot be digested properly because the intestinal wall is irritated by the protein allergy and loses its absorption ability. Most of the food eaten is passed directly into the feces because the intestine cannot absorb it. Loss of weight occurs as other tissues break down to supply the required calories and nutrients. This disease can be prevented very easily by feeding a gluten-free diet. Wheat flour that does not contain this gluten protein has been commercially produced. In many cases, celiac disease disappears after a few years. In others, the disease may be so mild that it goes unrecognized until later in life when it shows up again.

Some children and adults have an allergy to certain other proteins such as those in milk. In some rare cases, it can be so severe that consuming the protein can cause a type of shock reaction, which can close up the throat and windpipe and even lead to death from lack of oxygen. Reasons for these allergies are not well understood. In babies, the allergic reaction to cow's milk can be circumvented by using an infant formula based on soy protein.

SUMMARY

Protein is a major requirement in the human diet. Besides supplying energy at a rate of four Calories per gram, it is essential in the growth, repair, and maintenance of many tissues. Protein contains amino acids. Eight of these are essential to adult humans. A lack of certain essential amino acids in the diets of people of various countries has led to severe deficiency diseases, especially among young children. The essential amino acid profile of a protein and various animal tests such as the protein efficiency ratio (PER) can be used to estimate protein quality, that is, its potential for performing the needed functions in the body. Different foods may be eaten together to get a high-quality protein mix in the diet.

When protein is utilized, the nitrogen is incorporated into urea, which is excreted in the urine. People with liver or kidney failure cannot do this efficiently, so they must decrease protein intake. In the United States, excess consumption of protein is the norm, especially for those undergoing physical training. A little less protein in our diets would probably be beneficial.

The protein deficiency disease kwashiorkor is prevalent in areas of the world where high-quality weaning foods are lacking.

*Multiple
Choice
Study
Questions*

1. Proteins are polymers composed of

A. fatty acids
B. nucleic acids
C. citric acid
D. amino acids

2. The approximate number of different amino acids that make up proteins is

A. 8
B. 10
C. 12
D. 20
E. 40

3. The waste product of protein catabolism is urea, a substance that

A. is recycled into fatty acid
B. is diluted with water by the kidneys and excreted in the urine
C. is concentrated by dehydration and removed from the body primarily via the feces
D. is broken down to amino acids
E. both a and b are correct

4. Enzymes present in the foods we eat are

    A. important since they help digestion
    B. important sources of protein value
    C. digested as a source of amino acids
    D. helpful to reactions occurring in the body

5. The adult body requires about ___ essential amino acids.

    A. 12
    B. 6
    C. 8
    D. 21

6. Which amino acid is felt to be required only by children?

    A. histidine
    B. tryptophan
    C. threonine
    D. lysine
    E. methionine

The following is a list of amino acids that are present in protein. Use this list to answer questions 7 through 10.

    A. lysine
    B. methionine
    C. glycine
    D. tryptophan
    E. phenylalanine

7. This amino acid is the most limiting one in wheat.

8. This amino acid is the most limiting one in soybean.

9. This amino acid is the most limiting one in corn.

10. This amino acid is not an essential amino acid for humans.

11. The chemical score is used to evaluate

    A. vitamin stability
    B. synthetic vs. natural
    C. protein availability
    D. fat digestability
    D. protein quality

12. PER stands for

    A. percent vitamin E requirement
    B. protein evaluation requirement
    C. protein efficiency ratio
    D. protein excretion ratio
    E. None of the above

A new protein isolated from soy has the following amino acid composition. (Egg and corn are shown for comparison.) Use this table to answer questions 13 through 18.

Amount (mg.) per g. Protein

Food Protein	Histidine	Methionine	Phenylalanine	Lysine	Tryptophan
Soy	15	10	30	40	9
Corn	13	12	29	20	4
Egg	15	20	35	40	10

13. Which amino acid is the most limiting in soy, based on this data?

A. histidine
B. methionine
C. phenylalanine
D. lysine
E. tryptophan

14. The chemical score of the soy protein would be ____.

A. 20
B. 40
C. 50
D. 86
E. 90

15. If the soy were supplemented with the most limited amino acid to the value found in egg, the next limiting amino acid would be.

A. histidine
B. methionine
C. phenylalanine
D. lysine
E. tryptophan

16. The new chemical score of the supplemented soy protein would be ____.

A. 40
B. 50
C. 86
D. 90
E. 100

17. If the corn shown above were mixed in equal parts with the soy, which amino acid would be limiting?

A. histidine
B. methionine
C. phenylalanine
D. lysine
E. tryptophan

18. What would be the new chemical score?

    A. 40

    B. 55

    C. 65

    D. 75

    E. 100

19. To balance out poor quality proteins in your diet you

    A. can eat a high-quality one at one meal and then a lower one at the next meal

    B. must take vitamin pills so the amino acids can be used more easily

    C. must mix the protein with meat, milk, fish, or eggs at the next meal

    D. should mix proteins that complement each other and supply missing amino acids

    E. none of the above

20. Vegetarians would have the most problems

    A. getting enough thiamin

    B. with endurance because they are underweight

    C. balancing their dietary amino acids

    D. in fulfilling their vitamin C intake

21. Which best describes the cause of kwashiorkor?

    A. lack of gelatin in diet

    B. lack of both essential amino acids and total protein

    C. lack of vitamin C

    D. lack of utilization of vitamin B_1

    E. lack of exercise

22. Celiac disease is a result of intolerance to

    A. phenylalanine

    B. tryptophan

    C. gelatin

    D. gluten

    E. galactose

Essay Study Questions

1. What functions do proteins perform in the body? How much is required by the adult human?

2. What is the difference between an essential and nonessential amino acid?

3. For what reason are complementing proteins used? Give an example.

4. Discuss PER as a measure of protein quality.

5. How is chemical score used to measure protein quality? Compare to BV and PER.

6. How can a vegetarian meet nutritional needs by using the Basic Four food groups?

7. What is celiac disease?

8. Discuss protein and calorie malnutrition on a worldwide basis.

9. Discuss the protein requirements of an athlete.

Things to Do

1. Using the values for essential amino acids (Table 6.5), calculate the intake of each one for one day from the diet survey.

2. Look in magazines and papers for ads on high-protein foods. Discuss the value of the product and the reliability of the claims.

3. Ask various people, including athletes, for their views on protein. Discuss these views in light of the evidence presented in the book.

4. Ask the school athletic coaches what they feel about the needs for protein. Discuss these in class.

Chapter 6. Answers to Multiple-Choice Study Questions: 1, D; 2, D; 3, B; 4, C; 5, C; 6, A; 7, A; 8, B; 9, D; 10, C; 11, E; 12, C; 13, B; 14, C; 15, C; 16, C; 17, B; 18, B; 19, D; 20, C; 21, B; 22, D.

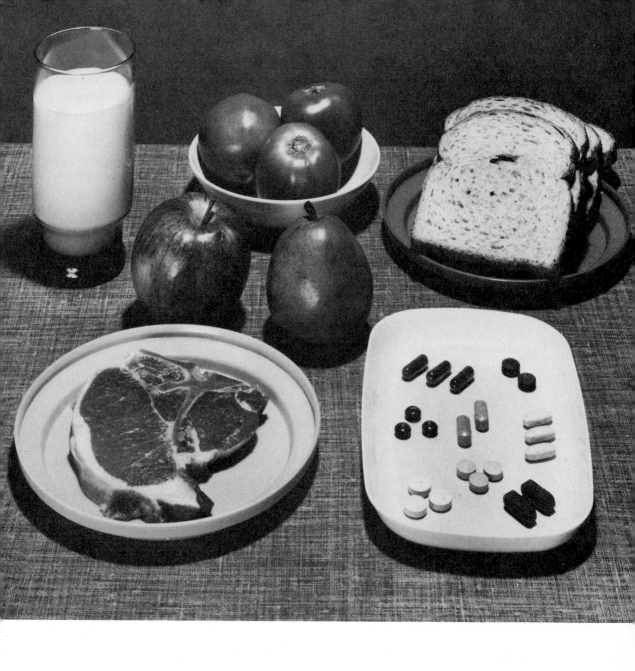

THE VITAMINS:
BIOLOGICAL
CATALYSTS FOR LIFE

7

THE TYPES OF VITAMINS IN FOODS

It has only been since the early 1900s that vitamins have been discovered, isolated, and chemically identified. Pasteur's discovery of disease-causing microbes in 1860 was largely responsible for the belief that all illnesses prevalent at that time were due to harmful microorganisms growing in the body. From 1860 until the early to mid-1900s scientists looked for germs or bacteria as the causes of diseases. Some diseases were actually the result of nutritional deficiencies. This search for bacteria hindered the probe into the nature and the functions of vitamins.

Many vitamins are utilized as organic catalysts to assist chemical reactions within the body. Others are incorporated into the membranes of cells. There are two categories of vitamins: water-soluble vitamins and fat-soluble vitamins. This nomenclature is based on the way in which they are isolated and does not mean that they function only in the water phase or in the fat tissues of the body. When the amount of a fat-soluble vitamin is measured in a food, for example, the food is extracted with an organic solvent that takes out fat and carries along any vitamins dissolved in it. The vitamin content can then be measured after separation from the solvent and fat. Water-soluble vitamins are usually extracted with an aqueous solution. It is interesting to note that any excess intake of water-soluble vitamins is usually excreted rapidly in the urine while an excess intake of fat-soluble vitamins is stored in the fat tissues of the body for later use.

Most of the vitamin deficiency diseases that plagued human beings for centuries have been severely reduced or alleviated throughout the world due to better choice of foods, food preparation practices, and food fortification programs. Many people, even in this country, still ingest marginal levels of some vitamins. The food industry must continue to increase the availability of a variety of nutrient-dense foods at affordable cost to all.

THE WATER-SOLUBLE VITAMINS

Vitamin B₁

A lack of vitamin B_1 (also called thiamin) in the diet produces a disease that was evident as early as 2600 B.C. called beriberi. The disease causes muscular weakness and leads to polyneuritis, which is a form of paralysis. In adults it prevents movement of limbs and in children it causes retardation of growth.

The disease was found primarily in the Orient where people ate diets based on polished rice. A rice kernel contains a bran layer around the outside, and the primary location of the thiamin is within the bran. Rubbing the rice between stones to polish it breaks this bran off and removes the brown color leaving attractive white rice. At the same time the thiamin is lost along with other B vitamins. The polishing of rice was an ancient practice that served as a method for cleaning the rice. In many parts of the Orient people felt that brown rice was dirty and therefore polished rice was much more desirable. In addition, the polished rice was more digestible. Beriberi became prevalent in the 1700s and 1800s as improved techniques for polishing rice were invented. This resulted in the removal of even greater amounts of thiamin.

In the 1880s the Japanese were losing great numbers of sailors to malnutrition because of their polished rice diets. Dr. K. Takaki, a Japanese doctor who had worked in the British Navy, decided to experiment to see if these losses could be reduced. Two ships were sent out with 276 men on board each ship. On one ship the traditional Japanese white rice diet was used, but on the other ship he administered the British Navy Diet, which consisted of meat, milk, eggs, and rice. At the end of nine months, almost 200 of the 276 men on the rice diet had developed beriberi. On the other ship only 14 crewmen developed the disease. Interestingly, these 14 men did not like the British diet. They had smuggled their own familiar supply of white rice on board and were not eating the British diet. Unfortunately, the Japanese doctor did not realize the relationship between polishing white rice and beriberi, and instead attributed the malady to a bacteria present in the white rice.

In 1886, a Dutch physician, Dr. Christian Eijkman, went to an Indonesian hospital to study beriberi. He noticed that chickens kept on the grounds for the purpose of supplying eggs gradually developed the symptoms of beriberi when consuming their white rice diet. He observed this for about three months, when the chickens suddenly recovered. Eijkman discovered that the camp had changed cooks after the three-month period and that the new cook was feeding the chickens brown rice, or peasant's rice. The cook felt he could not feed the more expensive rice to the chickens. Based on this observation, Dr. Eijkman concluded, as had Takaki, that there was a disease organism in white rice, and he searched for it unsuccessfully. However, he did get people to eat the brown rice to cure the disease.

In 1911 Casimir Funk, a Polish scientist, extracted about 800 pounds of the bran hulls from rice, and, after isolation, produced six ounces of pure white powder. He found that this powder could cure beriberi and he originally classified it as Vitalamine. This name was later changed to vitamin B_1 or thiamin.

Thiamin is found in meats, especially pork, liver, whole-grain cereals, and inactivated dry yeast. One serving of pork, in fact, contains about 0.6 mg., which is about 50% of the RDA for an adult. People have acquired vitamin B_1 deficiencies by eating raw clams and raw fish as a major part of their diet. These raw seafoods contain an enzyme, thiaminase, which destroys thiamin in the food as it is digested. Alcoholics can develop symptoms of beriberi, especially if they consume distilled wine because the thiamin originally present in the grapes does not carry over into the finished product. Alcoholics' diets are usually very low in most essential nutrients, including thiamin.

When foods are properly cooked and processed, about 10% to 20% of the thiamin is lost because it is slightly sensitive to heat. Excessive heating of foods can result in losses in excess of 40%.

White rice is a good source of thiamin if it is enriched or parboiled. The bountiful effects of parboiling can be traced back to the times when the Indonesians, Chinese, and Japanese all had beriberi, but people from India did not. The Indians had developed a process for easier removal of the hull by parboiling the rice: Rice is boiled for 10 minutes or so, and then taken out and dried. This allows the hulls to break off more easily when ground. When the dry rice is in the boiling water, water penetrates the hull and hydrates the rice kernel. The movement of water through the hull allows water-soluble vitamins to move from the hull into the rice kernel. At the present time most commercially processed white rice is handled in a similar manner. High-pressure steam is used to force the thiamin into the rice kernel. Some white rice contains higher percentages of thiamin than does brown rice because of this processing method and also because extra B vitamins are usually added as an enrichment technique.

It should be pointed out that the water-soluble nature of thiamin and other B vitamins causes them to be easily leached into the cooking water, especially if excess water is used in cooking or if cooking time is prolonged. It is far better to use a small amount of water for a short period to cook vegetables than to cover the vegetables with water and boil for a long period of time. More B-complex vitamins may end up in the cooking water (which is usually discarded) than in the cooked vegetables.

A major role that thiamin plays in metabolism is to catalyze enzyme reactions involved in removal of carbon dioxide (CO_2) from certain intermediates in carbohydrate metabolism. One such reaction is the transformation of pyruvic acid, a metabolic product of glucose, into acetyl COA. (Refer to Figure 4.2 and note that acetyl COA enters the Krebs Cycle and during its breakdown to water and CO_2, ATP is produced.) In thiamin deficiency, less acetyl COA is produced and thus not enough ATP is produced to supply the energy needs of the body for muscular movement or nerve transmission.

The RDA for thiamin, as shown in Table 2.1, is based on human biochemical studies. The need for this vitamin increases with greater caloric intake. If we consume 0.12 mg. per 1,000 Calories or less than 0.25 mg. per day for an extended period of time, muscular weakness in adults and growth retardation of children could occur. In addition, one might have speech difficulty, loss of memory, anorexia (a loss of appetite and body wasting), and edema (tissue swelling). Twice this level in the diet alleviates most of these symptoms. The body tissues become saturated with the vitamin if 0.5 mg. are consumed daily for several weeks. Any additional thiamin in the diet is excreted in the urine. Most people consume 1.0 to 1.5 mg. per day from their normal foods. This is around the RDA value. Thus the tissues are always saturated if all the vitamin is absorbed during digestion and the excess is excreted in the urine. If you stopped consuming thiamin, in about 9-18 days some symptoms of deficiency would begin to show because in that time about one-half of the thiamin that is stored in the tissues is used up. The average American diet is quite sufficient in vitamin B_1. In studies on the ingestion of excess quantities of thiamin, no deleterious or beneficial effects have as yet been found.

Vitamin B_2

Vitamin B_2, or riboflavin, is usually found in foods wherever thiamin is present. Riboflavin's main function is in the manufacture of ATP in the Krebs oxidation cycle. No real riboflavin deficiencies are found in the United States. However, where it has been found, this deficiency is recognized by cracks in the corners of the mouth, skin disorders, and a red swollen tongue. These deficiency signs may show up when consumption falls below 0.25 mg. per 1,000 Calories. Tissue saturation occurs at about 0.6 mg. daily intake. Slightly more riboflavin is needed during pregnancy, as indicated in Table 2.1.

Riboflavin is found in liver, milk, meat, and green vegetables. Vitamin B_2 is much more stable when heated than vitamin B_1, but can be destroyed by light. Milk is no longer stored in clear glass bottles so as to protect the riboflavin from light-induced breakdown. The same is true for packaging cereal in paperboard boxes. There is no known toxicity for riboflavin.

Vitamin B_6

Vitamin B_6 is chemically found in foods in three forms, pyridoxine, pyridoxamine, and pyridoxal. Although there is no known specific deficiency disease for this vitamin, in some studies with infants on a formula diet deficient in B_6, nervous disorders developed. B_6 is involved as part of enzyme systems used for synthesizing nonessential amino acids from the essential ones. Tissue saturation occurs at about 0.5 mg. per day, but the RDA is set four times higher (about 2.0 mg. per day). If a diet is completely deficient in B_6, about half the stored B_6 is used in 15 to 20 days.

Recent evidence indicates that some women taking oral contraceptives may require more vitamin B_6. At low intakes, especially when taking contraceptives, anemia, weight loss, and depression may occur. Vitamin B_6 is often administered to pregnant women to relieve nausea and vomiting. As with the previous vitamins, there are no known toxic effects at high doses. Although high doses of six to eight grams per day (or 3,000 to 4,000 times the RDA) have been used to treat schizophrenia, there are no properly controlled studies to show that this practice is effective.

Vitamin B_{12} (Cobalamin)

The lack of vitamin B_{12} in the diet or poor absorption of it can result in pernicious anemia. Poor absorption is usually caused by a rare genetic disease in which the human lacks a protein- and carbohydrate-containing substance (intrinsic factor) that can aid in the absorption of B_{12} from the gastrointestinal tract. For these people B_{12} must be given by injection. In true vegetarians, pernicious anemia can result because B_{12} is present almost exclusively in foods of animal origin. Without B_{12} not enough healthy red blood cells are formed and anemia results. Red blood cells in blood take up oxygen in the lungs and carry it to the cells where it is needed so glucose can be metabolized to form ATP. Without sufficient oxygen transport to cells, not enough ATP is formed and therefore one becomes weak and has a low resistance to disease.

As seen in Table 2.1, the RDA for B_{12} is very small (3 μg. for an adult). The actual requirement is actually only 0.1 to 1.0 μg. per day. The higher RDA accounts for the biological differences in absorption by people. Today B_{12} can be made in the laboratory through fermentation processes, but previously it had to be extracted from beef liver; one ton of liver yielded only one gram.

Vitamin B_{12} is found in all animal foods. The average diet supplies 5 to 15 μg. per day or two to five times the RDA. Although B_{12} is not present in vegetable foods, B_{12} deficiency takes three to five years to appear in a pure vegetarian who consumes no meat, fish, poultry, or dairy products because the vitamin is stored in the liver. This vitamin is unique compared to other B vitamins since they are poorly stored and lost from body tissues at a far greater rate than is B_{12}. The liver can supply the needed B_{12} this long because only about 0.1% of the initially stored quantity is used per day. Thus pernicious anemia would be a slowly developing disease in pure vegetarians unless they took dried yeast occasionally, or had a B_{12} injection.

Niacin

Niacin (nicotinic acid or nicotinamide) is another water-soluble vitamin that is found in foods in several forms. Pellagra, the disease caused by lack of niacin, is still very common in some parts of the world, especially in Africa. The word pellagra means rough skin. In niacin deficiency, parts of the body exposed to sun suffer from a severe reaction; the exposed area becomes covered with lesions that are red and very rough. A smooth, red tongue is another sign of the disease. Niacin deficiency can also cause severe diarrhea. A lack of niacin may eventually lead to mental confusion. It is sometimes referred to as the disease of 3 Ds: dermatitis (skin disorders); dementia (mental confusion); and diarrhea. A forth D—death—can result if pellagra is not treated with niacin.

Pellagra was first described in detail in the medical literature in the 1700s and became more well-known during the United States Civil War. The disease became epidemic around the turn of the century among the poor in the South who at that time consumed corn meal and grits as the major part of their diet, along with pork fat. This diet caused pellagra. In 1914, Dr. Joseph Goldberger of the United States Public Health Service found that adding milk or meat to this minimal diet solved the problem. Since this treatment did not follow the germ theory, scientists looked for some antipellagra factor in milk for many years but did not find it. Niacin is present in milk, but in very low quantities (about 0.1 mg. pint). Milk cured the disease because the essential amino acid tryptophan present in milk (and meat) can be converted to niacin by the body. This process will occur if niacin is lacking in the diet. The efficiency of this conversion is only 60 parts tryptophan making one part niacin, but it is high enough to prevent pellagra. Niacin, and the mechanism of its conversion from tryptophan, was finally discovered by research workers led by Dr. Conrad Elvehjem at the University of Wisconsin in 1937. Pellagra still occurs in parts of the world where the diet is inadequate in niacin, especially if the major food in the diet has a low protein or tryptophan content as does a staple diet of corn products or cassava.

The major niacin-deficiency disorders show up when the dietary intake of niacin falls below 4 mg. per 1,000 Calories or 8–9 mg. per day. The RDA is set at about twice this level. In the average American diet tryptophan supplies some of the niacin needs. The average diet contains about 8–17 mg. of niacin and 50–1,000 mg. of tryptophan daily or more than twice the equivalent level of the RDA. The major dietary sources of niacin are enriched breads, cereals, pasta, and rice. Some niacin in whole-grain cereals is bound and poorly available for humans' use. Meat and fish supply on the average from 2–4 mg. per 3.5-oz. serving. Consumption of high levels of niacin has caused flushing of the skin and headaches in some individuals.

Folic Acid

Folic acid (sometimes called folacin or folate) has the chemical name pteroyl monoglutamic acid (PGA). Folic acid is present in a wide variety of foods including liver, fresh fruits, and leafy vegetables. Some of it is bound, however, so it cannot be totally utilized. It has been estimated that the average human needs about 50 micrograms per day. The RDA has been set at 400 micrograms, as shown in Table 2.1.

Dietary intake studies show that we ingest about 40 to 350 micrograms of folic acid daily. In addition, some bacteria in our intestinal tract synthesize folic acid that we can partially absorb. In spite of this, some diets, especially in children, young girls, and pregnant women are low in this water-soluble vitamin. As with vitamin B_{12}, lack of folic acid results in poorly formed red blood cells. Women who take oral contraceptives may require additional folate. Folic acid is lost in heating of foods. People who don't consume many fresh fruits and vegetables may be obtaining low levels of folic acid from their diets.

Pantothenic Acid

This vitamin is part of the enzyme system that is involved in the metabolism of glucose, fats, and proteins in the step where their breakdown products are brought into the Krebs Cycle. Pantothenic acid also contributes to steroid hormone synthesis. It is found widely distributed in animal foods, whole-grain cereals, beans, and nuts.

A deficiency disease has not been found in human beings. Removing it from the diet of experimental animals creates a wide range of problems and can result in death. Deficiency is unlikely in people as the average diet in the United States supplies about 5–20 mg. per day. The estimated safe and adequate dietary intake (Table 2.3) for pantothenic acid is 4–7 mg. for adults.

Biotin

This vitamin is usually found bound to a protein. It is important for the synthesis of fats. The average intake is about 100–300 μg. per day; but about three to six times more biotin is excreted in the urine. This suggests that biotin is also synthesized by bacteria in the intestine and we can absorb some of it. The only deficiencies that have been found are caused by consuming large quantities of raw egg white. A protein in the egg white (avidin) prevents biotin from being absorbed. When the egg is cooked, the protein has no effect on biotin.

Vitamin C (Ascorbic Acid)

As with thiamin, lack of the water-soluble vitamin C in their diets caused trouble for ancient sailors. The disease that results from a deficiency of vitamin C is called scurvy. The failure of early sea explorers to carry along a balanced diet led to the death of many seamen. In those times scurvy was thought to be caused by cold, damp conditions on board the ship. Analysis of the records kept by many of the early sailors from Europe revealed that the seamen consumed diets basically composed of dried beans, cheese, and some salted, dried beef. There were no fruits or vegetables for the common sailors, yet the officers always had supply of these foods. The officers were much less prone to scurvy. However, the dietary factor was not associated with the disease until much later.

Early symptoms that appear with a vitamin-C deficiency are lesions in the mouth, weak and bleeding gums, and loosening of teeth. A prolonged deficiency can lead to convulsions and death can result from poor resistance to infection. Occasionally mild scurvy still shows up in the United States. Dentists sometimes treat gum problems as periodontal disease when it is actually scurvy. The most amazing fact about scurvy is that in advanced stages it can result in old wounds reopening. James Cook, the famous explorer, wrote about some of his sailors in their late 60s who had 50-year-old wounds reopen. This is because vitamin C is necessary in the crosslinks of tissue proteins that hold tissues together. When vitamin C is deficient, the links weaken and the tissues separate.

James Lind, a British medical officer and one of the first men to study scurvy, was interested in the difference between the diet of the officers on board ship and the common sailors. In 1710 he ran an experiment on one of the ships he was assigned to in which he fed the sailors their normal fruit-free diet plus different diet supplements including cider vinegar, garlic, salt, alcohol, and other foods. In one diet some of the sailors were fed two oranges a day. This diet cured their scurvy, whereas sailors on the other tested diets were not cured. Upon his return to London, Lind went before the Royal Medical Society and presented the results of his experiments. Unfortunately, he was laughed at for the simplicity of the results. No one believed that a disease could so easily be cured by a change in diet.

The British Navy forbade Lind to continue these experiments on other ships. It was not until 1795 that the British Navy finally concluded that the results of Lind's experiment were meaningful. They then ordered that lemon juice be added to the diets of the sailors. At that time, lemons were called limes, and the British sailors receiving the daily dose of lemon juice became known as limeys.

The mission of Adamson Scott, the explorer who went to the North Pole in 1912, ended in death for everyone because there were no fruits and vegetables in the diet of his men. Autopsies of the victims revealed that they had developed scurvy. It should be noted that in 1535 when Jacques Cartier was exploring North America, many of his men were suffering from scurvy. American Indians he met gave the men pine-needle broth, which cured them, but of course they did not realize the broth contained vitamin C and was the cure of the disease.

Scurvy is not fatal in itself. It lowers the body's resistance to other disease, which can eventually be fatal. The exact relationship of vitamin C in lowering resistance is not known.

It was not until 1932 that ascorbic acid (vitamin C) was isolated, and identified and named by Dr. Albert Szent-Gyorgyi, a Hungarian scientist, and Dr. Charles G. King of the University of Pittsburgh.

Vitamin C is found mostly in fruits and vegetables. Orange juice is an excellent source; six ounces at breakfast supplies about 60 mg., which is the RDA. Fresh young potatoes are also an excellent source. Some of this vitamin C is lost in storage, but stored potatoes are still high in vitamin C. A medium-sized baked potato contains 20 mg. of vitamin C, one-third of the RDA. More vitamin C is lost, however, when french fries are made because of the higher temperature used in frying.

Ascorbic acid is the least stable of all the vitamins. Heat processing, such as the overcooking of vegetables, can result in a 30% to 100% loss of vitamin C. The industrial canning of vegetables, which is needed to make them safe from botulism (see Chapter 17), destroys about 10% to 20% of the vitamin C in the process. Vitamin C is easily leached from foods with water. Proper preparation and cooking techniques are needed to maintain vitamin-C content in foods.

Vitamin C is involved in many different mechanisms in the body. It is part of the protein linkages that hold tissues together. Thus, in a deficiency the body will easily bruise and bleed if slightly injured. Vitamin C is also involved in the formation of some hormones. Vitamin C enhances iron absorption from foods and utilization in the body. Some scientists also feel that it acts as an antihistamine that provides some resistance to stress.

The average requirement for adults has been set at 60 mg. per day. This maintains the tissues below the saturation level of about 80 mg. per day. However, one would have to drop consumption to less than 10 mg. per day to have scurvy result. Based on the fact that about one-half of the vitamin-C store is used up in 20 days, early symptoms of scurvy could appear after 30–45 days on a diet that had no vitamin C.

Some people believe vitamin C helps prevent colds. Others feel that vitamin C prevents cancer as well. Linus Pauling, who won the Nobel Prize in Chemistry and the Nobel Peace Prize, wrote a book on the usefulness of vitamin C as a preventive for the common cold. However, conclusive evidence supporting this concept has yet to be uncovered. A study conducted by the University of Toronto Medical School used a double-blind experiment to test the vitamin C cold prevention theory. A double-blind experiment is one in which the doctors who administer the doses and who check the patients do not know if the subjects in the experiment are receiving a placebo (something that looks, tastes, and smells like the drug but has no effect) or the actual test drug. Only the researcher who sets up the experiment is aware of the doses and who is getting what. In this experiment involving about 2,000 students, there was no significant difference in the number of colds people caught, but there was a 40% reduction in the duration of colds for people who were given vitamin C. (For example, instead of having a cold for three days, it may have only lasted one and one-half days.) When this experiment was repeated, the results were less dramatic. The National Institute of Health also conducted an experiment and found no effectiveness for vitamin C in cold prevention or treatment. Thus, vitamin C probably has little effect in preventing colds for most people.

More recently, vitamin C has been promoted as a cancer preventive agent. People are being urged to consume several grams of the vitamin daily. No solid evidence exists to support the theory that vitamin C prevents cancer. Even if there were, consumption of several grams of vitamin C daily is a therapeutic dose level and would have little to do with the nutritional role of the vitamin.

One problem with taking too much vitamin C occurs in people who are susceptible to gout. Gout results from the deposition in joints of the metabolic breakdown products of some of the large molecules that form the genetic material in the cells. These large molecules are known as RNA and DNA. Uric acid is one of the products formed when DNA or RNA decomposes. Under certain conditions, when the pH of the blood changes, deposition of uric acid in the joints of the body can occur. One of the first joints affected is the big toe. Gout is more prevalent in men, appearing at 30 to 35 years of age as a sudden pain in a big toe lasting for a very short time. A gout condition can be made more acute by an excess intake of vitamin C, which can change the acidity of the blood and cause uric acid deposition. About 5% of the male population of the United States has a tendency to develop gout. At high levels of vitamin C, oxalic acid, a breakdown product of ascorbic acid, may also crystallize out of the urine leading to kidney stones. Thus one should be careful in taking too many vitamin-C tablets. Some people have been using one to four grams per day for cold prevention. At about four to nine grams per day, the problems discussed above may occur. In addition, stomach upset and diarrhea may occur.

In one study with women taking high levels of vitamin C (six grams per day), severe menstrual bleeding occurred. Pregnant women may also induce a condition of high vitamin C requirement in the child if they take too much ascorbic acid. When the child is born, the normal infant diet does not supply this higher need, and scurvy can appear. This condition is known as rebound scurvy.

THE FAT-SOLUBLE VITAMINS

Two of the fat-soluble vitamins, A and D, are important historically because of the worldwide prevalence of diseases caused by dietary deficiencies of these vitamins. The other two fat-soluble vitamins, E and K, one rarely deficient in human diets.

Vitamin A

Vitamin A (retinol) is associated by the public primarily with maintaining eyesight, but it has many other roles in the body. For centuries thousands of children, especially children in the Orient, the Middle East, and Africa have become blind each year because of a dietary deficiency of vitamin A. In World War I the Danes sold much of the butter they manufactured to England in order to get money to buy armaments. Consequently, children at that time were forced to drink skim milk. Since the butter fat had been removed and the vitamin A that was supplied by milk remained in the fat, many of them became blind because of the lack of the vitamin. The Scots and Canadian fishermen in the early 1900s found that by eating fish liver they could prevent night blindness, but it was not until 1930 that vitamin A was isolated at the University of Wisconsin.

Vitamin A is required for proper growth for most tissues in the body. It is particularly important for maintenance of the cells of the eye, skin, and gastrointestinal tract. Another function of vitamin A is to help us see in dim light. Pilots were told during World War II to eat lots of carrots to help their night vision. Vitamin A is also necessary for proper bone growth and for reproduction functions in both men and women.

Vitamin A values are expressed in terms of International Units (IU) or retinol equivalents (RE) since there are many different forms of the vitamin in foods. One RE is equivalent to 3.3 IU of vitamin activity from retinol. At a daily intake of less than 150 RE, night blindness occurs. With lower levels the tear ducts stop up and eventually the smooth cells of the eye are replaced by rough cells leading to blindness. Above 400 RE per day symptoms of vitamin A deficiency are absent.

Vitamin A is found as carotenoids in dark green leafy vegetables, in some orange vegetables, such as carrots, and in fruits. In animal tissue, such as liver and butter fat, it is in the form of retinol, which has the greatest biological activity. Table 7.1 lists the equivalent vitamin A content of some foods based on the conversion of carotenoids to the active form of vitamin A in the body. The RDA for vitamin A is 800 RE for women and 1,000 RE for men. Since vitamin A is partially stored in the liver, one serving of liver every other week should just about meet the RDA as would a serving of carrots every third day.

Vitamin A is a vitamin that can be very toxic if taken in large amounts. If 10 to 20 times the RDA daily is consumed over a period of time, anorexia, headache, blurred vision, hair loss, muscle soreness, flaky skin, and cracked lips can occur. In fact, inter-cranial pressure can be so high that some people have been operated on for a brain tumor when the pressure was due to an excess vitamin-A intake. At 70,000 IU of β-carotene daily, skin yellowing can occur, but the other toxic effects have not been shown to occur because carotene itself is not toxic. Thus one cannot overdose on carrots or other vegetables.

On the other hand, it is not difficult to overdose on vitamin pills. Most health-food stores sell vitamin A pills in 25,000 IU tablets. Two such tablets daily contain ten times the RDA. This level has been

TABLE 7.1 Foods high in vitamin A

Food	Serving size	Amount vitamin A	
		IU	RE
Cantaloupe	½ medium	7,000	2,100
Carrots	4 oz.	10,000	3,000
Liver	3½ oz.	40,000	12,100
Milk	8 oz.	300	90
Spinach	3½ oz.	1,000	300
Summer squash	3 oz.	3,000	900
Sweet potato	3½ oz.	8,000	2,400
Winter squash	3 oz.	3,000	900

IU = International Units
RE = retinol equivalents
Adapted from USDA Handbook No. 456

recently shown to be toxic to some individuals when ingested daily over a long period of time. Levels of 50,000 to 125,000 IU of vitamin A are sometimes prescribed for prevention of acne and cancer. This level of intake is extremely dangerous and unwise. Researchers are currently testing synthetic derivatives of retinol which are far less toxic than vitamin A for their potential as acne and cancer prevention agents. These vitamin-A derivatives act as drugs and not as vitamins. Self-treatment with vitamins is very unwise and should be discouraged for all.

Interestingly, polar bear liver has about one million IU of vitamin A as retinol in a three-ounce serving. Eskimos had learned through experience that polar bear liver had to be excluded from their diet because it resulted in death due to the vitamin-A toxicity. Unfortunately Artic explorers learned the same lesson from consuming polar bear liver.

In 1975 an Englishman who consumed high quantities of carrot juice and vitamin A capsules died of vitamin-A toxicity. He was consuming over two million IU per day. What can be learned from this is that moderation in vitamins is important.

Vitamin D

Vitamin D deficiency is called rickets when it occurs in children. The disease began to occur more frequently in the late 1600s when people began migrating from farms into the cities, such as London, where they encountered fog made worse by high levels of smoke caused by the burning of wood and coal in their shelters and homes. Levels of available sunlight were thus reduced. Because sunlight causes a conversion of a chemical in the skin into vitamin D, the conversion was inhibited, and rickets resulted.

Rickets usually affects children and causes malformation (bowing) of the legs because vitamin D is important in the absorption of calcium and phosphates from the intestinal tract. If insufficient vitamin D is present in the diet, not enough calcium is absorbed, and the bones will not form properly. In adults, the deficiency disease is called osteomalacia, which results in bone softening. Vitamin D is also important in reabsorption of calcium from the kidneys so that the mineral is not lost in large amounts in the urine.

The early study of rickets led to many controversies. The children of Scottish people who lived in small towns usually did not get rickets. The parents attributed this to the fact that the children drank cod-liver oil every week. Medical people, however, could not believe something as simple as fish oil could cure disease. The issue was also complicated by the fact that people living in the city slums in the Orient did not show signs of rickets. The fact that they received much more sunlight than did the Europeans was not taken into consideration since the mechanism occurring in the skin was unknown. It was not until 1922 that vitamin D was isolated from cod-liver oil by Dr. E.V. McCollum. At the same time it was also discovered that a sterol, which is similar to cholesterol, present in the fat just below the skin, was converted to vitamin D upon exposure to sunlight.

As a public-health measure, in many states, milk is required to be fortified with about 400 IU (international units) of vitamin D per quart. An international unit is used as it is with vitamin A, since vitamin D comes in many forms. Margarine, which has become a popular substitute for butter, is often fortified for the same reason. One egg supplies 40 IU, which is 10% of the RDA.

The RDA for vitamin D for adults over 19 years of age is lower than it is for children because bone growth is minimal. In children, 100 IU per day prevents rickets and 300 IU gives maximum bone growth rate even with no sun exposure.

Vitamin D is more toxic than vitamin A. Symptoms such as fever, irritability, vomiting, and diarrhea occur with 2,000 IU per day. At 4,000 IU daily over a period of time, soft tissues of the body can become calcified. This means that calcium begins to get deposited in arteries, muscle, and the kidney, leading to loss of their function.

Vitamin E

There have been no recognized human deficiency diseases caused by a lack of vitamin E (tocopherol) as has been found for other vitamins. Rats fed an oil-free diet containing no vitamin E develop a hemolytic anemia, pregnant rats have an increase in the number of stillborn births, and male rats become sterile. In some cases, when human infants were put on a very low fat diet, edema, anemia, and fragility of the capillaries occurred, but no clinical effects have been shown in adults.

Chemically, vitamin E protects polyunsaturated fats in body cells from being broken down by oxidation. Vitamin E also protects vitamin A from oxidation. Because it is hard to determine any adverse effects at low dietary levels, the RDA has been set based on normal consumption patterns. For adults the RDA in Table 2.1 has been set at 8 to 10 IU per day, although in some studies measured intakes are less. An international unit is used again because of the several different forms found in foods which have different biological activities.

Table 7.2 shows the major sources of vitamin E in the diet. Also shown is the ratio of vitamin E to unsaturated fats. This value is considered an index of the degree of protection of the body from

TABLE 7.2 Good sources of vitamin E

Food	Tocopherol content per 100 g.	Ratio of vitamin E (mg.)/g. polyunsaturated fat
Soybean oil	11 IU	0.6
Corn oil	20 IU	0.5
Safflower oil	24 IU	0.35
Margarine	15 IU	0.83
Cottonseed oil	80 IU	1.0

oxidation. A level greater than 0.6 mg./g. unsaturated fat consumption is considered adequate. This can be achieved if soybean and cottonseed oils and margarine supply 20% of the calories in the average diet. This is about 450 Calories or 50 grams of the unsaturated fats. The rest of the diet, especially whole-grain cereals, supplies the remaining vitamin E. In general, those vegetable oils that are high in polyunsaturated fats are also high in vitamin E. Thus, vitamin E is probably acting as a natural antioxidant in the soybean or wheat germ to protect against oxidation of unsaturated fatty acids.

Some clinicians have made unrealistic claims for the use of vitamin E in treating arthritis, healing burns, preventing heart disease, and improving sexual powers. These claims have not been scientifically substantiated. It is possible that the high levels prescribed (220–500 IU/day, or 20 to 40 times the RDA) can be dangerous. Some recent studies have shown that 300 to 800 IU per day caused fatigue and blurred vision in males but other studies have shown no effects from an excess.

Vitamin K

Vitamin K is an essential cofactor for several steps of the complex set of reactions necessary for blood clotting. Outright deficiency of this vitamin would lead to uncontrolled bleeding and a quick death. Deficiency of this vitamin is rare because not only is it found naturally in dark-green leafy vegetables and in other food, but it is synthesized by bacteria in the large intestine. About half of our daily needs are supplied by the intestinal synthesis. Newborn infants, whose intestinal tracts are not yet inhabited by bacteria, and persons who have taken antibiotics over a long period of time are at risk for vitamin K deficiency. Vitamin K is usually administered in these cases to prevent uncontrolled bleeding. The rest of the population is at little risk of vitamin-K deficiency. For this reason no RDA has been established for vitamin K. It is, however, listed on the estimated safe and adequate daily dietary intake list (Table 2.3).

SUMMARY

Vitamins are the trace organic compounds that perform many essential functions in the body, especially as parts of the enzyme systems. They are classified as being either water-soluble or fat-soluble. Because of poor diets or the improper storage or processing of some foods, worldwide deficiency diseases can develop. This chapter shows that a wide variety of foods must be consumed to attain a diet sufficient in all of the vitamins. The RDAs established for each vitamin are based on historical and biochemical evidence, tissue saturation studies, and levels in the normal diet. Certain vitamins, such as A and D, have toxic effects if taken in excess. Thus, overindulgence in vitamin pills is not a good practice. Vitamin C, thiamin, and folic acid can be destroyed if foods are overcooked. The major vitamins are distributed in the foods included in the Basic Four food groups.

Multiple Choice Study Questions

1. Which of the following is not a water-soluble vitamin?

A. niacin

B. thiamin

C. riboflavin

D. tocopherol

E. folacin

2. Which of the following is not a fat-soluble vitamin?

A. carotene

B. vitamin D

C. niacin

D. tocopherol

E. vitamin K

3. The B vitamins as a class are

A. soluble in food fats

B. important as energy foods

C. cofactors for various enzymes

D. low in meats and liver

4. Which is not a good source of niacin?

A. enriched bread

B. converted rice

C. whole-grain cereals

D. meat

E. orange juice

5. Tryptophan, present as an amino acid, can replace the vitamin requirement for

   A. niacin
   B. pyridoxal phosphate
   C. riboflavin
   D. ascorbate

6. A lack of vitamin B_{12} depresses the level of

   A. cholesterol
   B. bilirubin
   C. trypsin
   D. white blood cells
   E. hemoglobin

7. Women using birth control pills may have an increased need for

   A. B_1
   B. B_2
   C. B_6
   D. vitamin A
   E. vitamin E

8. Which vitamin is prevented from being absorbed by raw egg white?

   A. B_1
   B. C
   C. riboflavin
   D. folic acid
   E. biotin

9. A good source of vitamin C is

   A. milk
   B. baked potato
   C. meat
   D. rice cereal
   E. french fries

10. The "sunshine" vitamin is

   A. carotene (vitamin A) since it gives the skin a rosy color
   B. especially needed by adults
   C. produced from sterols
   D. formed when vitamin C is exposed to ultraviolet light

11. Vegetarians generally will have a problem in maintaining their intake of

   A. B_{12}
   B. niacin
   C. phosphorus
   D. potassium
   E. vitamin A

12. The best source of vitamin E is

   A. safflower oil
   B. cottonseed oil
   C. soybean oil margarine
   D. wheat germ
   E. raw almonds

13. This vitamin is needed for blood clotting.

   A. thiamin
   B. folacin
   C. choline
   D. vitamin K
   E. vitamin A

The following is a list of five essential vitamins. Match the one that best prevents the disease deficiencies described in questions 14 through 23.

   A. niacin
   B. ascorbic acid
   C. α-tocopherol
   D. β-carotene (retinol)
   E. vitamin D

14. A lack of this vitamin led to a disease that plagued many ships' crews and ancient explorers, causing old wounds to reopen.

15. Infants put on a formula diet low in fat content easily develop evidence of cell fragility (that is, the capillaries are easily broken).

16. The disease rickets, which causes weak, soft, misshapen bones in young children is prevented by adding this vitamin to the diet.

17. A disease described as the 3 Ds (diarrhea, dementia, and dermatitis) is caused by an absence of this vitamin from the diet.

18. Consumption of this nutrient at levels below 80% of the RDA causes a loss of balance and a decreased sensitivity to taste and smell.

For the same vitamins listed above, certain toxic effects become evident when they are consumed in excess. Questions 19 through 23 list these conditions. Which vitamin, when taken in excess, causes the described condition?

19. There is no clear toxic effect for this vitamin. However, symptoms of flushing of the skin, nausea, cramps, and headache may develop.

20. When taken in high levels by children, calcification of tissues, especially the kidney, can result.

21. In men at about 800 mg./day signs of fatigue and irritability develop.

22. This vitamin, in excess, causes pigmentation of the skin, hair loss, nausea and vomiting.

23. At high levels may cause diarrhea and may lead to kidney stones.

24. Pregnant and lactating women

   A. should increase calories only

   B. have greater needs for all nutrients

   C. should not increase ascorbic acid intake as it may result in infant scurvy

   D. should decrease iron so as to prevent hemochromatosis in the fetus

   E. should never gain more than 10 pounds

Essay Study Questions

1. What are vitamins and how are they categorized?

2. For vitamins B_1, A, D, and C discuss

   A. The specific nutritional disease caused by a lack in the diet.

   B. The RDA.

   C. The major food sources in the American diet.

   D. The effects of processing.

   E. The effects of an excess.

3. Relate the various theories associated with excess vitamin C in relationship to colds.

4. Discuss the various misconceptions people have about vitamin E.

5. What is a double-blind experiment?

6. What is the historical significance of beriberi and rice?

7. How are the RDAs established for vitamins?

8. What vitamins are most easily destroyed or lost during food processing?

Things to Do

1. Collect ads for vitamin pills from magazines and newspapers. What do they promise? Are they reliable?

2. Using the seven-day dietary survey, evaluate your nutritional health for two vitamins. If problems exist, how can they be solved?

3. Make charts showing the equivalent amounts of foods needed to be consumed compared to commonly available vitamin pills. Discuss the significance of your findings.

4. Examine and discuss the vitamin content of fortified cereals and bread. Do you feel it is necessary to add vitamins to these foods?

5. Ask people for their viewpoints on various vitamins. Discuss them in class.

6. Evaluate your vitamin-A intake. Is it sufficient?

Chapter 7. Answers to Multiple-Choice Study Questions: 1, D; **2,** C; **3,** C; **4,** E; **5,** A; **6,** E; **7,** C; **8,** E; **9,** B; **10,** C; **11,** A; **12,** B; **13,** D; **14,** B; **15,** C; **16,** E; **17,** A; **18,** D; **19,** A; **20,** E; **21,** C; **22,** D; **23,** B; **24,** B.

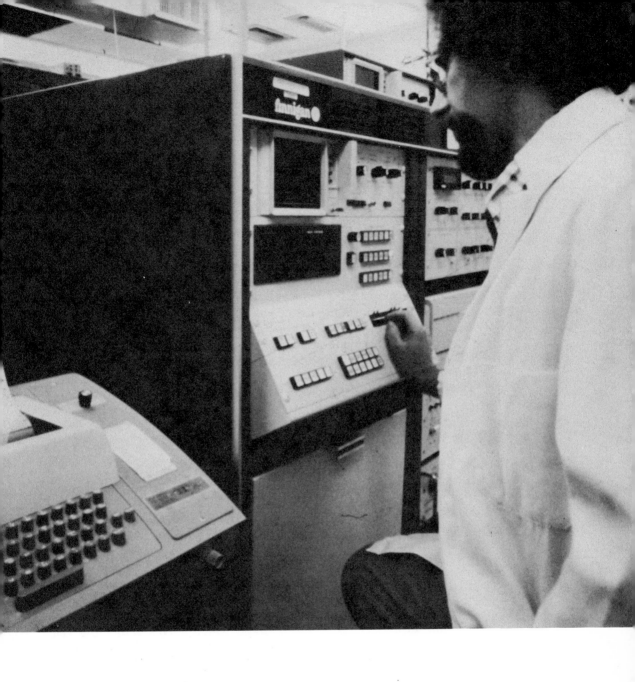

THE OTHER NUTRIENTS: MINERALS AND TRACE ELEMENTS

8

The nutritional significance of many minerals and trace elements is under extensive research today with new discoveries constantly being reported. Frequent breakthroughs in our knowledge of mineral nutrition remind us of the infancy of this field of nutrition research. In this chapter several essential elements will be discussed from the standpoint of (1) their distribution in the body and foods, (2) their function, and (3) the daily requirements.

MINERALS

Some minerals are required in large amounts. For example, the calcium recommendation is about 0.8 grams per day (800 mg.), whereas an average person needs less than 1/10,000 of that level for iodine. These elements may become part of cell structures or act as cofactors with the myriad of enzymes in the metabolic process. It should be noted that some marginal mineral deficiencies exist in the typical American diet. Calcium, iron, and possibly zinc, copper, selenium, and chromium are deficient in many diets partially due to poor dietary habits. There is concern that increased consumption of highly refined foods has reduced mineral intake. In addition, some people feel that depleted soil results in reduced trace mineral intakes.

Sodium and Potassium

These two elements are found in many foods and are important in maintaining the electrical, fluid, and chemical balance between the tissue cells and the blood. Sodium (Na) is found in higher concentrations outside the cells in the extracellular fluid while potassium (K) is located primarily inside the cell. Maintenance of proper concentrations of sodium and of potassium on each side of the cell membrane insures cellular equilibrium. Maintenance of sodium and potassium balance is also essential for nerve transmission. When a muscle undergoes contraction or an impulse travels along a nerve, there is a rapid exchange of these two elements across the cell membrane. The exchange creates the electrical impulse that controls the contraction.

Potassium is also involved with the function of many intracellular enzymes. A deficiency of potassium can lead to nervousness and, more seriously, irregular heartbeats and in some cases sudden heart failure. Cases of severe potassium deficiency and heart failure have been reported during prolonged fasting for weight loss and with some imbalanced diet plans. The chloride ion is usually associated with both sodium and potassium ions in the body. There have been no RDAs established for either sodium or potassium although both are listed on the estimated safe and adequate daily intake list (Table

2.3). We consume much more than the "safe and adequate" amounts, however, as determined in nutritional balance studies where intake and excretion are accurately measured.

The excessive intake of salt (sodium chloride) has been implicated in hypertension (high blood pressure) and as a risk factor in coronary heart disease, as will be discussed in Chapter 11. As the sodium concentration increases in the bloodstream, more water leaves the cells to dilute it so that chemical equilibrium can be maintained. This increased blood volume helps cause an increase in the blood pressure. Because of this many physicians and nutritionists suggest that people should decrease their salt intake. The high levels of salt could also lead to congestive heart failure if the ion balance is upset. In some cases, potassium chloride can be substituted for some of the sodium chloride in table salt to achieve the same flavor. Products like this are now on the market.

Those with kidney disease or kidney failure have to reduce consumption of all salts because the kidney cannot remove these ions from the blood efficiently. Since urinary excretion is the major way excess ions are naturally removed from the body, the person with severe kidney disease must be placed on a kidney dialysis machine or get a kidney transplant.

People in the United States consume from 2 to 7 grams of sodium per day, which is equivalent to about 5 to 18 grams of table salt. Some Oriental populations consume large quantities of salted fish, monosodium glutamate (MSG), and soy sauce, which results in intakes of up to 40 grams of salt daily. These populations also have higher incidences of high blood pressure than most others. High intakes of sodium should be discouraged. Most animal foods contain higher amounts of sodium than potassium, whereas the reverse is true of vegetable foods. The intake of these foods should be modified to achieve a better balance. Orange juice, bananas, and dried fruits are quite high in potassium. Some processed foods, such as pickles, canned hams, and some cheeses are very high in sodium, which is needed for processing and stability. Unfortunately, potassium does not have the same function. Some research has tentatively indicated that the sodium and potassium intake ratio should be 1:1 to prevent hypertension, but more work is needed to verify the theory. Therefore, the best way to reduce sodium intake is to stop using the salt shaker. Eventually people get used to less salty flavors.

Calcium and Phosphorus

The roles of calcium and phosphorus are also closely related. These two elements, which make up 70% of the mineral weight of the body, are found mainly in a mineral complex in the bones and teeth.

Over 99% of the calcium in the body is found in the structure of the bones and teeth. In a 70-kg. (154-lb.) person this amounts to almost three pounds (1,400 grams). The remaining calcium is involved in the nerve excitation process, muscle contraction, the maintenance of the acid/base balance of the blood, blood coagulation, and for many enzymes. The RDA for calcium is 800 mg. per day. The RDA is based on the fact that not all dietary calcium is absorbed by the body. Dairy products such as milk and cheese supply 85% of the dietary calcium for most Americans. The amount absorbed depends on the amount of phosphorus in the diet and on the nutritional status with respect to vitamin D. In addition, the adsorption of calcium from certain foods is prevented by some natural chemical constituents. One of these is phytate found in cereals. With calcium these materials form insoluble salts that cannot be absorbed. The Food and Agriculture Organization (FAO) of the United Nations has set the RDA for calcium at about one-half the United States RDA value because the calcium requirement is also related to protein intake. The higher the protein intake the more calcium is needed. Most of the world consumes much less protein than we do and thus the calcium RDA in the United States is higher.

The RDA for phosphorus, which is readily absorbed from the diet, is also set at 800 mg. per day although most people consume over 1,500 mg. per day. Phosphorus is present in all foods and thus no known dietary deficiencies have been found.

Phosphorus is a major part of the energy-rich compounds formed in the body, such as ATP. It also is part of the structure of the bone mineral complex and is found as a constituent of phospholipids (see Chapter 5). If antacids are used continuously, weakness and anorexia can occur because the chemicals in the antacid combine with phosphorus making it unavailable nutritionally. This results in phosphorus deficiency symptoms even though there is enough phosphorus in the food.

The ratio of calcium to phosphorus (Ca/P) in the diet may also be important, as was mentioned for the Na/K ratio. A ratio of 1:1 has been recommended. Unfortunately, due to a gradual decrease in the consumption of milk and most other dairy products except for cheese in the last decade, the American dietary calcium to phosphorus intake ratio is less than 1:1 with the average being about 0.7:1. This change is also partially due to the fact that the phosphorus level in some processed foods (for example, certain soft drinks and cured meats) is high. Phosphorus is used in cured meat to retain water and to help the meat keep a juicier texture during cooking. It is also used in some soft drinks to create an acid taste and to prevent microbial growth (lowers pH). Some soft drinks, such as the colas, use phosphoric acid as their primary acidulant and therefore contain high levels of phosphorus. Meats, as do all animal tissues, have a naturally high phosphorus content. It is hard to increase calcium in the diet while keeping calories down. Thus cutting back on consumption of foods with high phosphorus content will help reduce the Ca/P ratio to get it closer to the desired 1:1.

Contrary to most people's conceptions, the bone is an active tissue. Calcium, once deposited as a part of the bone, does not remain there forever. When calcium is needed somewhere else in the body for other functions, it can easily be resorbed from the bone, transported, and used. Bone is also under continual breakdown and repair. Therefore, we need to continue our consumption of calcium even after bones are fully developed. After the age of 30, if not enough calcium is consumed, the bones will slowly become depleted of this element. Osteoporosis, a major nutritional disease in the elderly, results from slow mineral loss from bone. It is prevalent in older women and may be the result of several decades of demineralization of bone. With osteoporosis the bones become thinner, shorter, brittle, and weak. They fracture quite easily. In elderly people, bone mineral loss can be so severe that bones such as the hip may just snap with normal walking or standing. Women are thought to be more prone to osteoporosis than men for several reasons. Large quantities of calcium and phosphorus from bone are used during the growth of the unborn child as well as during lactation if the mother breastfeeds her child. If the mother gets inadequate dietary calcium, a net loss of bone calcium may occur. Multiple or closely spaced births may accelerate bone losses. Women frequently diet,

TABLE 8.1 Calcium to phosphorus ratios in some foods

Food	Serving size	Calcium mg.	Phosphorus mg.	Ca/P
French fries	3½ ounces	9	86	1/9
Hamburger	3½ ounces	12	192	1/16
Rolls	medium size	74	85	1/1.05
Cheese	1 ounce	280	166	1.7/1
Milk	6 ounce	236	182	1.3/1
Above items together as a meal		611	1,231	0.5/1
Oranges	medium	40	20.	2/1
Orange juice	3 ounces	11	20	1/2
Sardines	3½ ounces	437	499	1/1.1
Sauerkraut	3½ ounces	36	18	2/1
Butter	1 ounce	7	5	1.3/1
Beans	3½ ounces	56	44	1.2/1
Seaweed	3½ ounces	1,100	240	4.6/1

Calculated from USDA Handbook No. 456.

and high-calcium foods such as milk and cheeses are often eliminated from the food choice list. Also, the hormonal balance in women changes after menopause, which either reduces calcium absorption or accelerates excretion. All these changes are not thought to be beneficial for bone calcium status.

There has been a great debate as to whether one can reverse osteoporosis by dietary changes. Most researchers agree that increasing dietary calcium intake during middle age can delay bone calcium losses, and therefore osteoporosis. However, it is not clear whether one can ever reverse osteoporosis and effect remineralization of the bone through dietary means. It must be recommended that people continue to consume foods such as dairy products and certain vegetables and beans from age 20 onward to reduce the chance of osteoporosis. Reduction of phosphorus intake may also be wise, as noted earlier.

Table 8.1 lists some foods and their Ca/P ratios. This table can be used to increase the amount of calcium in relation to phosphorus in the diet.

Magnesium

Magnesium (Mg) is also found in high concentrations in the body. Its distribution is similar to that of phosphorus; about 70% is in the bone and 30% in other tissues. Magnesium is required in muscle contraction and as a cofactor for some of the enzymes that take part in the Krebs Cycle. This mineral is also involved in nerve transmission.

The RDA for magnesium is about 350 mg. per day, based on balance studies. A magnesium deficiency is rarely found because magnesium is present in all foods. It is highest in cereals and vegetables. In the latter it is part of the green pigment, chlorophyll. Two or three servings of whole-grain bread and vegetables a day supplies all the magnesium the body needs. The only reported deficiencies have been found in children fed strictly on a cow's milk diet, since cow's milk is low in magnesium. Also, persons with severe fluid losses from prolonged diarrhea or vomiting or from alcoholism have been shown to have signs of magnesium deficiency. In extreme cases of magnesium deficiency, tetany, an uncontrolled contraction of muscles, can take place.

TRACE ELEMENTS   Iron

Iron (Fe) is one of the most important trace elements for humans. It is found in high concentrations in red blood cells. In the blood cell it is part of the hemoglobin molecule, which picks up oxygen in the lungs. The hemoglobin carries oxygen to the cells where it is needed for the utilization of glucose, fats, or proteins to produce ATP. Iron is also part of numerous enzyme systems. It is also part of myoglobin, a molecule similar to hemoglobin that is found inside muscle cells. Myoglobin binds to the oxygen that was transported through the blood to the muscle cells. There it holds the oxygen until needed for energy production. Myoglobin with bound oxygen gives meat foods and human muscles a red color. After slaughter, stored meats age, the iron in myoglobin reacts with the additional oxygen, oxidizes, and turns the meat brown. The consumer associates the red color with fresh meat and the brown color with meat that is not fresh, although the brown product can still be perfectly edible and of high quality.

The amount of iron required in the diet is affected by various factors. Iron is usually recycled very efficiently in the body. Only with blood loss do we deplete body iron rapidly. Women lose considerable iron as a result of blood loss during menstruation. Men lose only about 1 mg. per day and women 1.5 mg. per day if the loss is averaged out over the month. The RDAs for men and women in Table 2.1 were set according to these average losses; only 10 mg. per day are recommended for men whereas the recommendation is 18 mg. a day for women. The RDA for iron is about 10 times greater than the amount lost daily from the body because iron is so poorly absorbed from the food in the digestive tract. The higher RDA accounts for the poor absorption. The efficiency of iron absorption from the diet depends upon the individual's needs, the form of iron in the diet, and the makeup of a particular meal. Unfortunately for women, the RDA of 18 mg. is extremely hard to meet through a normal diet without overconsuming calories. Because of the wide distribution in individual requirements, however, not all women develop anemia. For those who do, an iron supplement is recommended that can be taken in food form such as a fortified cereal.

Individuals deficient in iron tend to absorb the element better than those individuals with normal iron stores. Because only about 10% of iron is usually absorbed by a non-deficient person, there is considerable room for improvement for absorption by a deficient person. The extent of actual increased absorption depends upon the form of the ingested iron and the makeup of the rest of the meal. In general, iron in meat is better absorbed than iron from other sources. The iron in hemoglobin and myoglobin (heme iron) is more efficiently absorbed than iron not associated with the heme group (non-heme iron). Iron from plant products is consequently less efficiently absorbed than iron from animal tissue. Absorption of iron from iron salts is greatly dependent on the form of iron, especially when taken other than with a meal. Ferrous sulfate and many other ferrous (Fe II) salts are highly absorbable, whereas ferric

(Fe III) salts may be less absorbable. The choice of iron source for food fortification presents an interesting dilemma for the food scientist. The most efficiently absorbed sources catalyze oxidation and thus tend to cause flavor and color problems, whereas the more chemically inert forms of iron are not as well absorbed. One reasonable compromise is the use of very small particles of elemental iron (sometimes called iron reductum or reduced iron).

The interaction of components of a meal influences the efficiency of iron absorption from the meal. Absorption of iron from iron salts is generally lower when the iron is taken with a meal. An unidentified factor in meat enhances the availability of iron from plant products in the same meal, whereas the tannins of tea can exert an inhibitory effect. Vitamin C greatly enhances absorption of non-heme iron if consumed at the same time as the iron.

Iron deficiency anemia may be one of the most prevalent forms of nutritional disease in the United States. If not enough iron is consumed, the number of red blood cells, which contain the hemoglobin, is reduced, and not enough oxygen can be brought to the cells to permit even moderate exercise. A person with this condition becomes lethargic. Iron deficiency anemia can be caused by too low an intake or by consuming foods that prevent iron from being absorbed from the digestive tract. There are other dietary deficiency problems that can cause anemia. Lack of copper, folic acid, vitamin B_{12}, and other deficiency problems can cause anemias. Also, certain hereditary problems can decrease the efficiency of the absorption process. Not all anemias result from a deficiency in iron intake; the cause must be diagnosed by a physician. Self-diagnosis is often wrong and always foolish.

One of the biggest problems of iron deficiency occurs with women in their childbearing years. During this time if their monthly loss of blood through menstruation is large, they will have a reduced hemoglobin level in the blood and can become tired and weak. Infants are also susceptible to iron deficiency. Thus iron supplements, especially for infants, are often prescribed.

Iron deficiency was recognized as a big problem in the 1930s. As a result of nutritional health surveys, especially of Army recruits, the government, during World War II, required by law that bread, cereals, and rice be enriched with iron. (The addition of thiamin, riboflavin, and niacin was also required.) Bread at that time was a major part of everyone's diet, so this was the easiest way to get the iron (and other deficient nutrients) into the diet of those who needed it the most. After the war this requirement was dropped and left up to the states. Today only 26 states require enrichment. In addition, people today consume less bread and fewer cereal products (about 20% of the diet compared to 40% previously) so fortification of bread and cereal is less effective in alleviating the iron-deficiency problem.

In 1974, the Food and Nutrition Board of the National Academy of Science recommended that the level of iron in bread be increased by three times to reduce iron deficiency. The Food and Drug Administration was still considering this recommendation in 1984. Two major problems could result from an increased level of iron: first, the iron could cause the bread to have a shorter shelf life because iron causes fats to rapidly become rancid (this would tend to increase food waste); second, a very small number of people have a disease called hemochromatosis in which a high iron intake (about 40 mg. per day) causes the liver cells to be destroyed. The decision to increase fortification levels thus will have to be based on the risks involved versus the benefit to the population as a whole. Perhaps proper education and labeling could help those at risk avoid the high iron cereal products.

Iodine

Iodine (I) is another essential trace nutrient. It also has a very low daily requirement, about one ten-millionth of a pound per day. One would expect that since the body intake requirement is so low, no major worldwide nutritional deficiencies of iodine would occur. However, goiter, which is a manifestation of iodine deficiency, still exists today in many areas of the world where the iodine level in the soil is low or where seafood, a major source of dietary iodine, is not consumed on a regular basis.

The chief role of iodine is in the formation of the hormone thyroxine in the thyroid gland. This gland is located in the neck. Thyroxine is intimately related to caloric metabolism, especially in controlling the basal metabolic rate (BMR). Underproduction or overproduction of thyroxine can lead to problems in maintaining weight because the BMR can be upset.

When iodine is deficient in the diet, the thyroid gland enlarges to try to capture more iodine from the blood to produce more thyroxine. This can be observed as a large swollen area protruding from the neck. In some parts of the world, especially in mountain regions like the Andes and the Alps where soils are low in the mineral, goiter may still be a serious problem. Some South American Indians, in fact, sell wooden doll souvenirs that have enlarged necks because they think the condition is aesthetically pleasing. Old art works of Europe portray subjects with goiter, as it was a common condition at that time. Today goiter can be prevented by eating salt to which iodine has been added (iodized salt) or by eating ocean fish regularly. Until table salt was iodized in the 1930s as a public-health measure, goiter was prevalent in several midwestern states in the United States. Some cases of goiter were reported in

Michigan as late as 1969. One problem, of course, is that if people reduce salting their foods to control hypertension, some other food vehicle for iodine supplementation will be needed.

Excess iodine intake can be caused by consumption of milk products containing residues of iodine compounds (iodophores) that are used as sanitizing agents in the dairy plant. If the pipes in the plant are not thoroughly rinsed, the next batch of milk will be contaminated. Drinking this milk will result in goiter enlargement. Excess iodine intake has also been reported in Japan where iodine consumption from seafood is quite high.

The RDA for iodine is about 150 μg. per day for adults. Iodized salt provides around 76 μg. per gram of salt. Since we consume from 5 to 18 grams of table salt (sodium chloride) a day, this could supply much more than our needs, in fact a large excess. However, all sodium chloride is not iodized. Food processors, for example, generally do not or cannot use iodized salt because of federal regulations. In addition, as with iron, iodine enrichment can create stability problems. The rest of the iodine in the normal diet comes basically from dairy products (due to carryover from sanitizing solutions) seafoods, and bread. During processing of bread by some methods, an iodate salt is used that increases the elasticity of the protein to help in dough texture.

Iodine can be toxic, as are some of the vitamins. The safe level is about 1,000 μg. per day, a level easily reached with too much salt consumption. Therefore, we are concerned both with persons who consume too little iodine and with those who consume too much. The symptom (goiter) for both problems is the same. Recent surveys by the USDA show that the average U.S. intake is four times the RDA.

Zinc

Zinc (Zn) is the last trace element listed in Table 2.1 for which an RDA has been established. This metal is associated with many enzymes. For example, zinc is an important part of the enzymes that help to manufacture stomach acid, the enzyme that breaks down alcohol in the body, the enzyme involved in vitamin-A utilization, and an enzyme that is involved in the metabolism of the nucleic acids.

Zinc is found in meats, liver, eggs, and shellfish at about 2–6 mg. per 100 grams. As with iron, its bioavailability varies with the food. Oysters are the richest source of highly available zinc. Cereals contain about 0.5 mg. per 100 grams. However, the presence of phytate and the fiber in cereals and oilseeds has been shown to somewhat reduce zinc absorption during digestion. In areas of the country where the soil is deficient in zinc, both the foods that are grown and the animals that forage on these soils have low zinc contents. Therefore, zinc is usually added to both fertilizers and animal feed.

The RDA has been set at 10 mg. for children and 15 mg. for adults, based mainly on consumption patterns. A deficient intake of zinc can cause a loss of appetite and a decrease in taste acuity (hypogeusia). In severe zinc deficiency, growth failure leading to dwarfism and delay of puberty in boys will occur. This has been observed in certain populations that live along the river Nile as well as in Iran. Zinc deficiency may also impair wound healing. A concern exists today that many people may have marginal zinc deficiency because of the lower consumption of whole-grain cereals, the general source of zinc. Mean consumption of zinc in the USA is lower than the RDA. Supplementation of some food with zinc may be advisable.

OTHER TRACE ELEMENTS

Several other elements have been found to be necessary in the diets of humans and animals. Because so little is known about the requirements of these elements, no RDAs have been set for them. However, each of them (other than cobalt) is included on the "Estimated Safe and Adequate Daily Dietary Intake List" (Table 2.3). For many of these trace elements the toxic levels of intake may only be a few times higher than the usual intake, so care must be exercised in their consumption.

Copper

Copper (Cu) is a trace element that is part of many enzyme complexes. The body contains from 75 to 150 milligrams of copper, mainly in the brain, heart, and kidneys. This level decreases by 80% to 90% during aging. Experimental diets deficient in copper fed to animals cause skeletal defects, degeneration of the nervous system, loss of skin pigmentation, reproductive failure, and anemia. Copper is necessary for iron utilization in red blood cells. It is possible that some of the symptoms of the disease "marasmas," which is a calorie malnutrition in children, are due to copper deficiency.

Some copper is found in most foods. Nuts, shellfish, and liver are excellent sources whereas milk and beef have low copper contents. There is some concern about deficient copper intake by some populations of Americans. It has been suggested that a high zinc to copper ratio in the liver increases cholesterol production. Cereal, phytate, and fiber inhibit zinc absorption, which might lead to a lower blood cholesterol level by decreasing the dietary zinc to copper ratio. Vitamin C inhibits copper absorption, which appears to cause an increased cholesterol level in experimental animals. In the same regard low dietary copper also increases the zinc to copper ratio and may result in increased cholesterol production.

Cobalt

Cobalt (Co) is a critical component of vitamin B_{12}, the vitamin that is essential in the formation of hemoglobin. A moderate intake of meat and dairy products supplies all the needed cobalt in the form of B_{12}. There is no other known role of cobalt in humans other than its essentialness for the vitamin B_{12} molecule.

For animals, evidence of a deficiency of cobalt itself has been documented in certain coastal areas of New Zealand. Adverse health effects were observed in grazing animals that ate grasses devoid of cobalt, due to its absence from the soil. These animals get their B_{12} by bacterial synthesis in their rumen. Without the cobalt, however, the B_{12} is not formed.

Chromium

This trace element (Cr) is part of a complex that works closely with insulin to facilitate the uptake of glucose by cells. For some people with glucose intolerance, chromium supplementation has been shown to be helpful. In other people, chromium status is sufficient, but the functioning of insulin is impaired. Medical tests are necessary to determine if chromium supplementation might be helpful. In experimental animals it is clear that a deficiency of chromium is associated with adult-onset diabetes. Chromium is found in most meats as well as in yeast and beer. Rats on a chromium-deficient diet have an impaired growth rate.

Fluorine

Fluorine (F) is found in almost all foods. It is incorporated into the mineral structure of the teeth and bones. When supplied in adequate quantities in the water supply it can reduce dental caries by 50%. The dietary intake other than that from water is variable, ranging from 0.3 to 3.1 mg. per day. Tea is an excellent source whereas meat has only 0.1 mg. per 3.5-oz. serving. Many communities fluoridate their water to a level of one milligram per liter (1 ppm). Thus drinking two to three pints of water per day supplies slightly over one 1 mg. Toxicity occurs if 20 to 80 mg. are consumed per day for a period of several years. If water contains above 2 ppm fluorine, symptoms of toxicity may appear. The first symptoms are a mottled, darkened appearance of the teeth. Although many communities oppose fluoridation of water, they are doing a disservice to the nutritional well-being of their children. The overwhelming scientific evidence shows that fluorine protects children's teeth from decay. Fluorine may also make older people's bones more resistant to osteoporosis.

Manganese

This element (Mn) is essential in the structural information of the bone, in the reproductive process, and in enzymes of the nervous system. Nuts, whole-grain cereals, fruits, and vegetables are the main sources. They supply three to seven milligrams per day in an average diet.

Molybdenum

The amount of molybdenum (Mb) in the diet varies from 45 to 500 mg. per day. It is part of some enzyme systems. A molybdenum deficiency disease has never been produced in animals or humans.

Selenium

The trace mineral selenium (Se) has an antioxidant role in metabolism. It is part of an important enzyme system that protects cells from oxidation. In animal studies, selenium can be shown to substitute for vitamin E in some of the vitamin's antioxidant activities.

Recently, there has been interest in selenium's possible effect in cancer prevention. As in the cases of vitamin C and vitamin A, we should await research results before consuming selenium supplements. Selenium is quite toxic to animals in dose levels just above the safe intake levels. Therefore, consumption of large quantities of selenium supplements is not wise.

Others

Several other trace elements have been identified as part of the normal metabolic system of animals. These include cadmium, nickel, tin, vanadium, and silicon. They are all most likely required by humans, but deficiency diseases have never been found even experimentally. The study of essential trace elements is one aspect of nutrition that still needs a great deal of research.

SUMMARY

Like vitamins, certain minerals are essential for growth and functioning of the human body. Some, such as calcium and phosphorus, are utilized for many functions, including formation of the bone structure. As with the vitamins, some trace elements, such as iodine and iron, were and still are the focus of worldwide nutritional problems due to deficient intake. On the other hand, excess consumption of some elements produces toxic symptoms. For example, excess ingestion of sodium is linked to hypertension in humans. For many trace elements, the amount of the mineral that produces toxic side effects is very close to the level needed for normal body function.

Of primary importance in today's diets are the intake of sodium, the calcium/phosphorus balance, and iron intake for women. High dietary intake of sodium exacerbates hypertension. A low calcium/phosphorus ratio may lead to osteoporosis. Increased consumption of dairy products will increase calcium consumption and increase the calcium/phosphorus ratio. A low iron intake can lead to anemia. Women and infants are especially prone to anemia.

Another important element is iodine, a lack of which leads to goiter. Iodized salt is the best preventive for this condition, but occasionally iodine deficiency occurs in the United States. Over-intake of iodine also produces a goiter-like condition. Zinc is another element for which an RDA has been established. Its significance in terms of a deficiency in the American diet is still under investigation. Other trace elements are essential in human nutrition, and "estimated safe and adequate daily dietary intake" levels have been recently established for them.

*Multiple
Choice
Study
Questions*

1. The RDA for calcium was set high because

   A. the U.S. consumption of phosphorus is low
   B. calcium is very soluble and therefore cannot be absorbed
   C. the U.S. consumption of protein is high
   D. it had to match the zinc intake
   E. more people consume vitamin C

2. The major mineral in the body is

   A. phosphorus
   B. zinc
   C. iron
   D. calcium
   E. potassium

3. Which mineral is mainly found in the fluid outside the cells?

   A. potassium
   B. iron
   C. sodium

D. calcium

E. magnesium

4. The calcium/phosphorus ratio of hamburger is approximately

A. 1:20

B. 1:16

C. 1:1

D. 2:1

E. 5:1

5. The calcium/phosphorus ratio of cheese is approximately

A. 2:1

B. 2:5.1

C. 1:1

D. 1:2

E. 1:5

6. With careful planning a pure vegetarian diet can be as nutritious or more nutritious than most American diets. The nutrients of major concern in this planning are

A. calories

B. calories and iron

C. calories and B_{12}

D. B_{12} and calcium

E. calcium and niacin

7. Which food component added to many processed foods may be creating a nutritional problem?

A. potassium

B. phosphorus

C. linoleic acid

D. calcium

E. zinc

8. A major nutritional deficiency in the U.S. diet is

A. vitamin D

B. vitamin C

C. iron

D. protein

E. fat

9. Goiter is a major nutritional disease caused by a lack of

A. salt

B. selenium

C. zinc

D. iodine

E. copper

10. An excess of this mineral can cause hemochromatosis in some people
  A. calcium
  B. potassium
  C. magnesium
  D. iodine
  E. iron

11. One type of blood anemia that affects many women is
  A. due to deficiency in vitamin B_{12}
  B. caused by a poor level of protein in the diet
  C. due to hemoglobin loss during menstruation that cannot be resupplied by the average iron intake from foods
  D. due to high dietary iron causing hemochromatosis

12. Which element is probably not required by humans?
  A. nickel
  B. silicon
  C. vanadium
  D. argon
  E. tin

13. The Zn/Cu ratio may be related to
  A. coronary heart disease (CHD)
  B. cancer
  C. diabetes
  D. hypoglycemia
  E. mongoloidism

14. The nickel requirement of humans
  A. is zero since it is not required
  B. is not met by the diet
  C. is not known at this time
  D. is 20 mg. per day
  E. none of the above

The following is a list of elements felt to be essential. Use the list to answer questions 15 through 19.
  A. iron
  B. zinc
  C. copper
  D. cobalt
  E. iodine

15. Which element forms part of vitamin B_{12}?

16. Which element is the major element in the pigment of beef and is part of the oxygen-carrying system of blood?

17. Which element is part of many enzyme systems and blood cholesterol may increase when it is deficient?

18. Which element is essential for the formation of certain hormones that control the metabolic rate?

19. A deficiency of which trace mineral has led to dwarfism in certain areas of the world?

Essay Study Questions

1. Discuss the calcium/phosphorus balance and the problems in maintaining it.

2. Relate the consumption of table salt to possible diseases injurious to health.

3. Discuss the problem of iron deficiency in the United States and how it could be alleviated.

4. Why is it difficult to determine trace element requirements for humans?

5. How has the iodine deficiency problem been solved in the U.S.? Is this applicable to other parts of the world?

Things to Do

1. Collect ads for mineral supplements from magazines and newspapers. What do they promise? Are they reliable?

2. Using the seven-day dietary survey, evaluate your mineral nutritional status. How could it be improved?

3. Make charts showing the amounts of foods needed to be consumed to obtain the equivalents of common mineral supplements.

4. Examine and discuss the mineral fortification of cereals and bread.

5. Ask people for their nutritional viewpoints on various minerals. Discuss them in class. Try to find someone who is consuming very high levels of minerals to improve health.

6. Try to find foods in the market to which phosphorus is added. Is this phosphorus also listed in Handbook No. 456 or in Appendix I.

Chapter 8. Answers to Multiple-Choice Study Questions: 1, C; **2,** D; **3,** C; **4,** B; **5,** A; **6,** D; **7,** B; **8,** C; **9,** D; **10,** E; **11,** C; **12,** D; **13,** A; **14,** C; **15,** D; **16,** A; **17,** C; **18,** E; **19,** B.

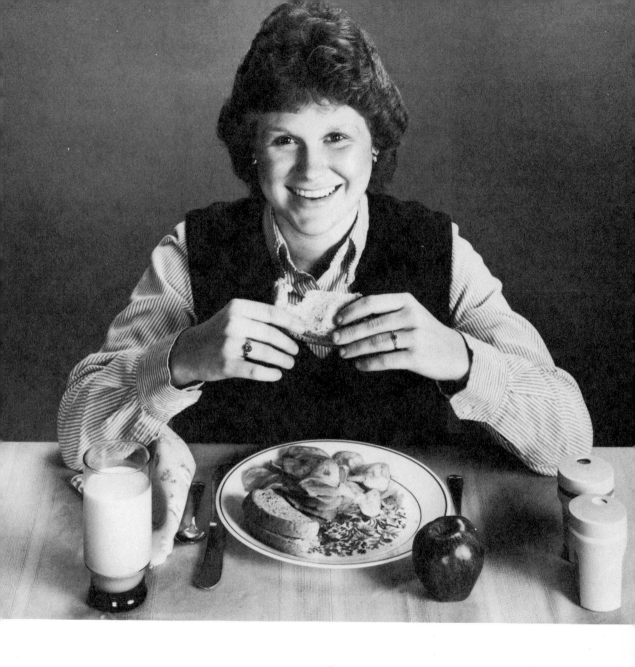

THE PROCESS OF DIGESTION AND THE FOODS WE NEED

**THE PATHWAYS
OF DIGESTION
IN HUMANS**

The Upper Digestive Tract

The process of digestion consists of the mechanical, enzymatic, and chemical actions that result in the breakdown of foods into basic subunits. These small molecules can then be absorbed through the intestinal wall and be utilized by the body. Some foods cannot be digested entirely unless they are heat-processed in some way. For example, cooking solubilizes starch to make it more available to enzymatic digestion. The same is true for the elastic protein fibers in meat such as collagen. Slow cooking makes them more soluble and thus digestible. Cooking can also destroy some antinutritional factors, such as avidin in egg white, which prevents biotin from being absorbed, and the antitrypsin factor in soybeans that prevents protein digestion.

The digestive pathway is shown in Figure 9.1. Mechanical and salivary activities in the mouth make up the first step in digestion.

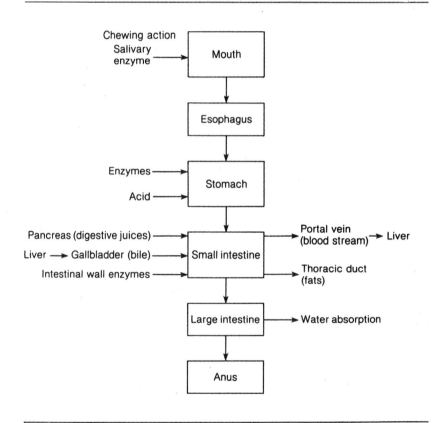

FIGURE 9.1 General process of digestion and absorption

The mechanical activity of chewing is important in reducing the size of food particles to facilitate their movement to the stomach. About two quarts of saliva are produced in a day to aid in the movement of food from the mouth to the stomach. The only enzymatic activity that occurs in the mouth is the action of amylase present in the saliva. Amylase begins to break down large carbohydrate polymers into smaller chains.

The esophagus, through a squeezing action, forces food down into the stomach. The small amount of digestion that takes place in the esophagus is the continued action of the salivary enzyme on starches.

The Stomach

The next major area in the digestive pathway is the stomach. The basic function of the stomach is to produce acid (hydrochloric acid) and enzymes for digestion. The stomach continually churns up the stomach contents and functions as a digestion vat. The pH or acidity of the stomach (gastric juice) is equal to about 1.0 to 1.5. This acid is enough to eat holes in an iron plate. The high acid level in the stomach is necessary for proper digestion of foods. Between meals, acid is normally not released into the stomach and the acidity of the stomach may rise to pH 5 or 6. However, as soon as food enters the stomach the gastric glands in the stomach wall start releasing the hydrochloric acid to lower the pH.

Pepsin is an enzyme released from the stomach wall that breaks down protein into smaller units. Pepsin can only function under the condition of high acidity such as is found in the stomach. The churning of the food that occurs in the stomach plus the high acid conditions cause some of the food to separate into smaller particles that can be acted upon more easily during later stages of digestion.

Depending upon the amount of fat taken in, food will remain in the stomach from about 20 minutes to almost four hours. Fluids such as carbonated beverages can go through the stomach in less than 20 minutes, while a meal high in fats will remain much longer. This is why a meal high in fat makes a person feel full. A less fatty meal may remain in the stomach for only one hour. The average residence time for most foods is about two hours.

For the most part, no absorption of dietary constituents takes place in the stomach. Some drugs, such as aspirin and alcohol, can be absorbed directly through the walls of the stomach into the bloodstream. This occurs especially when the stomach is empty. There are also some mechanisms for absorption, in both the mouth and stomach, of larger molecules such as proteins. However, the amount absorbed is very small.

The Small Intestine

The small intestine is extremely important for proper digestion of food. The small intestine is separated into three sections: the duodenum, the jejunum, and the ileum. The duodenum, which is the first section beyond the stomach, is about 10–12 feet long and is the location of many of the major digestive processes. The partially digested food entering this section from the stomach is immediately acted upon by sodium bicarbonate, a weak base released from the pancreas. The bicarbonate helps neutralize the acid from the stomach and raises the pH to about 5 to 6 in the first portion of the duodenum.

The gall bladder also releases bile into the top of the duodenum. Bile salts and bile acids are produced in the liver from cholesterol and are stored in the gall bladder until digestion begins. When released in the bile, they help emulsify the fats into small droplets, which can then be acted on by enzymes released into the intestine. These enzymes, known as lipases, break down the triglycerides into the fatty acids and glycerol for absorption. The bile also contains bilirubin, which is a breakdown product of hemoglobin. It is excreted from the body through the bile duct into the small intestine.

Many enzymatic digestive reactions occur in the duodenum. These enzymes are excreted by the intestinal wall and by the pancreas. The major digestion of protein occurs in this region, where it is broken down into single amino acid units. These units then pass across the intestinal wall of the small intestine and enter the bloodstream. The blood acts as a transport system that brings the amino acids to the cells where they are needed. The starches and other complex carbohydrates are broken down in the duodenum to form glucose, fructose, and other simple sugars that can also be readily absorbed across the intestinal wall. Some of the enzymes released in the duodenum are: trypsin, which comes from the pancreas and digests proteins to smaller units; lipase, which also comes from the pancreas, digests triglycerides into glycerol and fatty acids; sucrase, which comes from cells in the intestinal wall, breaks down sucrose into glucose and fructose; amylase, which comes from the pancreas, breaks starches into smaller units; and lactase, a second enzyme from the intestinal wall that breaks down lactose to glucose and galactose.

The jejunum and the ileum make up the next 20 feet of the small intestine and are the primary absorption sites for many nutrients. Some absorption of rapidly digested materials occurs in the duodenum but most of the material passes to the jejunum and ileum and is digested and assimilated through the intestinal wall there. In the jejunum, absorption of calcium, phosphorus, iodine, and vitamin A takes place. In addition, most of the glucose and amino acids are absorbed in this region. Fat absorption will also take place here as well as in the upper ileum.

The absorption process is a highly selective and controlled process. Normally the basic building blocks of the carbohydrates, proteins, and fats, i.e., the simple sugars, amino acids, free fatty acids, monoglycerides, and glycerol, are absorbed by passive transport; since the concentration is lower in the bloodstream they easily pass across the intestinal wall. However, some nutrients, such as amino acids, glucose, and some vitamins, are absorbed by a special transport mechanism called active transport. This means that if the concentration of a nutrient is higher on the bloodstream side of the intestinal wall, it can still be absorbed. High energy phosphate bonds from ATP provide energy for active transport of nutrients. Fat is absorbed by passive transport, where absorption occurs only when the concentration of fatty acids is higher within the intestinal contents than in the intestinal cell wall.

The water-soluble components, such as the simple sugars, amino acids, and other chemicals, pass into the portal vein of the bloodstream, which goes directly into the liver. They are acted upon in the liver. It is also in the liver that many poisonous chemicals that are absorbed are detoxified.

The fat components reassemble into triglycerides on the inside of the intestinal wall. They are transported in the body by the lymph system until they enter the bloodstream near the heart.

The last part of the small intestine, the ileum, is the major site where cholesterol, bile salts, some fat, potassium, chloride, vitamin B_{12}, and some other nutrients are absorbed. Some of the water used in digestion is also reabsorbed here. Total time from ingestion of food through this absorption period is about 16 to 28 hours, depending on the diet.

The Large Intestine

Undigested foods, as well as undigestible food components such as dietary fiber, leave the ileum and pass into the large intestine, which is about five feet long. This area is also known as the colon. In the large intestine there is a high concentration of bacteria that further digest these materials. Vitamin K produced by some of these bacteria can be absorbed into the body through the walls of this tissue.

Some people believe that yogurt should be consumed because the bacteria present in yogurt will accumulate and proliferate in the large intestine somehow producing some magical health effect. Also, it is thought that these organisms produce many desirable vitamins and nutrients that might be absorbed. This theory has been disproven in several clinical studies. One particular study showed that at the pH of stomach acid, 99.9% of all yogurt bacteria are killed. Any remaining bacteria, as other studies showed, could not proliferate in the small intestine or large intestine because the numbers are too small. The claims for yogurt are based on the effects that large gelatin capsules of billions of yogurt-type bacteria had on people after intestinal surgery and administration of high levels of antibiotics. The use of antibiotics kills off many of the organisms found in the large intestine. In some cases doctors give large, dry pellets of a strain of *Lactobacillus*, an organism similar to the one used to make yogurt, to help re-establish the microbiological conditions in the intestine necessary for good health. But once foods are consumed again, the other types of bacteria present in the food will invariably overtake the yogurt organisms and become predominant, since they are more efficient under the conditions present.

The major function of the large intestine is to reabsorb the water that was used for digestion. The amount of water can be quite large. When intestinal disorders occur, the water is not reabsorbed and diarrhea results. If a high-fiber diet is consumed, some of this water is retained to make a large soft stool that can be quickly eliminated from the body.

FOOD AND REQUIREMENTS

Up to this point we have concentrated on nutrients, not on food. We have discussed the structure, function, digestion, and health aspects of nutrients. However, since people eat foods, not specific nutrients, it is important for us to develop a working knowledge of the nutrient content of foods. To aid the reader, Appendix I lists the composition of 615 common foods, Table 9.1 shows where the average American obtains specific nutrients, and Table 9.2 lists those foods that are good sources of specific nutrients.

An easier way to design a balanced diet is with the use of the Basic Four food groups that was introduced in Chapter 2. This system can work well, and does not require one to have a calculator or home computer and a USDA notebook to check one's dietary status.

Unfortunately, today we eat many combination foods that do not fit into any specific one of the four or five categories. A pizza with sausage, cheese, onions, peppers, and mushrooms is a good example. However, if we look closely at the pizza we see that this food fits all the food groups and is actually a fairly balanced meal if consumed with milk. One should learn to look at foods this way in order to achieve the proper nutritional status.

We have often heard that the typical fast foods we eat are not nutritious. The late Dr. Howard Appledorf of the University of Florida, Gainesville, often pointed out that proper food choices made in a fast food establishment could result in quite nutritious meals.

TABLE 9.1 Average nutrient supplies available for an individual from various food groups

Food groups	Food energy (%)	Protein (%)	Fat (%)	Carbo-hydrate (%)	Cal-cium (%)	Phos-phorus (%)	Iron (%)	Magne-sium (%)	Vita-min A value (%)	Thia-min (%)	Ribo-flavin (%)	Niacin (%)	Vita-min B-6 (%)	Vita-min B-12 (%)	Ascor-bic Acid (%)
Meat (including pork fat cuts), poultry and fish	20.2	41.5	34.7	0.1	3.5	26.2	29.1	13.7	21.5	28.1	24.5	45.6	45.8	69.7	10
Eggs	2.0	5.1	2.9	0.1	2.3	5.4	5.1	1.3	5.8	2.2	5.1	0.1	1.9	8.3	0
Dairy products, excluding butter	11.1	22.5	12.4	6.6	75.7	36.1	2.3	21.6	12.9	9.0	41.0	1.6	10.2	20.5	4.0
Fats and oils, including butter	17.8	0.1	42.6	a	0.4	0.2	0	0.4	8.1	0	0	0	0	0	0
Citrus fruits	0.9	0.5	0.1	1.9	0.9	0.7	0.8	2.2	1.5	2.8	0.5	0.9	1.2	0	26.3
Other fruits	2.2	0.6	0.2	4.7	1.2	1.1	3.3	3.9	5.5	1.8	1.5	1.7	5.5	0	11.4
Potatoes and sweet potatoes	2.7	2.4	0.1	5.3	0.9	3.9	4.4	7.1	5.3	6.2	1.7	7.1	11.2	0	18.0
Dark green and deep yellow vegetables	0.3	0.5	a	0.5	1.6	0.7	1.6	2.1	21.2	0.9	1.1	0.7	1.7	0	8.3
Other vegetables, including tomatoes	2.5	3.3	0.4	4.7	4.9	5.0	9.0	10.4	15.5	6.9	4.5	6.1	9.2	0	27.6
Dry beans and peas, nuts, soy flour	3.2	5.4	4.0	2.2	2.8	6.2	6.4	11.7	a	5.7	2.0	7.6	4.3	0	a
Flour and cereal products	19.2	17.8	1.3	34.8	3.3	12.5	28.2	17.9	0.4	36.3	17.4	24.0	8.9	1.5	0
Sugars and other sweeteners	17.3	a	0	38.4	1.5	0.3	7.4	0.2	0	a	a	a	0	0	a
Miscellaneous [b]	0.7	0.4	1.2	0.6	1.0	1.8	2.4	7.6	2.3	0.1	0.7	4.8	0.1	0	3.5
Total [c]	100.0	100.0	100.0	100.0	100.0	100.0	100.0	100.0	100.0	100.0	100.0	100.0	100.0	100.0	100.0

[a] Less than 0.05%.

[b] Coffee and chocolate liquor equivalent of cocoa beans and fortification of products not assigned to a specific group.

[c] Components may not add to total due to rounding.

Source: U.S. Dept. of Agr. (1974), Preliminary data.

TABLE 9.2 Foods that contain important nutrients

Protein Sources	Amount
Cooked meat and poultry	20–30% protein
Fish	20–30%
Cheese (American)	25%
Cottage cheese	13–17%
Nuts	16%
Eggs	13%
Dry cereals	7–14%
Bread	8%
Beans	7–8%
Milk (whole)	3.5%
Milk (skim)	4.0%

Fat Sources	Amount
Oils	100% fat
Butter and margarine	80%
Mayonnaise	80%
Walnuts	65%
Chocolate	50%
Peanut butter	50%
Cheese	25–35%
Meats	20–40%
Ice cream	10–16%

Carbohydrate Sources	Amount
Sugar	100% carbohydrate
Chocolate creams	85%
Cereals	70–80%
Cookies	70%
Jams	70%
Cake	60%
Bread	50%
Rice, spaghetti	20–35%

Calcium Sources	Typical Serving	Amount
Cheese	1 slice—processed	150–200 mg.
Dark green, leafy vegetables	spinach—1 ounce	10–25 mg.
Milk	whole—1 cup	300 mg.
Sardines	per fish	50–80 mg.
Iron Sources		
Beans and peas	peas—1 cup	2–3 mg.
Beef	3 ounce—cooked	2–3 mg.
Chicken	1 slice—cooked	0.7 mg.
Dark green, leafy vegetables	spinach—1 cup cooked	4 mg.
Eggs	one—cooked	1–1.3 mg.
Liver	cooked—3 ounce	8–12 mg.
Pork	cooked—3 ounce	2.5–3 mg.
Prune juice	4 ounce	5 mg.
Enriched bread and cereals and pasta	bread—1 slice	0.7 mg.
Whole—grain cereals	wheat—1 cup cooked	1.2 mg.
Niacin Sources		
Salmon, tunafish	Tuna—one 7 ounce can	18–20 mg.
Liver	3 ounce—cooked	14 mg.
Meats	beef—3 ounce cooked	4–5 mg.
Peanut butter	1 tbs.	2.4 mg.
Poultry	2 medium slices	5–6 mg.

TABLE 9.2 Foods that contain important nutrients *(Continued)*

	Typical Serving	Amount
Niacin Sources (Cont'd)		
Enriched bread, pasta, and cereals	one slice bread	0.7 mg.
Peas	one cup—cooked	14 mg.
Whole-grain cereals	wheat—one cup cooked	1.5 mg.
Peanuts	10 nuts—shelled	3–4 mg.
Vitamin A Sources		
Cantaloupe	½ melon	8000 IU
Carrots	1 carrot—medium	8000 IU
Dark green, leafy vegetables	broccoli—1 medium stalk	4500 IU
Liver	3 ounce—cooked	35000 IU
Spinach	1 cup—raw	4500 IU
Squash	Acorn—½ baked	2200 IU
Sweet potato	baked—one medium	9200 IU
Fortified butter, margarine, Milk	butter—1 tbs	140 IU
Thiamin Sources		
Liver	slice—3 ounce—cooked	0.22 mg.
Nuts	10—shelled	0.06 mg.
Peas	1 cup—cooked	0.22 mg.
Pork	lean—3 ounce—cooked	0.5–0.92 mg.
Pork sausage	one link—fried	0.20 mg.
Veal	3 ounce—cooked	0.06–0.08 mg.
Beans	snap—1 cup—cooked	0.04 mg.
Whole-grain cereals	1 cup—wheat—cooked	0.15 mg.
Enriched bread	one slice	0.07 mg.
Fortified cereals	1 cup—corn type	0.11 mg.
Enriched pasta	1 cup—spaghetti	0.20 mg.
Vitamin C Sources		
Cabbage	1 cup cooked	40–45 mg.
Citrus fruits	1 medium orange	50–66 mg.
Potato	1 medium—baked	30 mg.
Tomato	1 medium	20–25 mg.
Green peppers	3 strips—thin	20–30 mg.
Brussel sprouts	½ cup cooked	60 mg.
Orange juice	6 ounce—glass	90 mg.
Fruit drinks	6 ounce—grape drink	30 mg.
Riboflavin Sources		
Cheese	1 slice—processed	0.06–0.09 mg.
Fish	1 cod filet	0.07 mg.
Liver	3 ounce slice cooked	3.5–4.0 mg.
Meats	3 ounce beef patty	0.15–0.2 mg.
Milk	1 cup	0.41 mg.
Poultry	2 slices chicken	0.04–0.05 mg.
Whole-grain cereals	1 cup cooked	0.05 mg.
Enriched cereals, pasta, and bread	1 slice bread	0.07 mg.
Soy flour	1 cup—defatted	0.34 mg.
Spinach	1 cup leaf—raw	0.11 mg.
Beans	1 cup—drained	0.07 mg.
Vitamin D Sources		
Eggs	1 cooked	25–30 IU
Fish oil	cod—1 tsp	400–800 IU
Fortified milk, margarine,	margarine—1 tbs	20–80 IU

Since Americans are consuming, on the average, one-third of their meals outside the home, food choice at restaurants is extremely important. Appendix II contains the nutrient analysis of foods from a number of fast food franchises. If one assumes that a meal should supply about one-third the RDA for a nutrient, one can compare the values in Appendix II to those in Table 2.1, after adjusting the values in Table 2.1 to one-third RDA.

When analyzing fast food meals, one notes that including milk or a milk shake instead of a soft drink in a meal will usually round out the nutrient profile of the meal. However, fast food meals are generally high in calories and salt and low in vitamins A and C. Despite these problems, proper choice of foods can result in a nutritious meal.

With any meal choices, whether inside or outside the home, we should aim for a balance over a one-or two-day period. If the fruit and vegetable group is neglected at one meal, increase the serving size at the next meal. Eating an unbalanced meal once in a while is not going to cause a nutrition deficiency. If you have a balanced diet, there is no need for vitamin pills. Many people take them for insurance because they do not realize that their meals actually supply all their needs. These people will end up with more vitamins in their urine than many people in the world have in their foods. One should be aware by now that consuming a vitamin pill instead of a meal is not a sound practice since food contains more than vitamins.

Now that we have related food to nutrients, in the next chapters we will examine the American diet, diet and heart disease, obesity, and organic and natural foods. Finally, we will discuss processing and storage of foods for nutritional value and how we can increase food shelf-life to maintain quality and nutrient value.

SUMMARY

Digestion is the process that converts foods into basic subunits that can be absorbed by the body. During digestion enzymes break down the constituents of food into smaller units. Mechanical action and addition of saliva in the mouth, acid and pepsin in the stomach, and bile and enzyme action in the small intestine all work to digest food. These smaller units are absorbed in the lower part of the small intestine. Most of them enter the portal vein and are transported to the liver for further processes; however, fats are transported to the bloodstream by the lymph system.

This chapter has also listed the various foods that are important sources of nutrients. With a working knowledge of these tables and the use of the Basic Four concept, we can improve our dietary practices.

*Multiple
Choice
Study
Questions*

1. The major area for absorption of nutrients is the

 A. large intestine
 B. esophagus
 C. stomach
 D. small intestine

2. Which enzyme breaks free fatty acids off of triglycerides?

 A. pepsin
 B. trypsin
 C. chymotrypsin
 D. amylase
 E. lipase

3. Fats are absorbed from the intestine into the

 A. portal vein
 B. liver
 C. pancreas
 D. bloodstream
 E. thoracic duct

4. The gall bladder excretes ____ to help digestion.

 A. enzymes
 B. lactase
 C. trypsin
 D. bile salts
 E. vitamins

5. Triglycerides are broken down to fatty acids in the

 A. mouth
 B. esophagus
 C. stomach
 D. small intestine
 E. large intestine

6. Water is mainly reabsorbed in the

 A. stomach
 B. duodenum
 C. ejunem
 D. ileum
 E. colon

7. Which vitamin has been shown to be produced and absorbed from the intestinal tract in man?

 A. vitamin B_1
 B. vitamin K
 C. vitamin B_6
 D. vitamin A
 E. vitamin D

8. Which enzyme breaks down proteins in the stomach?

   A. pepsin
   B. trypsin
   C. chymotrypsin
   D. amylase
   E. lipase

9. Which enzyme breaks down complex starches into smaller units?

   A. pepsin
   B. trypsin
   C. chymotrypsin
   D. amylase
   E. lipase

10. The major acid present in the stomach is

    A. lactic acid
    B. hydrochloric acid
    C. ascorbic acid
    D. fumaric acid
    E. sulfuric acid

11. The major detoxification steps of a food component occurs in the

    A. small intestine
    B. liver
    C. bloodstream
    D. kidney
    E. stomach

Essay Study Questions

1. Discuss the steps of food digestion for each section of the digestive tract.

2. Name some important enzymes that help in the digestive process.

3. Elaborate on the use of yogurt to improve the health of the digestive tract.

4. Discuss the importance of water and pH during the digestion process.

5. What value does the typical fast food meal have in a person's diet?

*Things
to Do*

1. Obtain a copy of Handbook No. 456 and make a list of the nutrients for those foods not compiled in Appendix I that you consume regularly.

2. Find a book on animal nutrition and compare the digestive process between a ruminant (horse, cow) and humans.

Chapter 9. Answers to Multiple-Choice Study Questions: 1, D; 2, E; 3, E; 4, D; 5, D; 6, E; 7, B; 8, A; 9, D; 10, B; 11, B.

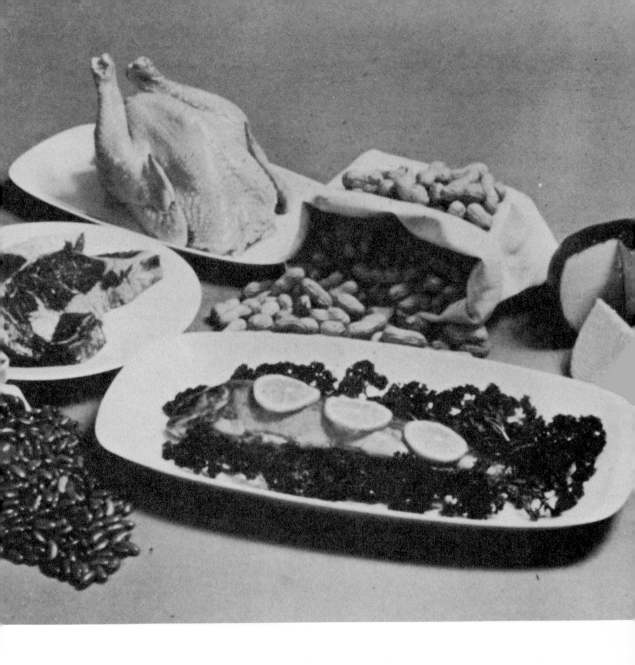

THE AMERICAN DIET: IS IT ADEQUATE?

10

GENERAL PROBLEMS

The United States is one of the most affluent countries in the world, yet nutritional problems exist in this country. Deficiency diseases can still be found in some individuals. As much as 30% of the population is overweight or obese. Americans are spending 14% of their total food and beverage dollar on alcoholic beverages. People with little knowledge of nutrition are constantly trying fad diets and other special diets with hopes of miraculous weight loss, weight gain, or disease cures. Various scientific groups argue over the validity of diet change with respect to heart and artery disease and cancer. Many groups decry the use of food additives, which they suggest are leading to the pollution of our inner ecology. It is hoped that better research and education of the public will bring some of these problems into perspective.

MALNUTRITION

Malnutrition in the United States is a particular problem in low socio-economic areas. The problem is due to both the lack of money to buy food and the lack of education in choosing a proper diet with the money available. But malnutrition is not confined to poor people. The rapid pace of today's society has virtually eliminated breakfast from many people's diets. The proliferation of snack foods can detract from eating a balanced diet even when money is available. Aged people find it hard to get around so they just don't often shop for food. Retired persons on fixed incomes often have reduced buying power. They also may not be able to eat the same things they did when they were younger. As a result, consumption of certain necessary foods may decline.

An indication of the low level of intake of certain nutrients by a significant number of the U.S. population can be found in Table 10.1. The table reports selected findings of three-day dietary reports from over 10,000 individual respondents from the Nationwide Food Consumption Survey of 1977–78. From Table 10.1 it is clear that although many persons consume diets containing levels of nutrients in excess of the RDA, for many Americans some nutrients are being consumed at levels that can be considered marginal or deficient. These "at risk" nutrients are calcium, iron, vitamin A, vitamin B_6, magnesium, and vitamin C. For iron, vitamin A, and vitamin C, a large proportion of people also consume amounts greater than the RDA. Although not listed in Table 10.1, it was also found that many blacks had a deficiency in iron intake. The reasons for this were related to both diet choices and economics.

The reader should be reminded that the RDA is a standard that does not have to be precisely met on a daily basis. However, persons who continue to consume levels of nutrients below 60% of the RDA for a long period of time are considered at risk. Population

TABLE 10.1 Selected results from the nationwide food consumption survey (1977/78)

Nutrient	Percentage of Population consuming 100% or more of RDA	Percentage of Population below 70% of RDA	Percentage of Population below 60% of RDA
Calcium	32	42	30
Iron	43	32	19
Vitamin A	50	31	23
Vitamin B$_6$	20	51	35
Magnesium	25	39	23
Vitamin C	59	26	19
Energy	24	32	16
Protein	88	9	1

groups at risk must then be evaluated for clinical symptoms of nutritional deficiencies.

Severe vitamin deficiency diseases that occurred 30 to 40 years ago are not found to be a problem today. In 1967, health statistics for the United States showed only 13 cases of pellagra, 10 cases of rickets, no scurvy, and almost no goiter. The Ten-State Survey from 1968 to 1970 found that many people had bleeding gums, and, as shown in Table 10.1, that some Americans consume marginal levels of vitamin C. Since some people do not practice good dental care habits, it was hard to determine how much of the gum problem was due to scurvy. The gum problem could however be correlated with reduced consumption of fruits and vegetables by children. Even in school lunch programs where vegetables, fruits, and salads were served, a survey of consumption showed that children left half the vegetables, over one-third of the fruits, and almost all of the salad.

A USDA survey in the mid-1960s showed that poor diets were found in 20% of the families and good diets in only 50%. It is hoped that this trend is reversing as a result of better education, but no data exist to prove it. Income is not the only answer for poor diets, because in 1965 10% of the poor diets were found in families in the top income bracket. Of real concern is the fact that in 1976 the United States Office of Education reported that although most people in the United States could read words, close to 20% were functional illiterates because they could not understand what they read. Another 30% of the American adult population were on the borderline of illiteracy. This means that nutrition education programs may not be useful unless they are developed on a very low level.

The Ten-State Survey pointed out that adolescents between 10 and 16 years of age had the highest evidence of unsatisfactory nutritional status of any age group studied. The Type A school lunch program (Basic Four hot meal subsidized by USDA money) has helped somewhat to improve nutrition in this area. It is usually pointed out that school-age children are better off nutritionally than they were 20 years ago.

One of the problems in making comparisons between today's surveys and the earlier data is that the RDAs have changed. In 1941 the protein RDA for a 15-year-old girl was 80 grams; today it is only 46 grams. Thus, many of the girls deemed inadequate in 1941 would be adequate today, according to the 1980 RDA.

Students in the College of Liberal Arts at the University of Minnesota participated in a seven-day dietary survey in 1974/1975. About 375 students were involved. Table 10.2 depicts the results of the data collected. It shows that the averages for all nutrients meet or exceed the RDA for every category except for iron in women. However, the average or mean value is deceiving because those with high consumption balance out those with low consumption. Table 10.2 also indicates those below 80% and 60% of the RDA. The latter value is more meaningful and can be compared to the data in the Ten-State Survey or National Household Food Consumption Survey. As seen in almost every category, there is some small percentage of the group that could have a nutritional inadequacy. Of course this is dietary survey data and not biochemical evidence.

What is of concern is the high percentage (61%) of women below 60% of the RDA for iron. Follow-up studies of these women by the Student Health Service found only a few with possible true iron deficiency; however, many of the women probably had little or no iron reserves. To illustrate the data better, Figures 10.1 and 10.2 show the distribution for iron and for protein intake for the student group. Both curves are very similar to Figure 2.1 in that they show a bell-shaped curve. These graphs give a better indication of nutrient intakes of various segments of the population. The protein graph shows very high intake as was discussed in Chapter 5, and the iron graph shows that iron deficiency is a female problem that is related to the higher requirement for women.

Another concern in Table 10.2 is the high percentage of both men and women whose diets are below 60% of the RDA for vitamin A. This could be due to the fact that vegetable consumption was low for this group and very few students consumed liver. Unless they can be taught to eat more vitamin A-rich vegetables, fortification of ketchup or mustard used in fast food chains could be used to raise the vitamin A levels, since this is a usual part of their diet. Lastly, the calcium intake is below 60% for 14% of the women. This indicates a low consumption of dairy products, which could easily be reversed.

TABLE 10.2 University of Minnesota 1974/1975 seven day dietary survey M (90 Males) F (285 Females)

Nutrient	Minimum value % of RDA	Maximum value % of RDA	Mean value % of RDA	% below 80% of RDA†	% below 60% of RDA†	RDA 1968	RDA 1974	RDA 1980
Calories								
total	34	217	96	26	6			
M	51	168	98	23	3	2800	3000	2900 (KCal)
F	34	217	96	26	7	2000	2100	2100 (KCal)
Protein								
total	40	370	146	4	2			
M	92	261	168	0	0	60	54	56 (g.)
F	40	370	139	5	2	55	46	44 (g.)
Calcium								
total	22	309	124	22	11			
M	38	309	166	10	2	800	800	800 (mg.)
F	22	275	111	26	14	800	800	800 (mg.)
Phosphorus								
total	55	367	172	3	0			
M	110	367	235	0	0	800	800	800 (mg.)
F	55	342	152	5	0	800	800	800 (mg.)
Iron								
total	19	357	78	71	47			
M	90	357	147	0	0	10	10	10 (mg.)
F	19	159	56	93	61	18	18	18 (mg.)
Vitamin A *								
total	11	641	94	55	34			
M	20	319	96	51	23	5000	5000	5000 (IU) *
F	11	641	94	56	38	5000	4000	4000 (IU)
Thiamin								
total	34	219	94	32	9			
M	35	178	99	29	9	1.4	1.5	1.5 (mg.)
F	34	219	93	33	9	1.0	1.1	1.1 (mg.)
Riboflavin								
total	14	330	120	18	6			
M	45	268	143	8	1	1.6	1.8	1.7 (mg.)
F	14	330	113	22	7	1.5	1.4	1.3 (mg.)
Niacin								
total	43	304	107	21	5			
M	46	217	117	9	1	18	20	19 (mg.)
F	46	304	104	25	7	13	14	14 (mg.)
Vitamin C								
total	16	1504	219	12	6			
M	19	603	212	16	4	60	45	60 (mg.)
F	16	1504	221	11	6	55	45	60 (mg.)

* For Vitamin A the 1980 RDAs are listed in Retinol Equivalents (RE).
For college-age men the RDA is 1000 RE and for college-age women it is 800 RE.
† Based on the 1968 RDA Values

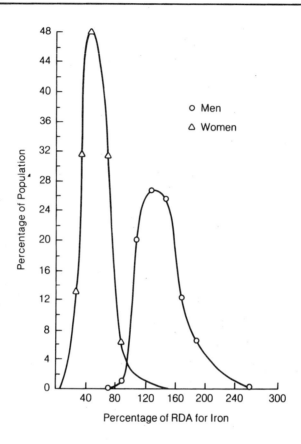

FIGURE 10.1 Iron consumption levels as a percentage of RDA for a University of Minnesota student population

Table 10.3 indicates intake values in the same student survey for nutrients that do not have established RDAs. Consumption of sodium and potassium covered a broad range. The estimated safe and adequate daily dietary intakes for adults were set at 1.1–3.3 grams of sodium and 1.9–5.6 grams of potassium, respectively, in the 1980 RDA book. The mean value for sodium intake for men exceeds the estimated safe level. Some very high intakes of sodium were noted. This intake pattern for sodium reflects the entire U.S. population, many of whom consume excess quantities of the mineral.

The percentages of calories from fat, protein, and carbohydrates come very close to those recommended by the American Heart Association and other health groups who are concerned with heart disease and health maintenance. It is interesting that this group of students achieved these ratios with little to no nutrition education.

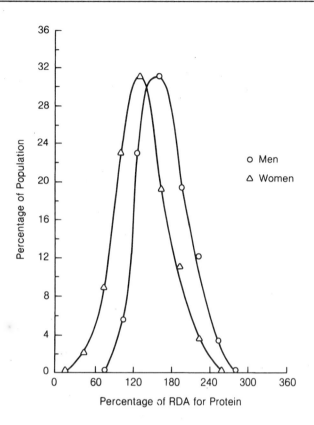

FIGURE 10.2 Protein consumption levels as a percentage of RDA for a University of Minnesota student population

More data like these on various population groups is needed so that education about proper dietary changes and legislation on food fortification can be initiated. By education and dietary modification, it is hoped that the marginal nutrition inadequacies can be eradicated from our population.

FOOD DISAPPEARANCE DATA

Table 10.4 shows data that is used to predict general food consumption patterns in the United States. It is based on food disappearance. The USDA has been publishing estimated food disappearance data since 1909. Food disappearance is based on how much food was produced in this country and entered warehouses or storage facilities plus any imports of the product minus any exports. It is

TABLE 10.3 University of Minnesota seven-day dietary survey food consumption data 1974/75

Nutrient	Minimum value	Maximum value	Mean value
Sodium			
Total	0.7g.	14.2g.	2.7g.
M*	1.3g.	14.2g.	3.6g.
F**	0.7g.	11.0g.	2.5g.
Potassium			
Total	0.8g.	9.4g.	2.5g.
M	1.1g.	5.2g.	3.3g.
F	0.8g.	9.4g.	2.3g.
% of calories as Protein			
Total	9%	30%	16%
M	11%	27%	16%
F	9%	30%	16%
% of calories as Fat			
Total	15%	52%	35%
M	26%	52%	37%
F	15%	48%	35%
% of calories as Carbohydrate			
Total	22%	63%	48%
M	22%	59%	47%
F	34%	63%	48%

* M—male
** F—female

not based on how much is consumed by the population but the total amount from above is divided by the population to get an average amount of food available to each citizen. Obviously, some of this food decays before consumption occurs and some of it is wasted in the home, fed to pets, or thrown out in the garbage. Estimates of these losses run from 10% to 20%. Infants and children would also not eat as much of each of these foods. Despite these limitations disappearance information is useful because it shows the trend in food availability for the United States population since early this century. As can be seen, potential meat consumption has increased while egg consumption increased in the 1940s and then has dropped. The changes in eggs are due in part to price, education, and health concerns. Consumption of dairy products has dropped significantly in recent years. Total dairy consumption has decreased by 24% since 1960. This decrease and the increase in meat consumption have led to changes in the calcium/phosphorus balance. The mean calcium/phosphorus ratio from Table 10.2 is 0.72, which is close to that projected from the national average in Table 10.5.

It is interesting that total per capita fruit and vegetable (fresh and processed) consumption decreased between 1949 and 1980, although it has been slowly increasing recently. Again, however, we must realize that this is disappearance data for the total population. Table 10.4 does not separate the data for various population groups. The decrease in fruit consumption correlates well with the low vitamin-C intakes in the Ten-State Survey but not with the college-student data.

TABLE 10.4 Food disappearance weight of the U.S. food supply (per capita per year)

Food Group	Years		
	1909–13	1947–49	1980 [a]
	lbs. retail wt.		
Meat, poultry, and fish			
Beef	54	52	78
Pork	62	64	69
Poultry	18	22	62
Fish	13	13	17
Total	172	176	245
Eggs	37	47	35
Dairy products			
Whole milk	265	299	171
Lowfat milk	61	36	106
Cheese	5	10	22
Total	381	507	469
Fats and oils			
Butter	18	11	4
Total	41	46	61
Fruits			
Citrus	17	66	77
Non-citrus	159	142	119
Total, fresh	168	164	107
Total, processed	8	44	89
Total	176	208	197
Vegetables			
Tomatoes	43	48	55
Dark green, deep yellow	14	31	24
Other	146	157	141
Total, fresh	186	184	143
Total, processed	17	52	77
Total	203	236	219
Potatoes			
White, fresh	182	110	51
White, processed [b]	0	[c]	62
Sweet, fresh	23	12	4
Sweet, processed [b]	0	[c]	1
Total	205	123	118
Dry beans, peas, nuts, soy products	16	17	18

TABLE 10.4 Food disappearance weight of the U.S. food supply (per capita per year) *(Continued)*

Food Group	Years		
	1909–13	1947–49	1980 [a]
	lbs. retail wt.		
Grain products			
Wheat flour	213	137	119
Corn flour and meal	50	13	8
Total	291	171	154
Sugar and sweeteners			
Refined cane/beet sugar	77	95	88
Other sugar and syrup	14	19	54
Total	91	114	143
Coffee	8	15	9
Total Beverages [d]	10	19	12

Adapted from Welsh and Marston. J.Am.Diet.Assn. 81:122, 1982

Totals include some foods not listed in this table; components may not add to a total due to rounding.

[a] Preliminary data.

[b] Fresh equivalent weight

[c] Less than 0.5 lb.

[d] Includes coffee, tea, and chocolate liquor equivalent of cocoa and chocolate products.

The United States Department of Agriculture calculated the nutrient content of the available food for the same three time periods; the values are presented in Table 10.5. As can be seen, there is more than 100% of the RDA available for the average man or woman even if we accounted for 10% to 20% waste. Our problem obviously, is that some people consume much more and some much less than the RDA of some nutrients. We must do a better job of educating the public to choose food properly.

OVERNUTRITION

Close to 30% of the population is overweight to some degree. The reasons for this will be discussed in Chapter 12. The problem is compounded by lack of good education on nutrition and loss of control by some individuals of the quantity of their food intake. Americans spend over 40% of their food dollars for meals away from home, many of which are being served without a vegetable or salad. We also increased our consumption of soft drinks by 151% between 1960 and 1976. In addition, such foods as candies, chips, pretzels, and so on amount to 50 pounds consumed per person per year, close to 3% of the diet. This is a small percentage, but a small percentage every day adds up to a lot of weight if it contributes only excess calories. Some individuals consume large quantities of these and other foods that supply few nutrients and many calories. There

TABLE 10.5 Nutrient content of the U.S. food supply, based on per capita per day disappearance.

Nutrient	Years		
	1909–13	1947–49	1980[a]
Food energy (kcal)	3,480	3,230	3,540
Protein (gm.)	102	95	104
Fat (gm.)	125	141	169
Carbohydrate (gm.)	492	403	408
Minerals			
Calcium (gm.)	0.82	1.00	0.94
Phosphorus (gm.)	1.56	1.55	1.56
Iron (mg.)	15.0	16.2	17.6
Magnesium (mg.)	408	368	349
Zinc (mg.)	12.6	11.5	12.5
Vitamins			
Vitamin A (I.U.)[b]	7,600	8,800	8,400
Thiamin (mg.)	1.64	1.91	2.23
Riboflavin (mg.)	1.87	2.31	2.45
Niacin (mg.)[c]	19.0	21.0	26.8
Vitamin B_6 (mg.)	2.17	1.89	2.06
Vitamin B_{12} (g.)	8.4	8.9	9.7
Ascorbic acid (mg.)	104	114	123

Adapted from Welsh and Marston. J.Am.Diet.Assn. 81:122, 1982

[a] Preliminary data.

[b] "Vitamin A" refers to the vitamin A value of foods calculated from data for preformed vitamin A, beta-carotene, and other carotenoid precursors of vitamin A.

[c] Excludes niacin equivalents of trypotophan.

is nothing wrong with these foods as a part of a balanced diet; the problem is to learn to balance one's diet.

We have also become obsessed with vitamin pills. Many feel that as long as they take their vitamins, they are getting all the needed nutrients. This can lead to an imbalance in food intake since people then don't eat what they should. It also really wastes money because a good diet can supply the nutrients needed. It should be obvious from the early chapters that vitamins alone do not supply good nutrition and the results in Table 10.5 show that our food can supply us with the needed vitamins.

Often forgotten in evaluation of dietary patterns is our overconsumption of alcohol. Americans spend in excess of 40 billion dollars on alcoholic beverages yearly. The USDA estimates that for each man, woman and child in the United States, over 20 gallons of beer, 2 gallons of wine and 2 gallons of liquor are consumed. Since most children and some adults do not consume any alcohol, it is apparent that many Americans are moderate to heavy drinkers. Most of us are aware that the alcoholic has a whole series of nutritional and health problems. We usually are not aware, however, that "social" drinkers can significantly stress their nutritional status. Alcohol provides about seven Calories per gram consumed. This translates to about 150 Calories for eight ounces of wine, 125 Calories for a twelve-ounce can of beer, and 160 Calories for two ounces of 100-proof scotch. For a moderate drinker (two to three drinks daily), it is quite easy to consume 10–20% of one's daily calories from alcohol. Because alcohol contains few if any nutrients, this reduces the nutrient density of the diet. In addition, alcohol contributes to obesity as well as reduces the absorption and utilization of several vitamins and minerals.

SUMMARY

Although we have one of the best food supplies in the world, nutritional disease still exists in the United States. Part of the problem is poverty, but a main part is lack of education about food and nutrition. Surveys made of the United States population revealed some nutrition problems. For example, poor dental care and diets low in vitamin C are responsible for poor mouth and tooth conditions. In addition, adolescents between 10 and 16 years of age had the poorest nutritional status despite the Type A school lunch program.

A seven-day diet survey of college students (18 to 24 years old at the University of Minnesota) showed much better food intake patterns of vitamins and minerals than did the Ten-State Survey. The most significant problems were in iron levels for women and in vitamin-A intake for both sexes.

Food disappearance data from the U.S. Department of Agriculture correlates with the diet-survey information, especially with respect to decreased fruit and dairy product consumption. But we should be aware that the USDA average nutrient levels available are misleading because they are only averages and not specific for certain population groups. In many cases we have both overnutrition and undernutrition in various classes of people. Overnutrition is responsible for the high incidence of obesity in our population. High intakes of sodium and alcohol also place stress upon our nutritional status.

Multiple Choice Study Questions

1. The deficiency of nutrients in the U.S. diet stems from

    A. an inability to pay for the correct foods

    B. an inability to choose the correct foods

    C. there is no deficiency problem; the only problem is oversupply

    D. A and B above

    E. none of the above

2. Typical American diets are most frequently deficient in which one of the following nutrients?

A. protein
B. vitamin C
C. calcium
D. bioflavanoids
E. phosphorus

3. The black population surveyed in the Ten-State Nutrition Survey was most deficient in

A. iron
B. vitamin A
C. vitamin B_1
D. protein
E. calcium

4. The Ten-State Nutritional Survey of 1968–1970 showed the highest prevalence of deficiencies in

A. iron, calories, vitamin A, riboflavin
B. vitamin A, riboflavin, fiber
C. iron, riboflavin, fiber
D. iron and fiber
E. iron, vitamin A, and riboflavin

5. In the University of Minnesota student diet survey the two most lacking nutrients for women, besides iron, were

A. protein and vitamin C
B. calcium and phosphorus
C. calcium and vitamin A
D. vitamin A and thiamin
E. thiamin and vitamin C

6. Food disappearance in USDA tables is based on

A. actual food consumption per capita
B. U.S. food production statistics per capita
C. the food balance of payments per capita
D. per capita production plus imports
E. per capita imports minus exports plus production

Essay Study Questions

1. Discuss the major malnutrition problems found in the United States.

2. What is food disappearance data? How can it be related to nutritional status?

3. How does the government assess nutrition status?

4. Are fast food meals worthless to the human body?

5. Which age group has the worst nutrient intake status? How can this be improved?

6. Are there over nutrition problems in the United States? Discuss.

Things to Do

1. Compare your seven-day dietary averages with the survey results listed in this chapter.

2. Do a survey for a young child and an elderly person. What is their nutritional status?

3. Calculate the nutritional content of some fast food meals you consume. Are they adequate? (See Appendix II.)

4. Compare your dietary pattern to that recommended by the 1977 McGovern Senate Select Committee on Nutrition (Dietary Goals for the United States available from the Superintendent of Documents).

Chapter 10. Answers to Multiple-Choice Study Questions: 1, D; 2, C; 3, A; 4, E; 5, C; 6, E.

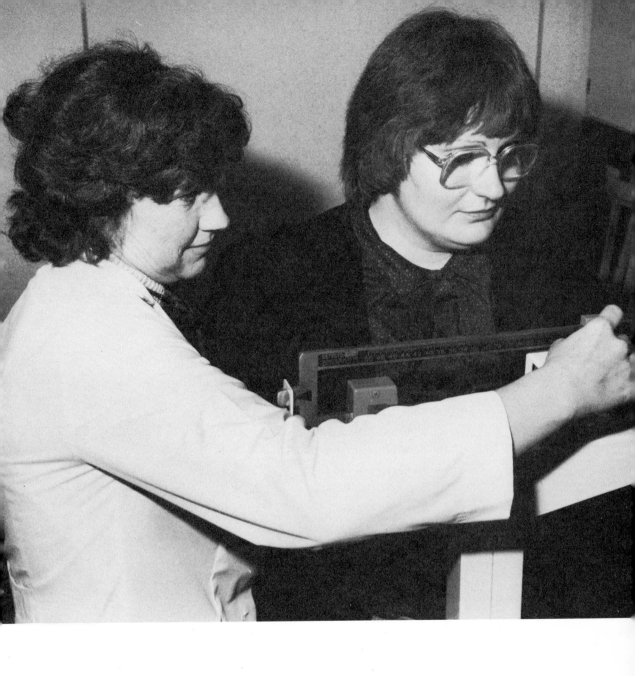

HEART DISEASE: RELATIONSHIP TO THE DIET

11

Over the past 25 years, coronary heart disease (CHD) and atherosclerosis and their various consequences have been major topics of conversation at the dinner table, on TV, at parties, and elsewhere. Almost every dietary ingredient imaginable has been implicated in causing heart disease. Here is a list of some factors that epidemiologists, scientists, and physicians have connected with heart disease. Next to each "cause" is a number that relates creditability of the factor in terms of "causing" heart disease and atherosclerosis. A value of 1.0 would suggest an absolute cause/effect of that factor in heart disease; zero would suggest no effect.

Cause	Factor
1. Homogenized milk	0.2
2. Cholesterol in diet	0.5
3. Degree of water hardness	0.5
4. Hydrogenated fats	0.5
5. Refined sugar	0.5
6. Zinc/copper ratio in diet	0.6
7. Lack of exercise	0.7
8. Lack of fiber	0.7
9. Obesity	0.7
10. Cigarette smoking	0.8
11. Hypertension	0.8
12. Saturated fatty acids	0.8
13. Stress of society	0.9
14. Hereditary factors	1.0

We will discuss how some of these factors are related to CHD. We will also discuss how changes in our lifestyle and dietary habits may improve and maintain our health status.

INCIDENCE OF HEART DISEASE

It is estimated that heart and related artery diseases cause over one million deaths yearly in the U.S., making these diseases the number one cause of death in the United States. These adverse health conditions account for almost 50% of all deaths. Other causes of death, in order, are: cancer—350,000 deaths; accidents—113,000 deaths; pneumonia and flu—61,000 deaths; and diabetes—40,000 deaths. All other causes total another 350,000 deaths. The major cardiovascular (heart and blood vessel system) diseases afflict close to 30,000,000 people, or almost 15% of the population, although many people may be unaware that they have such a condition.

In 1900 the major single cause of death in the U.S. was also cardiovascular disease (heart disease and stroke). However, only 14% of the population died from heart disease at the turn of the century. Since close to 50% of deaths are due to CHD today, one would initially conclude that today the rate of death due to CHD is extraordinarily higher.

This conclusion must be tempered by several facts. First, our life expectancy increased 26 years between 1900 and 1982—from 47 years to 73 years of age. We now live long enough to suffer from the consequences of the chronic diseases of CHD and cancer. Acute illnesses such as tuberculosis, acute rheumatic fever, smallpox, tetanus, and others have ceased to be principal threats to health. For example, 30,000 people between the ages of 15 and 44 died of tuberculosis in 1940 compared to 407 in 1973. Total acute illnesses now cause less than 2% of the health problems that they did in 1900. In short, we live long enough to die from chronic diseases.

The finite number of yearly deaths from CHD has increased about three-fold since 1900, but these crude death-rate figures are misleading because of the issues raised above. Due to the fact that the U.S. population has expanded, most survival statistics are now reported in terms of "age-adjusted death rates." Statistics from the U.S. government show that the age-adjusted heart disease death rate increased somewhat up to 1950 but decreased 15% from 1950 to 1969 and decreased another 20% by 1975.

The decline in age-adjusted death rates can be attributed to improved health and emergency care, better medical treatment, decreased smoking, increased public awareness, and perhaps improved nutrition. Thus, even though a great number of persons suffer and die from CHD, we are doing a better job at reducing the rate of death. We should take great pride in our increased life expectancy but should continue to investigate those factors in our diet that may decrease or increase incidence of heart disease.

PROGRESSION OF HEART DISEASE AND STROKE

Coronary heart disease is a progressive chronic disease that may continue over three or four decades of life without outward signs. Autopsies of American men from the Korean and Vietnam wars showed that 50 percent of soldiers in their early 20s had initial signs of atherosclerosis in their arteries. The first stage of development of CHD is arterial damage to the endothelial cells of the vessel. The cells of the endothelium are the outermost cells of the artery wall that are in direct contact with the blood. Lipids, especially triglycerides and cholesterol, penetrate and get trapped in the artery wall and form a fatty streak. In advanced stages of this artery disease fibrous plaques form and protrude into the center of the artery.

These plaques narrow the space that the blood flows through, forcing blood pressure to build up behind them. These vessels may become completely blocked. When this occurs in an artery supplying the heart, the loss of blood may cause the heart muscle to die, since the heart cannot get the fuel needed for muscular movement. In addition, the vessel walls may become so weak from the plaque growth that the high blood pressure (hypertension) can cause them to burst. This is what causes hemorrhaging of the artery. Small plaques may also break loose and plug up the arteries supplying blood to the brain or heart. This can lead to a stroke or a heart attack that can result in death.

TOTAL FAT, SATURATED FAT, AND CHOLESTEROL

Americans have dramatically and steadily increased their consumption of total dietary fat from 1900 until about 1975. In this period there was about a 25% increase in amount of fat consumed. Most of that increase was in the form of unsaturated fat from vegetable oils. Since 1975 there has been a decline in fat intake, probably due to increased public awareness of the undesirable nature of high fat intake. Today, for most people, probably more than 40% of food calories comes from fat. Health groups recommend that we reduce this to below 35% of calories.

Cholesterol consumption has increased only about 10% since the turn of the century. Cholesterol consumption has not increased as much as total fat consumption primarily due to the adverse publicity about cholesterol in the last 25 years. Consumption of eggs, lard, butter, and some dairy products, all significant sources of cholesterol, has declined in the last quarter century.

One of the three major risk factors for CHD is elevated serum cholesterol (the others are hypertension and cigarette smoking). The plaque material that develops on artery walls during the progression of CHD is high in cholesterol and fat. Therefore, it has been quite logical to relate high intakes of fat and cholesterol to CHD. However, the associations of dietary fat, saturated fat, and cholesterol with CHD is not clear-cut. After decades of conjecture and experimentation, few conclusions can be made and these associations are still highly controversial.

Although high serum levels of cholesterol and total lipids correlate rather strongly with CHD, dietary intake of cholesterol and fat by *individuals* do not correlate well with serum levels of those lipids. There are, of course, persons in our population with a strong genetic predisposition to high blood lipids (hyperlipemia). Persons in some families do not have the ability to regulate either blood cholesterol or triglycerides very well. For these families, control of dietary cholesterol, fats, calories, or even carbohydrates (and alcohol) is essential. However, for the majority of the population, reduction of or increased intake of, for example, cholesterol does not necessarily correspond to a decrease or increase in serum cholesterol. Dr. Michael DeBakey, an eminent heart surgeon, says:

> We found very little relationship between diet and cholesterol level, and coronary artery disease. Much to the chagrin of many of my colleagues who believe in this polyunsaturated fat and cholesterol business, we have put outpatients on no dietary program, no anti-cholesterol medications. We have found that 80 percent of our patients with severe occlusive coronary artery disease had had blood cholesterol levels comparable to the levels in normal people. When the levels are comparable, it doesn't make sense that elevated cholesterol levels are the cause of coronary artery disease. (Comments at the Cardiovascular Disease Seminar, Dandiger Institute of Menorah Medical Center, Kansas City, Missouri, 1971.)

Dr. R. Reiser of Texas A & M presented a controversial hypothesis in 1972 that high cholesterol levels among young people could be due to starting life with too little cholesterol in their diets. He felt it was possible that there was too little cholesterol available in infants' diets because of the use of synthetic formulas without cholesterol instead of mother's milk. Thus, during the first few years of growth and development, the body established mechanisms to overproduce the needed cholesterol. These mechanisms would then stay in effect during the remainder of one's life, providing unnecessarily high levels of cholesterol. Conversely, if infants are fed high levels of cholesterol in their early diets, the body would not develop mechanisms that would produce large amounts of cholesterol at later stages of life.

The results of two studies published in 1982 (Hulbron et al., *J.Nutr.* 112:1296; McMurray et al., *Am.J.Clin.Nutr.* 35:741) did not support the Reiser hypothesis, but conclusive human studies cannot be undertaken for ethical reasons. We would not want to place infants at risk for CHD by dramatically modifying their infant formulas to test the hypothesis.

Despite the lack of evidence for a direct role of dietary cholesterol in CHD, the American Heart Association (AHA) advises a drastic reduction in the intake of foods that are high in cholesterol, and recommends that foods such as eggs and meat, as well as saturated fats, be avoided. They recommend using margarine and vegetable oils instead of butter and animal fat for cooking and for spreading, and suggest that beef be replaced with chicken and fish because of their lower levels of saturated fats.

Recommendations of the AHA as well as of other groups include reducing the intake of fats to less than 35% of the total calories consumed. At the present time Americans obtain a higher percentage of their total caloric intake in the form of fats, although the students mentioned in the study in Chapter 10 were close to the recommended value. Using the AHA recommendations would lead to a greater intake of polyunsaturated fats, decreased intake of saturated fats, and decreased cholesterol consumption.

The American Heart Association also suggests that intake of saturated fats be reduced and that carbohydrates be consumed in their more complex forms, that is, as starches. An increase in fiber intake and a lower intake of dietary salt are also advised. All these recommendations seem desirable to some degree.

The Food and Drug Administration has regulations concerning the labeling of cholesterol and fat content on food packages that disallows any comment about the curing of heart disease. (See Chapter 24.) Unfortunately, this type of comment cannot be prevented in media advertising and may cause consumer concern about something that has not been proven.

We should avoid overresponding to fears about certain food ingredients such as cholesterol. Rejection of all foods containing cholesterol would be unwise and perhaps unhealthy. Eggs, for example, contain very high quality protein and an excellent profile of vitamins and minerals. Total rejection of eggs from the diet could decrease intake of many desirable nutrients.

OTHER DIETARY FACTORS

Refined Sugar

Some nutritionists have attributed heart disease to the consumption of highly refined sugars such as sucrose, but no direct biochemical mechanism has been elucidated. No conclusive experiments with humans have supported this hypothesis. Dr. John Yudkin of the University of London has been the major proponent of the sugar-CHD link. But the evidence is based mostly on epidemiological studies, that is, studies showing that most countries where sugar consumption is high have higher incidence of heart disease. This is not true for the West Indies, however, where sugar consumption is very high. In fact, there is a better statistical correlation between heart disease and owning a color television set for those who live in highly developed countries.

Sodium

High blood pressure or hypertension is a major risk factor in CHD. Approximately 17% of the American population is predisposed to high blood pressure. The predisposition is highly family-linked. About half the people with high blood pressure can lower their blood pressure by restricting salt (sodium chloride) intake. Reduction in weight is most desirable in hypertensive people.

High blood pressure may be the cause of the initial damage to the endothelial cells of artery walls. After damage occurs, high blood pressure may well accelerate deposition of lipid within the walls.

When excess salt is consumed by many hypertensive people, the sodium enters the bloodstream and acts to retain water in the blood. This is a protective measure by our body to maintain the proper osmolarity in blood. It results in a greater blood volume being contained in the same circulation system, thus exerting a greater pressure. The heart also has to pump harder. Early detection is as easy as having blood pressure measured, a very simple process. Treatment involves both reduction of salt in the diet and, in some cases, drug therapy. Few people realize how much salt they consume, yet when they slowly reduce their intake they find that foods still taste good and salted foods seem overseasoned. Most Americans consume far more salt than necessary. Many health groups recommend reduction in salt intake. The American Medical Association currently recommends that Americans restrict their intake to below 10–12 grams daily.

Recent reports in the literature suggest that persons with low calcium intake are far more prone to hypertension than are those with adequate intakes of calcium. Clearly, hypertension is a medical problem with many possible causes including diet. Dietary levels of sodium is only one of the factors—but one of the easiest to control. Many food companies are reducing the sodium content of their products in response to the growing concern about sodium and hypertension.

Protein

Dr. K.K. Carroll of the University of Western Ontario has published rather convincing evidence with experimental animals suggesting that feeding proteins from plant sources results in lower blood cholesterol levels than does feeding proteins of animal origin. We anxiously await further developments in this area.

Fiber

The relationship between fiber and heart disease has been pointed out by Dr. Denis Burkitt of London who has carried out extensive epidemiological studies in Africa. He found that tribes with high fiber consumption had very little coronary heart disease, and he suggested that fiber had a protective effect. Studies do show that pectin and some gums bind dietary cholesterol and bile salts in the digestive tract and prevent them from being absorbed through the intestinal wall. Most other forms of fiber such as cellulose and wheat bran have no such effect on cholesterol metabolism. Studies of individuals who are genetically prone to heart disease and who have extremely high blood lipids and cholesterol show that reducing cholesterol by eating a material that prevents absorption of cholesterol from the digestive tract has some positive benefits on blood cholesterol levels. However, whether the slight reduction in cholesterol absorption from pectin consumption can significantly affect the incidence of CHD is not clear. The use of various forms of dietary fiber to reduce blood cholesterol is currently being extensively researched. Because of the other benefits of fiber mentioned in Chapter 4, increasing fiber in the American diet would be prudent.

DEGREE OF WATER HARDNESS

Epidemiological evidence shows that in areas of the world where water has a high mineral content (hard water), the residents have a lower rate of CHD. Hard water contains higher amounts of calcium, magnesium, iron, sulfate, and other metal ions. The differences in hard versus soft water that contribute to the reduction of the incidence of CHD have been studied since the mid 1950s. There are many theories but there is still no clear-cut evidence that explains the positive effect of hard water in reducing CHD.

ZINC/COPPER RATIO

The dietary zinc/copper ratio is another factor currently undergoing extensive research. Dr. L. Klevay of the USDA Human Nutrition Laboratories in North Dakota was responsible for elucidating this factor. He concluded that human diets deficient in copper but high in zinc were more conducive to heart disease because a high zinc/copper ratio possibly induces the liver to produce more cholesterol. Fiber is related because it preferentially binds zinc, making it insoluble and thus unavailable to the body. This decreases the available zinc/copper ratio in the digestive tract, which should be beneficial. The degree of water hardness may also be related. In soft-water systems, fewer mineral salts are present. The mineral salts in hard water may bind zinc in the intestine, thus also lowering the ratio of available zinc to copper. Klevay also feels that exercise is related to CHD because sweating increases zinc excretion, thus lowering the zinc/copper ratio in the body and reducing cholesterol synthesis.

Copper consumption by many Americans is quite low, and inadequate copper consumption may be very unfavorable to CHD. High zinc intakes, especially by those taking zinc supplements, may aggravate the low-copper problem. It will be interesting to read about future investigations in this area.

OBESITY

Overeating is an unsound practice (see Chapter 12). Obesity clearly reduces life expectancy. Studies have shown that when the body mass exceeds 30% above average the mortality rate increases by about 40% in men and 30% in women due to increased CHD, diabetes, strokes, and various digestive diseases. Maintenance of ideal body weight is a principal factor in maintenance of health.

OTHER FACTORS

Genetics

Factors not related to the diet have also been correlated with CHD. The best correlation is that of a family history of deaths caused by heart disease. Children from families with high levels of serum cholesterol and other lipids generally also have high serum lipid levels. These families may have one of a group of genetic lipid disorders. High blood pressure is also genetically linked.

Persons with a family history of heart disease must be more cautious with their diet, their weight, and their lifestyle than other people. They must not neglect medical exams, a healthful diet, and appropriate exercise. We must all do a better job of listening to and monitoring our body signs.

Exercise

Dr. George Mann of Vanderbilt University has suggested that exercise is the most important factor in controlling CHD. In those areas of the world where people work hard at physical labor there is a lower incidence of CHD. The lower disease rate from CHD may be related to dietary factors, to the higher secretion of zinc in sweat, or simply to stronger heart and blood vessels that can withstand the ravages of the disease. Certainly a large part of our society exercises much less and leads a more sedentary life than it did 40 or 50 years ago. A medical study on the incidence of CHD in brothers, half of whom came to the United States from Ireland, showed that the Irish brothers did more hard physical work and had less CHD. The brothers in the United States ate less butter, consumed more unsaturated fats and calories, consumed less starch, and drank more whiskey and coffee than their Irish brothers. The United States brothers weighed more and had a significantly higher incidence of heart disease. Both groups smoked the same amount of cigarettes. It is believed that the harder physical labor of the Irish brothers could be one reason for their better health and lower incidence of CHD.

For the average person, a significant increase in exercise should be undertaken only after consulting a physician. Exercise must also begin gradually so as not to precipitate a heart attack. Strenuous exercise is not recommended for everyone.

Smoking

Cigarette smoking also correlates highly to heart disease as well as to many other diseases such as lung cancer. The exact cause-effect relationship is still unknown. Despite the evidence linking smoking and CHD people still smoke, to the detriment of their health as well as to the health of those around them. The National Academy of Science estimates that 17 out of 100 people who smoke will die of some disease related to smoking.

Behavior Stress

Lastly, the stress of society (*Type A Behavior and Your Heart,* M. Friedman and P. Roseman, Fawcett, 1975) has been highly correlated to heart disease. The type A-individual is one who is always striving to do well and who rarely relaxes. This individual is always on the move, is very intense, and continually worries about life problems. This type of behavior can cause great stress to all body systems and could well increase the incidence of high blood pressure, arterial damage, and CHD. Many of us must learn to relax for periods during the day and let our bodies rest.

HEART DISEASE, A MULTI-FACTORIAL DISEASE

Over the last ten years, there have been serious investigations of some three dozen risk factors of coronary heart disease. We have discussed only some of them in this chapter. CHD is not caused simply by one or two factors. Genetic predisposition, lifestyle, environment, diet, and exercise are all important factors related to this chronic disease. In one sizable experiment, known as the Framingham study, over 5,000 men and women have been followed over several decades in Framingham, Massachusetts, in an attempt to establish risk factors in CHD. Three major risk factors have emerged from this study: cigarette smoking, blood cholesterol levels, and blood pressure. Some of the results have shown that a person who smokes more than one pack of cigarettes a day has nearly twice the risk of CHD as does a nonsmoker. A person with blood cholesterol over 250 mg% has about three times the risk of a heart attack as a person below 194 mg%. Moreover, the risk factors are additive. A person who smokes, has high blood cholesterol (over 300), and high blood pressure (systolic over 180) has five times the risk of a person with none of these risk factors.

Coronary heart disease is a multifactorial problem. Reducing risk for CHD can be achieved by following a prudent life style. The age adjusted death rates due to CHD has been decreasing since 1950 in the U.S. but about 1,000,000 people die yearly as a result of this disease. Improvement of our life style is strongly suggested.

A PRUDENT DIET
Obviously we don't know all the causes of CHD. Some diet modification would be prudent despite the controversial nature of some of the evidence. The following diet and health plan can be recommended for those who wish to modify their food habits to help reduce their risk for heart disease and atherosclerosis.

1. Eat a variety of foods, eat in moderation, and maintain optimal weight.

2. Eat meats and eggs in moderation, but do not eliminate them from the diet. An egg every other day is a good rule of thumb, but once a day will probably do no harm.

3. Reduce fat consumption to about 35% of calories. Unsaturated fats can be increased but should not exceed a ratio of 1/1/1 for saturated to monounsaturated to polyunsaturated.

4. Increase fiber consumption by eating more fruit, vegetables, and whole-grain cereals.

5. Decrease the consumption of salt.

6. Maintain an exercise program.

7. Stop or never begin cigarette smoking.

8. Find time to relax in your life and begin to understand your body's needs and metabolism.

Multiple Choice Study Questions

1. The major cause of death in this country is
   A. auto accidents
   B. diabetes
   C. cancer
   D. smoking
   E. coronary heart disease

2. The highest correlation with CHD is
   A. dietary cholesterol
   B. Zn/Cu ratio
   C. hard water
   D. cigarette smoking
   E. hereditary factors

3. The plaque that forms in CHD does not contain

   A. cholesterol
   B. trace minerals
   C. saturated fat
   D. protein
   E. glycogen

4. The American Heart Association suggests reducing fat intake to

   A. 20% of the weight of food
   B. 20% of the calories
   C. 30–35% of the weight of food
   D. 30–35% of calories
   E. none of the above

5. The original experiments on coronary heart disease that implicated cholesterol were done with

   A. rabbits
   B. guinea pigs
   C. rats
   D. mice
   E. hamsters

6. Fiber is related to CHD through

   A. suppression of cholesterol production
   B. suppression of dietary cholesterol absorption
   C. reduction of fat metabolism
   D. increased zinc absorption
   E. none of the above

7. When one exercises hard

   A. blood pressure drops
   B. the copper level drops
   C. zinc is excreted in the sweat
   D. glycogen levels increase in the blood
   E. cholesterol excretion increases

8. In the study of the Irish brothers the primary difference that was implicated in the higher incidence of CHD was

   A. more cholesterol in the American diet
   B. more beer in the Irish diet
   C. less work and exercise in the American lifestyle
   D. more cigarette smoking for the Americans
   E. more whiskey in the U.S. diet

9. One factor that might be responsible for the correlation between soft water, hypertension, and heart disease is
   A. the presence of zinc in soft water
   B. the absence of copper in soft water
   C. the presence of cadmium in soft water
   D. the presence of sodium in soft water
   E. the presence of calcium in soft water

10. A possible deficiency of what trace metal may be partially responsible for CHD?
    A. cadmium
    B. stontium
    C. zinc
    D. chromium
    E. iron

11. Which has the least significant relationship to coronary heart disease from a scientific standpoint?
    A. cholesterol
    B. salt
    C. sugar
    D. homogenized milk
    E. soft water

Essay Study Questions

1. What is the significance of coronary heart disease as a cause of death in the United States?

2. How does atherosclerosis occur?

3. Discuss the pros and cons of cholesterol as a cause of coronary heart disease.

4. What did the Framingham study show?

5. What are the most important causative factors for CHD? Discuss each factor.

6. What dietary factors and nondietary factors might reduce the incidence of CHD for an individual?

Things to Do

1. Examine your dietary survey. What factors might be changed to decrease risk from CHD?

2. Make a list of foods available in the supermarket that are specifically developed for people who wish to control their cholesterol and fat intakes.

3. Do a dietary analysis of someone who has had a heart attack. Is the person following good nutritional principles?

4. Discuss dietary recommendations your physician should make for people with heart conditions.

Chapter 11. Answers to Multiple-Choice Study Questions: 1, E; 2, E; 3, E; 4, D; 5, A; 6, B; 7, C; 8, C; 9, C; 10, D; 11, D.

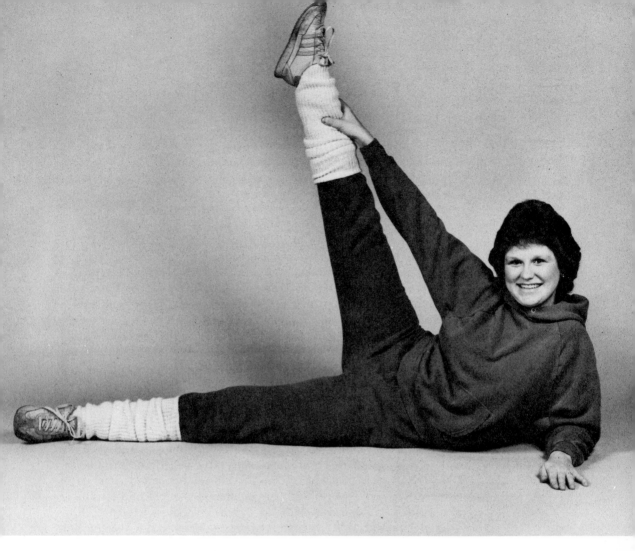

OBESITY, WEIGHT CONTROL, AND DIETING

12

During the past 25 years interest in weight reduction in the United States has grown from a moderate concern to an overriding preoccupation. At present, interest in obesity almost assumes the dimensions of a national neurosis. It would be a pleasure to report that this concern has resulted in new and more effective measures of obesity control or even in more effective use of old measures, but we have no evidence of any decrease in the incidence or severity of obesity. The major result of our national preoccupation has been to worry large numbers of mildly obese persons whose conditions present no real health hazard. It has done nothing about the prevalence of severe obesity among the poor.

The preceding statement was made by Albert J. Stunkard in his article, "The Obese: Background and Programs," one of the articles in the book *United States Nutrition Policies* edited by Jean Mayer (W.H. Freeman and Co., San Francisco, 1973). Obesity is not a new problem but has been with us for centuries. Many subjects in paintings of the fifteenth, sixteenth, and seventeenth centuries were obese. They were usually rich members of the ruling class. Plump ladies with large breasts were subjects for paintings that can be seen in any large art museum. Although today the thin look is in, it is not necessarily a healthy look.

THE OBESITY EQUATION

Overweight and obesity generally result from too much food in the diet or not enough physical activity. The principal formula for weight control is: calories in minus calories out equals change in weight. If the number of calories consumed is equal to the number of calories expended, generally no weight change will result. However, if "calories in" is greater than "calories out," weight will increase. Conversely, if "calories in" is less than "calories out" weight will decrease.

Unfortunately for 20% to 30% of our population, "calories in" has exceeded expenditure for a long period of time and these people have become clinically obese. Many others are slightly overweight, which is not necessarily a health risk unless additional weight is gained. About 40% of Americans report that they diet constantly. The vast majority are unsuccessful in maintaining weight loss.

AM I TOO FAT: DIAGNOSIS OF OBESITY

Many people do not feel that they are overweight or unable to control their eating. Those who do diet often do so on their own; very few seek the medical help they need.

A doctor treating an overweight person must decide if the excess weight is really due to excess fat. One of the most obvious criterion is appearance. However, appearance can be misleading because bulk is not always caused by more fat tissue. Increased muscle mass may give a person a bulky appearance. People who weigh up to 15% over the weight standard set by national insurance tables are considered to be overweight, and those who exceed the standard by 15% to 20% or more are considered to be clinically obese. This assumes that the extra weight in obese people is fat tissue. One way to measure fat tissue is to measure skin-fold thickness. By picking up a portion of flesh on various parts of the body and measuring the thickness of this fat layer with calipers, a health professional can estimate how much fat is on the body. This method of testing is not entirely valid because of variables in the amounts of flesh measured and in the area chosen to be measured, and because fat is not always evenly distributed over the body. But if done properly at several locations on the body, a good estimate of excess body fat can be made. For precise measurement of body fat, the person can be submerged in water and weighed, but few doctors have such equipment. Use of radioactive labels to measure lean body mass (muscle mass) can also be used.

Obesity can be classified into two types. Early-onset obesity starts with the young child. Only a few extra pounds are gained every year but by the teenage years a person could weigh over 200 pounds. The heaviest person ever recorded was Robert Earl Hughes who weighed almost 400 pounds when he was 10 years old, and 700 pounds at the age of 18. He continued to gain weight until he reached 1,069 pounds at age 32, when he died of kidney complications that were directly related to his obesity (*Guinness Book of World Records*, 1972). Fortunately most people do not gain even one-third this much weight. With most people, childhood-onset obesity gains of this type are not common. Weight gain may only be two to five pounds extra per year, but in 20 years this can result in up to 100 pounds overweight. It should be recognized that this weight gain is due to only about 50 extra calories a day, which could be less than a 5% extra calorie consumption per day. This type of obesity occurs among an estimated 5–10% of all teenagers. It has also been estimated that 25% of all obese adults were obese as children or teenagers.

The other major type of obesity is maturity-onset obesity. This usually begins at 20 to 30 years of age and can result with as little as a gain of about five pounds per year. In 10 years a person can be 50 pounds overweight by consuming only an extra 50 calories per day in relation to caloric expenditure. This is equivalent to about one half of a banana or one oatmeal raisin cookie a day. Usually we don't notice this happening because it goes so slowly and we are not growing as rapidly as in childhood. At this time in life people may exercise less yet keep the same eating habits they had when they were young and growing.

Interestingly, the body changes its composition beyond age 25 to 30. At age 20, men average 15% to 18% fat and women 20% to 23%. The amount of fat then generally increases significantly until age 60. In some cases the fat content may actually double without evidence of obesity.

CAUSES OF OBESITY: ENVIRONMENTAL AND SOCIAL FACTORS

The previous section states that the basic cause of obesity is an intake of more calories than are expended. In the majority of cases of obesity, overconsumption is a result of a number of environmental and social factors.

Eating pressures start as early as infancy. When a child is born, two questions are asked: Is it a boy or girl? How big is it? Bigness is better according to many, so the baby may be encouraged to overeat. The grandmother worries about the new mother not feeding the baby enough, if the baby is being bottle-fed. The baby is introduced to the first "food club," called the "empty bottle club." The baby is coaxed to finish up every bit of liquid in the bottle. If he or she doesn't, there must be something wrong. This then translates later on in childhood to the "clean plate club." This attitude may force young children to eat more than is needed because it supposedly is good for them. If this does not work, the child is told that leaving food is bad because so many people in Asia, Africa, and so on haven't enough food and would love to eat leftovers. If the child doesn't like to join the "clean plate club," he or she is then transferred to the "just desserts club." This means that if the children finish all their food, they are treated to a dessert that is often high in calories. These extra calories are probably not needed, but they taste so good that they are eaten.

Some researchers believe that eating patterns in infant and child feeding can lay down the foundations for future obesity. Studies with young rats suggest that excess calories in the diet may cause extra fat cells to be formed, which may then lead to overweight in later life. These studies have been difficult to perform experimentally in humans but they have been partially verified. The implications of excess food consumption in early life for adult health cannot be ignored.

Overconsumption at an early age sets the pattern for the rest of life with food as a means of rewards, socializing, and winning favors. Television constantly stresses foods and snacks to children and adults, many times without reference to balanced diets. Children spend many hours in front of the TV set being bombarded by these food advertisements and food reward situations. This imprints the use of food firmly in their minds.

If the child manages to make it through high school or college without becoming overweight, the environmental food game is not over. Money becomes more available as a job is taken. Food rewards during dating become an important part of male/female interaction. After graduating and taking a permanent job, less energy expenditure is usually needed as the pace of childhood and adolescence is left behind. In addition, the BMR drops slowly, so caloric needs are decreased. The new family enters the evening prepared for constant snacking in front of the TV. It is amazing that no more than 20% to 30% of us are obese.

The environment is even more difficult for the child of a fat family: 75% of obese children have obese parents, and 80% of obese children will be obese adults. Pregnancy can also be a problem because many women find it difficult to lose the weight they gain during this period.

Another important environmental factor is the availability of food. If food is readily available, the likelihood that "calories in" will be more than "calories out" is very great. The high standard of living in this country and in Western Europe has resulted in a great availability of food, which in turn can lead to a high incidence of obesity. Obesity is clearly not a major factor in African, Asian and many South American countries, where the food supply is at a bare minimum.

Food availability is also used to show hospitality. The extent of one's hospitality or friendship is frequently determined by the quantity and quality of the food served. Food serves essentially as a status symbol. If one wants to make friends feel welcome in the home, food is served. We have become accustomed to socializing over dinner. This is especially true around holidays when many cultural or special religious foods are served.

Lastly, the environmental factors of convenience and comfort of our surroundings contribute to obesity. We drive cars instead of walking, take elevators instead of climbing the stairs, use a snow-blower instead of a shovel, and sit in front of the TV all night instead of participating in some form of physical recreation. Advertising stresses that this device or that is easy to use and requires no effort. Our total environment stresses the ease of doing things.

On the whole, many environmental and social factors stress food and eating. Unless we control intake or increase energy expenditure under the onslaught of these factors, obesity will result.

CAUSES OF OBESITY: PHYSIOLOGICAL FACTORS

The genetic or biochemical factors that result in obesity in some people and not in others are complex and poorly understood. The basal metabolic rate of obese people can be lower than that of non-obese persons. Therefore, for equivalent caloric intake and energy expenditure, an obese person can gain more in weight than does a person with a higher basal metabolic rate.

A non-obese person generally produces more heat from a meal than does an obese one. Why this occurs is unclear, but it makes it more difficult for some of the obese to lose weight. This excess heat production suggests that the non-obese are actually less efficient than the obese in utilizing energy from food.

A normal person weighing 50 kg. has about 60 days' worth of energy available from fat, whereas the obese person has stored more fat and has a supply that can last much longer. Perhaps the biochemical system is induced to cause this fat deposition to protect the person for future times of starvation. Other obese people have lost their appetite regulation mechanism and respond solely to external factors such as the sight or odor of food, or the stress in their daily life. With loss of appetite regulation, people can actually eat themselves into obesity and a shortened lifespan.

In recent years a considerable amount of research has been performed investigating the body weight set point theory. Essentially, the set point theory suggests that each of us has an internal control mechanism that tells our body what weight it should be. In other words, each of us has a body weight set point. If we are below or above that set point the body strives to push or pull us back to that body weight. The set point can be affected by increasing age, weight suppressant drugs, various body stresses, components of our food supply, etc. For example, cigarettes or coffee may lower our body weight set point and if we give up either or both the body weight set point may increase and we tend to gain weight.

Some researchers feel that obese persons, for one reason or another, have very high body weight set points. Therefore, for those persons, dieting is a continuous downhill battle against the set point. They may lose 20 pounds but quickly gain it back.

BIOCHEMICAL AND METABOLIC CONSEQUENCES

Many different metabolic and biochemical changes take place as one becomes obese. For example, the levels of both cholesterol and fats increase in the blood. This could increase the incidence of atherosclerosis and heart disease.

There is also a larger prevalence of diabetes in the obese. For example, the population that is 30% overweight has about three times more adult-onset diabetes than does the normal-weight population. Many obese people become insulin-resistant. This means that the body's cells cannot take up glucose in the presence of insulin as easily as before. The pancreas, to overcome this resistance, increases the number of insulin-producing cells, which are known as the Beta cells of the Islets of Langerhans. This process is known as hyperplasia. A person who is 30% overweight has increased blood insulin levels as well as increased blood glucose levels.

TABLE 12.1 Effect of overweight on mortality

Percentage over normal weight	Increase in death rate compared to normal-weight population
10%	10–15%
20%	20–25%
30%	40–45%
40%	70%

Therefore people in this condition are less glucose-tolerant. This means that after a meal their blood glucose levels rise higher and stay elevated longer than blood glucose levels in a normal person.

Because of their diets, obese people frequently have a greater sodium intake. This fact may explain the high incidence of high blood pressure in obese people. Other adverse effects of obesity many also play a role. In any case, the higher blood pressure causes an increase in stress on the heart.

Obese people, especially women, have a four to five times greater incidence of gallstones and consequently gallbladder operations. This could be due to the greater need of the liver to convert the excess calories to fat. This increases the amount of cholesterol that is excreted in the bile. Excess cholesterol in the bile can crystallize out into gallstones blocking the bile ducts, although the process is not that simple.

Other problems that can occur with obesity include joint deterioration and kidney disease. Obese people find it more difficult to exercise and thus lose muscle tissue. Lack of exercise then promotes more obesity. Lastly, obesity precludes many people from having necessary surgery because it is difficult for the surgeon to work with all the fat that has to be cut through. Table 12.1 shows the dramatic increase in mortality due to overweight that is related to many of the metabolic problems discussed above.

TREATMENT OF OBESITY BY MEANS OTHER THAN DIET

Drugs

Many different drugs have been used to help people lose weight. Some involve hormone therapy. Since most cases of obesity are not due to major alterations in hormone balance, hormone therapy is of limited effectiveness and should be used only under carefully controlled medical supervision.

The most abused drug treatment for obesity has been the use of amphetamines—''speed'' in the street vernacular. These drugs work by suppressing the appetite, perhaps by modifying the body weight set point. Unfortunately, the side effects include nervousness, sleeplessness, and sometimes addiction. By the suppression of eating, the drugs promote the degradation of fat for energy. Since this induces ketosis, another drug, a diuretic, may be given to increase urine output. This also results in loss of body potassium. A drug to retain potassium may then be prescribed. Sometimes all these drugs are combined in one "rainbow" pill. The drugs result in weight loss, but the addiction problem is severe. For the most part, weight loss is largely water loss. Most persons quickly regain their lost weight when drug therapy is terminated.

Clinicians today recognize that they must spend more time in patient counseling rather than in just prescribing diet pills. Unfortunately, diuretics and diet pills are available for over-the-counter purchase. People can easily abuse these pills, especially since many people use them without doctors' advice or care.

Devices
The Food, Drug, and Cosmetic Act of 1938 (the law presently regulating medical devices) does not require proof of the effectiveness of a medical device before it is marketed. The device can be seized only if it is a health hazard. Because of this, newspapers and magazines are full of untested and ineffective devices that are reported to cure obesity by causing rapid weight loss.

Some of these devices are dangerous and have been seized. For example, using tight, whole-body sauna suits can induce bloodclots or cardiac arrest. These devices, as well as sauna belts, are reported to melt away fat. However, this is biologically impossible. The rubbing machines advertised in many health spas do not rub away fat as many think. Several books discuss how to get rid of cellulite, a supposedly special fat. In reality, these are just fat cells that have undergone hypertrophy due to overeating. Exercise and reduction of caloric intake are appropriate approaches to minimizing the so-called cellulite problem. The machines help somewhat by encouraging people to do something besides just sitting in front of a TV set.

Daily use of exercise machines increases caloric expenditure and can account for some weight loss. Unfortunately, advertisements for exercise machines, such as pedal devices, usually advertise rapid weight loss. This is impossible unless a strict low-calorie diet is followed. This diet is usually advertised in fine print at the end of the advertisement or in the printed matter a person receives. The major part of weight loss under this regime is water. However, since much weight gain is due to 50–100 extra Calories a day, a 10 to 15 minute interlude with a pedal bike at moderate speed would help reduce weight very slowly over a long period of time or at least prevent weight gain. This slow loss is probably the best way to minimize harmful effects to the body.

Surgery

Many different surgical procedures have been tried as methods of treating obesity. For example, some people have tried having their jaws surgically wired so they could not eat. All foods must be ground up in a blender and drunk through a straw. There are several instances of people who still gained weight with this method because they continued to overconsume, but this time through the straw.

In the mid 1970s intestinal bypass operations were performed to help massively obese people lose weight. In these operations, a portion of the small intestine was surgically bypassed with a shunt operation. The theory was that if the total absorptive area of the small intestine was reduced by the bypass, the obese person would not have to change eating habits because the food calories would be poorly absorbed and weight loss would occur. After about 10,000 operations in the U.S., it became clear that numerous physiological and nutritional problems developed some time after the operation. Vitamin deficiencies, mineral imbalances, and liver and kidney problems have not been uncommon. This type of operation is rarely performed today for treatment of obesity because of the serious nature of the side effects.

A type of surgery that is popular today is stomach stapling. In this procedure staples are used to reduce the stomach size to a very small pouch. Food entering the stomach from the esophagus quickly fills this pouch since it only holds about two ounces of food. Therefore, the person is severely restricted in the amount of food eaten at a sitting, and weight loss results. Unfortunately, the pouch will expand over time, so an obese person may initially lose weight, but can begin to regain weight if he or she overeats.

TREATMENT OF OBESITY BY FAD DIETS

In this country, fad dieting is the most common method used to lose weight. Dieting by various means is nothing new; it came of age in the 1920s. With the advent of movies, everyone wanted to look like the new Hollywood stars. The first major popular diet was the "Hollywood 18-Day" diet. It was based on eating only lamb chops and grapefruit for eighteen days. Not only was it boring, but it was nutritionally unbalanced. If people followed it they usually ate less and suffered ketosis, so rapid weight loss occurred initially due to water loss, but permanent weight change was most often not achieved.

Other fad diets have similar restrictions and promises. They are usually boring but promise rapid weight loss. Because people want to lose quickly, however, they religiously follow these diets for a while. Another point is that most fad diets suggest that you can eat all you want and still not gain weight. Since calories expended must exceed intake, this is obviously possible only if you decide to increase work and exercise activity.

Many people are also struck with the "Aunt Sophie's Daughter's Wedding Syndrome." This usually occurs about two weeks before a special event such as a wedding, when people suddenly realize that they are overweight. They want to lose 20 to 30 pounds to get into better-looking clothes, and they want to do it quickly. This can be done on a fad or starvation diet but weight loss is usually water. This rapid change can damage the body, especially since the weight is gained back even faster after the party or event.

Every week there seems to be a new crash or fad diet. You cannot walk past a newsstand or a checkout counter at a supermarket without seeing a newly discovered weight-loss program splashed across the cover of a paper or magazine.

There is no way that a textbook of this type can keep up with the latest weight-loss craze or evaluate all the types of weight loss clinic plans. Below are discussed a few of the popular fad diets. More will surface before the printing ink on this page has dried. A good rule of thumb is that major promises of weight loss—if they work—are only water losses. A true weight loss program should aim at a loss of only two to three pounds per week. Most likely a plan that is supervised by a dietitian in a hospital will be within the logical realm of safety and effectiveness.

Low-Carbohydrate Diets

There are many examples of the low-carbohydrate diet as popularized by Dr. Irwin Stillman in the 1970s. A low-carbohydrate regimen was first published as a diet by Banting in 1853. Dr. Stillman's diet suggests that you can eat all you want as long as you avoid carbohydrates. This is typical of the fad diet claim. Eating a low-carbohydrate diet in most cases means that you are consuming a high-fat diet. Since fat has a greater satiation factor, people will actually consume less food. A low-carbohydrate diet induces ketosis. Ketones in the blood also tend to reduce hunger and may result in lower food intake. Stillman recommended consumption of 8–10 glasses of water a day to dilute and wash out the ketone bodies through the urine.

Unfortunately, a low-carbohydrate diet is usually also low in vitamins A and C and in calcium so that a nutrient supplement should be provided. A loss of five to seven pounds occurs in the first three to four days, which seems miraculous to the average person. This is actually due to the effect of glycogen depletion and a shift to fat metabolism. One low-carbohydrate diet was said to result in a 25-pound weight loss in one week. To lose this much as fat tissue, a moderately active person normally consuming 2,000 to 3,000 Calories per day would have to avoid all food completely and exercise to burn eight Calories per minute continuously. This means the person would need to run rapidly for seven days straight without stopping. Large weight changes occur with a low-carbohy-drate diet because of the water loss and the satiation factor of the fat consumption; even so, 25 pounds of fat loss is impossible. Dr. Stillman also stated that his special diets could remove fat from particular zones of the body. This, unfortunately, is not true. There are no diets that can remove fat from a particular place. Exercise, however, can strengthen muscles such as those of the stomach to hold the fat in. Stillman also published other diets that are high in carbohydrates but low in fats and claimed that these are the only kind of diets that would work. It is interesting that he created his own paradox in suggesting exactly opposite types of diet.

The famous Scarsdale diet was also a low carbohydrate diet and thus was similar to the Stillman diet. This diet, like the Stillman diet or any low-carbohydrate diet, is dangerous to use without medical supervision.

Ketosis Diets

Since diets need gimmicks, a physician by the name of Dr. Robert Atkins, author of the best seller *Dr. Atkins' Diet Revolution,* intro-duced a diet gimmick that used the ketosis that occurs in low-carbo-hydrate diets to an advantage. Instead of recommending that diet-ers drink all the water prescribed to dilute the ketones produced by fat metabolism, Dr. Atkins suggested that ketosis is good and should be encouraged. Dieters are requested to buy ketone test strips used by diabetics. These strips can be used to check their urine; if the strip turns purple, they are in the state of ketosis, which is supposed to be beneficial since they are using fat to supply energy. This diet has many hazards and the American Medical Association and Ameri-can Heart Association have condemned it. Continued use can lead to nausea, increased blood lipids and cholesterol levels caused by high fat consumption, cardiac irregularities, fatigue, gout, and osteo-porosis.

The Beverly Hills Diet, Fruit Diets

The popular Beverly Hills Diet created by Judy Mazel is a good example of a poorly balanced fad diet. The author is neither a physician nor a nutritionist; her training was primarily in dramat-ics. For the first 11 days on this diet one eats nothing but fruit. The scientific merit of this diet was rigorously challenged in the *Journal of the American Medical Association.* Drs. Mirkin and Shore of the University of Maryland wrote *JAMA* on the potential hazards of the diet. They noted that hazards included severe diarrhea, potassium deficiency, and arrhythmia of the heart. The diet should be avoided.

Protein-Sparing Diet Plans

The Cambridge diet plan as well as many other plans provided by some weight loss clinics provides a total diet supplement or formula in powder form. One serving of powder in nine ounces of water taken three times a day generally provides 330 Calories daily, which is an extremely low calorie intake. The formula provides 44 g. of carbohydrate, 33 g. of high-grade complete protein, 3 g. of fat plus 100% of the USRDA for selected vitamins and minerals daily. The plan, if followed properly, does result in weight loss. The term protein sparing comes from the fact that enough carbohydrate is taken in to prevent muscle tissue from degrading to supply energy. However, the American Dietetic Association and the Food and Drug Administration, among other groups, have warned that diet plans like the Cambridge diet are not a common-sense approach to weight loss and should not be undertaken without strict monitoring by a medical professional. Although the label on the formula does advise that one should consult a physician before starting the Cambridge diet, few dieters actually do so.

Several deaths have been attributed to some protein-sparing diet plans, probably due to a minimal potassium intake. In fact, the FDA has proposed warning labels for any diet plan under 800 Calories a day. These deaths occurred with liquid products that were consumed as the only source of nourishment. The liquid protein was often a hydrolized collagen product with added vitamins, minerals, and flavorings. Daily intakes of about 300 Calories were usual on this diet. This diet resulted in large weight loss in obese people. Unfortunately, after several months on this totally imbalanced diet, many people experienced arrhythmias of the heart and some had heart failure, even when under a doctor's care.

We should learn a lesson from the liquid protein diet fad. Severe restriction of calories and dependence upon one or just a few ingredients in the diet during dieting is asking for severe metabolic problems.

Cider Vinegar/Lecithin/B_6/Kelp Diet

This diet has absolutely no scientific basis. In fact, it is not a diet at all, but a supplement containing four ingredients that are supposed to melt away fat. Vinegar is included because it has been used for centuries for all kinds of maladies. Lecithin is claimed to be able to melt away the fat and then carry it out of the body. Lecithin is indeed involved in fat metabolism as a phospholipid, but it cannot carry fat out into the urine. Fat only appears in the urine if the kidneys are severely damaged. Lecithin is an emulsifying agent used by the food industry. Vitamin B_6 is claimed to be able to stimulate the liver to burn fat. But the large excess consumed is probably excreted in the urine and does nothing to burn more fat. The kelp is high in iodine, which is claimed to stimulate the thyroid. But we usually get enough iodine in our diet; in fact, excess can be dangerous.

Other Fad Diets

There are many other diets that supposedly have similar magical powers for removing fat rapidly. The Mayo Diet, which has nothing to do with the Mayo Clinic in Minnesota, calls for eating a grapefruit before each meal. It is claimed that a grapefruit contains special enzymes that are absorbed into the body and that help dissolve fat cells. There is no scientific basis for this theory because any enzyme would be digested in the intestinal tract just like a protein. The grapefruit taste probably reduces the appetite so less food is eaten.

The "Calories Don't Count Diet" is similar to the Mayo Diet. A few tablespoons of oil are supposed to be eaten before a meal. This suppresses the appetite. Other unrecommended popular diets include the Air Force Diet (similar to Stillman's), the Stewardess Diet (first day seven eggs; next day seven hot dogs; next day seven bananas; repeat), The United States Ski Team Diet (high in eggs and meat), and the Drinking Man's Diet (low carbohydrate but includes alcohol). Finally, "Starch Blockers" should be mentioned. These are compounds extracted from beans that supposedly inhibit the intestinal amylases from breaking down starch. Thus, you could literally eat all the carbohydrates you want and not absorb calories. Several reports published in scientific journals have stated that starch blockers had no effect for humans. Moreover, severe medical problems in some people were attributed to use of starch blockers. They were the result of intestinal problems and some toxic reactions from other naturally occurring components in the pills that caused adverse effects on the pancreas. In 1982–1984 the FDA made a major effort to remove starch blockers from the market as an unapproved drug.

OBESITY TREATMENT BY STARVATION

Some popular magazines and some weight loss clinics have promoted starvation as a means of weight loss. However, the consequences can be very severe. Starvation initially causes euphoria due to the effects of the ketones on the brain. This makes the person happy and pleased with the initial losses, which, as we saw earlier, are due to water loss and glycogen depletion.

Prolonged starvation can result in renal impairment, hair loss, brain and nerve damage, weakness, and death. Starvation should be carried out only in a hospital but, even there, 500 to 800 Calories are usually given daily to prevent undesirable side effects. Glucose, for example, is supplied as an energy source and vitamins are given daily. Weight reduction clinics that use total starvation and claim 20- to 30-pound losses in a few weeks may be doing damage to the persons involved. In addition, scientific evidence shows that although some of the weight loss is water, only 30% to 35% comes from the fat deposits. The rest is from lean body mass, which means that the muscles can atrophy. Controlled hospital starvation diets limit weight reduction to two to three pounds per week and are used only on the severely obese, not on the 20 pound-overweight adult.

A GOOD WEIGHT–REDUCTION PLAN

To lose weight, the primary principles are to reduce caloric intake, increase caloric expenditure, or preferably do both. It is also important to consume a balanced diet to assure adequate micronutrient intake. In addition, in order to keep weight off, we should learn new eating habits. Based on knowledge gained from their studies, several psychologists feel that the latter is the most important factor for weight loss. They feel that many people are overstimulated by the food environment, which causes their overeating and that by controlling the environment and changing behavior, people can lose weight and keep it off. The techniques will be briefly discussed in the next section, but are pointed out here because maintenance of the new desired weight is difficult. Thus, a good weight-reduction program should teach new eating habits.

To lose weight the following factors should be used in the diet program:

1. The caloric intake should be between 800 and 1,200 Calories per day. Keep a daily diet diary to monitor all food consumed. An organization that supplies a computer analysis of the diet would be very helpful; the appendix in this book can also be used. A physician's help should be sought before attempting any regimen.

2. The diet must be pleasing and appetizing enough to satisfy desires. Diet plan type foods help if supplemented by other foods. Today a wide variety of reduced and low-calorie substitute foods and whole meals are readily available from a supermarket. One should make a list of them and use it to plan a diet.

3. The diet should be adequate in all nutrients but low in calories. It should emphasize nutrient-dense foods, that is, foods with a high concentration of nutrients per Calorie. Whole-grain cereals and green leafy vegetables are examples. So-called junk food such as potato chips or pretzels are generally low in nutrient density. By law, reduced or low-calorie foods now must be fortified to the level of the food they replace except for calories. This makes dieting much safer through easy choice of already prepared and processed foods (e.g., low-cal dressings, syrups, jam, lite beer). There are also available whole frozen meals controlled to about 300–400 Calories.

4. Three or more meals should be eaten per day. This helps maintain lower cholesterol levels because fat deposition is not induced by the body thinking it is going to be starved. Some studies suggest that faster and easier weight reduction can be accomplished if the same number of calories are spread out over the day rather than eaten in one meal. This also results in a better glucose tolerance.

5. The diet must be easily adaptable and use available foods.

6. It must be able to be used for a long time so desired weight loss can be attained.

7. Maximum weight loss should not be more than two to three pounds per week.

8. Exercise helps, even if it is only 50 extra Calories expended per day. There is some evidence that increased exercise will actually increase the BMR so there may be an additional advantage. It may also help to reduce the set point.

9. The diet should teach new eating habits. This can be accomplished in many ways. For example, one can learn to omit small portions of normally consumed foods. A good way to do this is to record all food consumed over a two-week period. Then, over a period of several months, a portion of a regularly consumed food is cut out. For instance, the third cup of morning coffee with sugar, a second helping of meat entree, or the third evening beer. These "littles" can amount to a large weight loss if caloric expenditure remains the same and no other food is substituted. One half-slice of toast less daily is a loss of four pounds in a year, while two fewer eggs per week is three pounds. Two fewer beers per week is equivalent to 20 pounds, while one less cup of coffee with sugar is two fewer pounds. All these "littles" together have the potential to amount to 30 or so fewer pounds, which would be a highly desirable weight loss for one year. It requires the right attitude and the knowledge of the caloric values of the foods consumed on a regular basis.

Another way to learn new habits is to go on an on/off diet. One day is the low-calorie day, the next is the day for you to eat at the caloric intake level calculated for your eventual desired weight and lifestyle. This is harder to do, but highly effective.

A simple but very difficult new eating habit is to avoid snacking entirely. This helps reduce calories but is impossible for many to follow. If snacks have to be used, a more lasting snack should be substituted for one that can be eaten quickly. For example, about 60 pretzel sticks have the same calories as one large pretzel. Snacking on fruit or vegetables (carrot sticks) or popcorn can reduce caloric intake when eaten instead of the usual high-calorie snacks.

10. The diet should be one that the entire family can help the person with.

BEHAVIOR MODIFICATION AND DIETING

Help in making behavioral changes is a necessary prerequisite to achieving desired weight loss and maintaining the loss. Most obese people will not stay on a diet very long. Of those who do, very few lose weight because they find it hard not to cheat or do not even realize they are cheating. Most of the people who lose weight will regain it. Most of us know of people who have lost 200 pounds over the last couple of years—20 pounds 10 times—yet regain them right back.

Many organizations have been formed to help people achieve their weight losses. Unfortunately, the results are not always as remarkable as may be claimed in advertisements. Some groups are far more successful than others. However, results show that only about 10% to 15% of the people joining in the purely social weight groups actually effect a sustained weight loss. Other groups that use behavior modification are more successful, but few statistics are available to determine the success rate five or more years later. Before joining any group, it might be advisable to ask for a documentation of their success rate.

Behavior modification is essentially based on change of the environment because many obese people respond to food differently than normal-weight people. The obese are more subject to smell, taste, and sight of food so control is needed. Controls involve elimination responses, suppression responses, and strengthening.

Elimination steps include the following:

1. Always eat in one place in the house or at work.

2. Don't do anything else when you are eating (never eat while watching TV, for example).

3. Don't buy problem foods.

4. Use a list when shopping.

5. Don't shop before dinner.

6. Don't put food bowls on the table.

7. Don't serve desserts.

8. Minimize eating out.

9. Cover all foods or place in opaque containers.

Suppression steps include the following:

1. Count mouthfuls when eating.

2. Use utensils for all eating.

3. Place the utensil down between each mouthful and completely chew the food.

4. Use smaller plates to make the food look bigger.

5. Record behavior as to why an eating episode occurred.

6. Don't skip meals; plan them.

7. Have low-calorie foods available, such as celery and carrots.

Strengthening steps include:

1. Provide a wide variety of foods.

2. Make foods more attractive by proper use of spices.

3. Save foods from meals for snacks.

4. Have a person help with and monitor your changes.

5. Learn something about nutrition.

There are many hospital groups that have used behavior modification techniques to achieve weight loss for very obese people. The results to date have been very encouraging.

ANOREXIA NERVOSA AND BULIMIA

The thin image projected in fashion magazines, on television, on the stage, and in films has probably increased the incidence of anorexia nervosa and bulimia. These are serious eating disorders that are seen primarily in teenage and young women who have a great fear of losing control of eating and getting fat.

Anorexia nervosa is estimated to occur in about 1 of every 200 high-school or college-age women. It is quite serious and can result in death of close to 10% of those who have the condition. Persons with anorexia deny themselves food, sometimes consuming less than 300 calories daily. They lose so much weight that a life-threatening situation develops and they need intravenous feeding. Anorexics rarely recognize the severity of their eating problems. Although they may be 25% or more below their ideal body weight, they will still insist that they are fat. Friends or relatives can provide lifesaving assistance by insisting that an anorexic seek counseling. Bulimia, a binge/purge eating disorder, is thought to be far more prevalent than anorexia nervosa, especially on college campuses. People with bulimia may consume 4,000 or more Calories at a sitting and then either vomit or use laxatives to purge the food out of the body. Treatment of these eating disorders requires simultaneous psychological and nutritional counseling in addition to hospitalization if the body weight is too low.

Although these eating disorders are not as prevalent as obesity in our population, they can be more dangerous. We must be careful how we approach obese patients with discussions of weight reduction. We do not want to solve one problem and create another by causing them to become bulimic or anorexic.

SUMMARY

In the United States, obesity and overweight are widespread overnutrition problems that can have serious health effects. This chapter has tried to explain some of the problems of weight control. By following the simple steps outlined and by learning good nutrition habits, one should be able to lose weight and keep it off. The major steps in losing weight are a reduction in caloric intake and an increase in caloric expenditure. This method works whether the overweight problem is due to maturity-onset or childhood obesity. Control of environmental factors through behavior modification techniques may also be of benefit. One should not follow fad diets or rely upon the use of drugs or diet foods. One must learn to develop new and better eating habits so as to improve health and maintain optimal weight.

Multiple Choice Study Questions

1. Childhood-onset obesity
   A. represents hypertrophic obesity only
   B. represents the plastic growth in size of adipocytes
   C. is initiated by overfeeding of infants that results in hypertrophy of fat cells

    D. is usually less severe than adult onset obesity

    E. results from hyperplasia of adipocytes from overfeeding during the first three years of life and includes hypertrophy of fat cells as part of the problem

2. To lose one pound of body tissue requires

    A. the burning of 4,000 calories

    B. three hours of vigorous exercise

    C. the burning of 3,500 calories

    D. special dietary foods

3. The percentage of the U.S. population that can be classified as obese is

    A. 5–10%

    B. 10–15%

    C. 20–30%

    D. 40–50%

    E. over 70%

4. Obesity is not generally caused by

    A. a glandular problem

    B. a change in BMR

    C. overeating

    D. high caloric intake

    E. underexpenditure of energy

5. Which disease is not known to be associated with obesity?

    A. CHD

    B. gallstones

    C. diabetes

    D. celiac disease

    E. kidney disease

6. People on starvation diets and diabetics have a common problem of

    A. high blood insulin

    B. depressed blood glucose

    C. ketosis

    D. high glucose in urine

    E. low BMR

7. Which reducing diet creates the dangerous state of ketosis?

    A. grapefruit diet

    B. Atkins diet

    C. Stillman diet

    D. Air Force diet

8. Obese people who want to reduce properly should

    A. reduce fat intake to a level equivalent to 1,000 calories/day

    B. reduce all calories to a level equivalent to 500 calories/day

    C. reduce calories to about 1,000 but maintain all other nutrients at a normal level

    D. remove all fat from the diet

    E. remove as many carbohydrates as possible from the diet

Essay Study Questions

1. What is the basic cause of obesity and how prevalent is it?

2. How is obesity diagnosed?

3. What is the difference between early-onset and maturity-onset obesity?

4. What environmental factors contribute to obesity?

5. Describe and discuss two popular dieting regimens that violate the rules of a sound diet program.

6. What adverse health consequences may occur if one is obese?

7. List at least nine rules to follow in a sound weight-reduction program.

8. How is behavior modification used in treatment of obesity?

9. What are the positive and negative effects of using drugs in obesity treatment?

10. What are starch blockers?

Things to Do

1. Collect advertisements for various weight-reducing schemes, diets, and devices. Discuss the relative merit of each one.

2. Try to develop a 1,000-Calorie diet plan using the guidelines of Chapter 12. Does it meet the Basic Four? Calculate the percentage of RDAs for several vitamins and minerals.

3. Discuss with various people the dieting schemes they have used. Were they using good dietary guidelines?

4. Examine the types of foods available in the supermarket for dieting. Discuss their composition and use in a diet plan.

5. Try to examine your behavior and feelings when eating. Make a list as follows:

Time	Food Eaten	Amount Eaten	Place Where Eaten	Hunger Level	Anxiety Level
—	—	—	—	—	—
—	—	—	—	—	—
—	—	—	—	—	—

Rate "hunger level" on a scale of 1 to 5 where 1 = no hunger and 5 = very hungry.

Rate your "anxiety level" on a scale of 1 to 5 with 5 being the highest.

Chapter 12. Answers to Multiple-Choice Study Questions: 1, C; 2, C; 3, C; 4, A; 5, D; 6, C; 7, B; 8, C.

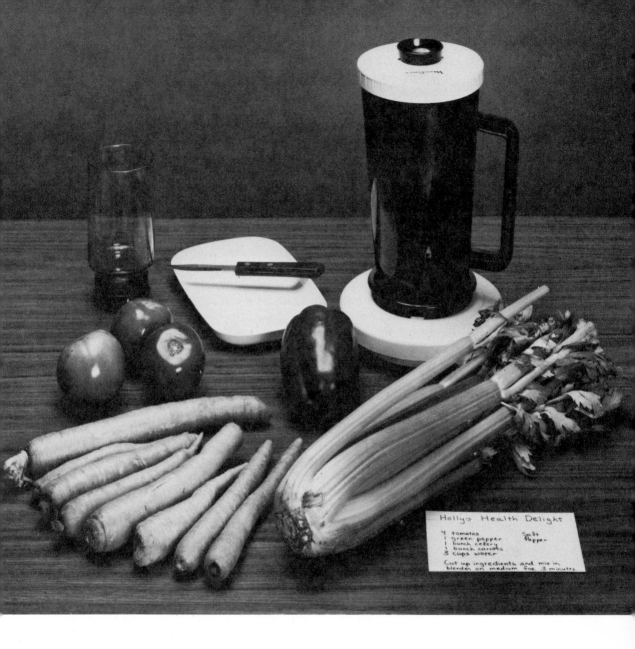

Holly's Health Delight

4 tomatos
1 green pepper
1 bunch celery
1 bunch carrots
3 cups water
Salt
Pepper

Cut up ingredients and mix in
blender on medium for 3 minutes

NUTRITIONAL IMPLICATIONS OF CURRENT DIETARY TRENDS: WE'VE COME A LONG WAY, AMERICA

13

For most of the existence of our human race on earth the major food concern has been to get enough to eat. In many parts of the world this is still an overriding daily drive.

Americans enjoy the most varied and bountiful diet in the world. We spend less than 20% of our income for our food supply. Most of us overconsume rather than underconsume. Achieving nutritional quality and balance of the foods we consume is now a major goal rather than just finding enough food to eat.

The average live expectancy for infants born in 1983 is 73 years. This is a remarkable increase from a life expectancy of 46 years at the turn of the century. Indeed, we have come a long way. Health care and the eradication of numerous acute childhood diseases have played a major role in the increase in life expectancy. Diet has also added to our longevity.

Should we be complacent with our progress and assume our goals have been reached? No! Especially not when 30% of Americans are obese; not when many people consume unbalanced diets; and not when diet is linked to numerous chronic and life-threatening diseases. We should, however, be quite proud of our progress. We should also avoid the monthly "panic" as the newspapers announce the latest link of some item in our diet to heart disease or cancer.

We need to put diet in perspective. Diet is one component of healthfulness. It is an important one and we must urge people to follow a balanced approach to diet. However, even an ideal diet will not guarantee optimal health.

Since the major source of malnutrition in the U.S. is overconsumption of calories, more effort must be directed towards balancing calories in (food) with calories out (exercise). Rapid weight-reduction diets must be avoided as they rarely result in permanent weight loss. These fad diets do not train a person to eat properly.

Eating should be an enjoyable part of our life, and it can be enjoyable without leading to overconsumption of calories—if it is approached properly. We should not feel guilty for eating certain foods that are low in nutrient density. These are foods that generally have high caloric value with little else in vitamins or minerals—snack or "fun" foods. There is room in diets for "fun" foods as long as efforts are made to include foods high in nutrient value along with those "fun" foods. Calories are of concern with these foods, but can be accommodated with proper menu planning. Snacking need not be a guilt trip, especially with proper choice of type and amount of a snack. As others have said, there is no such thing as a junk food, only a junk food diet. It's a matter of evaluating the entire food-intake pattern, not just of evaluating one can of cola or one bag of chips.

**CURRENT
TRENDS
(FADS) IN THE
U.S. DIET**

What are some of the trends in our food patterns, and are they for better or worse? Many of the trends and their potential impacts have been discussed in previous chapters. Below is a summary of some changes evident in our eating patterns. Some trends or fads may only be short lived, while others will be or have been of longer duration.

Nutrient Profile of General Diets

Total dietary consumption of fat, cholesterol, and sodium appears to be on the decline. Most professional and government groups that have issued dietary goals have urged Americans to reduce their consumption of these components of the food supply. Fiber consumption by Americans has been very low for several decades. In the last few years, Americans have become more aware of the health aspects of fiber and many have increased intake of foods (whole-grain cereals, vegetables, and fruits) containing fiber. Prudent diets should contain some foods high in fiber.

During this century intake of foods high in complex carbohydrates (and fiber) decreased markedly while consumption of simple sugars increased. A tendency to reverse this trend has become evident beginning in the late 1970s. Alcohol intake, which often has an adverse impact on health, is quite high for many Americans.

The vitamin and mineral content of our food supply has improved over the last few decades. Much of this can be attributed to the selective fortification of foods. This trend will probably increase. Intelligent use of food fortification can be quite beneficial to the population. Over-fortification must be avoided because it can lead to nutrient imbalances or outright toxicity.

Fast Foods and Eating Outside the Home

Since over one-third of our meals are consumed outside the home and about 40% of the food dollar is spent on these meals, their nutritional profile is of great concern (see Chapter 9 and Appendix II). Unfortunately, many fast food meals are high in calories, fat, and sodium. However, proper choice of food at restaurants can add to a good daily meal pattern. More nutrition education is needed to help people make good food choices both inside and outside the home.

Tailored Nutrition Foods

In the future we expect to see more and more foods that are designed for specific age or physiological groups. Today pet owners can purchase one of a series of foods for their dogs depending upon what "cycle" of life the dog is in. Puppy Chow is designed for puppies, etc.

Infant formulas and weaning foods have long been available in the marketplace. Low-calorie, low-fat, low-cholesterol, or low-sodium foods are available for those with weight or heart disease concerns. There is also a whole series of enteral (edible) and parenteral (intravenous) medical foods for persons with unique nutritional requirements. Foods designed specifically for the nutritional needs of elderly persons, pregnant or lactating women, and others are only a step away.

Other Dietary Trends

Vegetarianism Although the practice of vegetarianism involves only about 1 percent of the U.S. population, the trend is increasing, especially among young adults. Vegetarians can be classified as pure (Vegan) vegetarians—those who consume only plant foods, Lacto vegetarians—those who will consume dairy products, and Lacto-ovo vegetarians—those who eat dairy products plus eggs.

Many vegetarians are well educated about foods and nutrition and consume excellent diets. However, others consume diets that are a contradiction to optimal health. Nutritional risks to vegetarians can be overcome with adequate menu planning. The Seventh Day Adventists are a primary religious vegetarian group that has been able to achieve a longer lifespan than most people in this country. Whether this is due to diet or lifestyle is not known.

In comparison, Zen Macrobiotics is an example of a vegetarian diet associated with religious fanaticism. This diet of the counter-culture was quite popular in the early 1970s but has since faded, although Hare Krishnas and other groups sometimes follow it. The diet was designed by George Ohsawa, a Japanese person living in France. The goal of the Zen macrobiotic diet, as emphasized by Ohsawa, is the achievement of an inner peace through dietary practice. He professed that the diet, in conjunction with proper religion, could overcome any illness. His diet is based on the Oriental philosophy of Taoism, which includes the opposing forces of Yin and Yang. The diet has no connection with Zen Buddhism. Ohsawa felt that one's diet had to have a certain ratio of Yin to Yang and he classified various foods on this basis.

The Zen macrobiotic diet consists of ten levels (–3 to 7). The beginning level, –3, is a very well-balanced diet consisting of meats, vegetables, cereals, and so forth. Level 7 was designed to be used only in specific circumstances and consisted solely of cereal grains with very little water intake. Brown rice was the preferred cereal since Ohsawa ranked it as having the best Yin-Yang ratio. Brown rice lacks vitamin C and is low in protein content and protein quality. Unfortunately, many of those who follow the diet have abused this concept and profess that brown rice should be the only thing to be consumed all the time. This has resulted in some deaths and in the severe physical and mental retardation of some children. The *Journal of the American Medical Association* has also reported 20 cases of death due to pneumonia that resulted from the poor nutritional status and lower resistance to infection of the people on this regimen.

The Zen macrobiotic diet and philosophy is supposed to cure all diseases. If it fails to do so, Ohsawa stated that this was because there was not enough faith among the practitioners or because the person had not practiced the diet long enough. It is not the purpose of this book to criticize the religion per se but only to educate against the health hazards involved in a diet that does not supply the body with adequate nutrients.

Natural and Organic Foods Most foods are organic from a chemical standpoint since foods are basically composed of carbon, hydrogen, oxygen, and nitrogen, unless we consider the minerals, such as salt, which are a minor dietary component. "Organic" or "natural foods" are foods that are minimally processed or that have not been processed at all. In many cases, due to the lack of processing, organic foods may have a much shorter shelf-life than similar foods that are processed. The quality of organic foods may be worse, as good as, or better than other foods. Organic fruits and vegetables are those that are grown on soil that has not been chemically fertilized. They also must not have been sprayed with pesticides. The Organic Growers and Buyers Association (OGBA) investigates and certifies farmers and their produce if strict organic procedures are followed. Some Food and Drug Administration (FDA) investigations, however, have revealed that in some cases there are as many pesticides, or even higher levels of pesticides, on organic foods as there are on regular foods. This has probably been due to dishonesty among merchants of organic foods, who sell regular produce as organic. In addition, it is very hard to keep pesticides off crops if a neighboring crop has been sprayed or if the soil was previously used in normal production. The organic and natural food business has had a great growth rate in the '70s and '80s, expanding almost every year. Advertising and the media have turned some people off the supermarket-style food supply. There has also been an expanding interest in natural home-grown foods and, in some cases, in organizing food cooperatives to purchase and process foods in quantity so as to eliminate the cost of the normal distribution and food marketing system.

The ecology and antipollution movement has also increased the resistance to processed foods. People feel that the food supply is polluted with unnatural and poisonous additives. James Turner, author of *The Chemical Feast,* stated a similar idea in his book, which was inspired by Rachel Carson's *The Silent Spring.* Many consumers feel that the FDA is not doing an adequate job and that millions of Americans are being poisoned.

Some people join the organic food movement in a search for magic or miracle food cures. Many gullible people are fed information by quacks and unknowledgeable food faddists who take existing nutrition facts and bend them to suit their own selfish needs. In the 1500s and 1600s, country doctors had magic cures that greatly resemble many of the diets and dietary prescriptions advocated today by so-called nutrition experts. For example, vitamins from natural sources are extolled as being superior, yet there is no difference between synthetic and natural vitamins since they are the same chemical. The only difference may be the higher price paid for the natural variety. The use of an extract from apricot kernels to cure cancer has also been passed on to gullible people. The kernels contain a dangerous chemical that is converted into hydrogen cyanide in the body. Some children have died from overeating these kernels. In Mexico and Canada clinics treating people with this same chemical, in the form of a drug called Laetrile, are doing a medical disservice. Some persons have even called Laetrile vitamin B_{17}. To suggest that this substance is a vitamin is ludicrous and dishonest.

Health-Food Stores Most health food stores, especially those in shopping centers, are generally similar to supermarkets in that foods are well labeled and very commercial in appearance. The stores usually cater to those who are looking for special foods to cure or prevent some ailment. The main problem is that many stores also sell books that make health claims for various nutrient and non-nutrient supplements. Most of the claims are anecdotal—for example, my aunt cured her skin condition with product X. Few claims are based on scientific experiments. Therefore, the advice given is often not proven or factual. The most common cure prescribed is some type of vitamin taken in large doses. As pointed out earlier, this is either wasteful or dangerous. Prices for these vitamins (from natural sources) are usually several times higher than for a comparable vitamin at a department store. Protein tablets that are sold in some places are often nothing but compressed dry milk costing 50 to 100 times as much as a box of nonfat dry milk (instant powdered milk) from a supermarket. Other protein supplements are dried waste products from cattle slaughter houses such as organ meats, connective tissue, and skin.

The customer should be wary of fad products that are associated with amazing "cures." Millions of dollars are spent yearly on lecithin, kelp, bee pollen, and other such products. Scientific research cannot keep up with the claims made for these products. Government regulatory agencies do not have the staff, finances, or legislative power to monitor the safety or validity of the numerous "health-food" products.

Starch blockers were marketed simultaneously across the U.S. in the spring of 1982. No human testing had been done to prove their effectiveness. Millions of pills were sold before three separate groups of scientists showed in published research papers the complete lack of effect of starch blockers in reducing starch digestion in humans. In the spring of 1983, many stores were still selling the pills although the FDA had banned their sale. The FDA has been sued by several groups for banning the sale of starch blockers. Numerous other products are and will be sold to gullible people. Let the buyer beware. The reader is directed to *Nutrition Cultism: Facts and Fictions* by Dr. Victor Herbert (George F. Stickley Co., 1980) for further discussion.

YOUR NEXT DOOR NEIGHBOR— THE HEALTH EXPERT

Let the buyer also beware of his next-door neighbor. Your neighbor, or a member of your church or bowling team, may be a salesperson for one of those nutrition companies that markets health and beauty products. Your neighbor—the one who gives you good advice on where to plant your flowers—would never lead you astray on nutrition . . . or would they? There are well over one million salespersons of these types of products in the U.S. People may first buy products from someone they trust and then are recruited to sell to their friends. That's all well and good, but remember that these people probably know far less about nutrition than you do (especially if you have retained information from the first 12 chapters). They may believe in their product, but that belief does not mean that the product works or that it is even safe.

Again let the buyer beware. Don't fall for extravagant claims. Demand to see proof that the product actually works. Personal accounts are not adequate. Company claims are not adequate. Publications in peer-reviewed scientific journals are adequate.

SUMMARY

Yes, we have come a long way in this country toward providing the citizens with an opportunity to consume a varied and well-balanced diet. The life expectancy in the U.S. has increased over 35% since the turn of the century. Food availability and the nutritional balance of foods consumed have had an impact on increased lifespan. Educating the consumer about choosing balanced diets has fallen somewhat behind the availability of foods. As a result, overeating is the major food/nutrition problem in the U.S. Recently, Americans seem to be reducing intake of calories, fat, cholesterol, and salt and increasing complex carbohydrate intake. Whether these trends continue may depend, in part, upon our educational efforts.

Natural and organic foods are foods that have been minimally processed. They exist as alternatives for those who do not wish to consume foods that have been processed to a greater extent or that contain additives. In addition, some specific foods are eaten for religious or health-cure reasons. Fast foods are a more and more frequent choice due to our rapid lifestyle. Proper choice of foods in restaurants is important. Some natural-food diets can be dangerous because of imbalanced nutrition. Some nutrient supplements are unnecessary and can be dangerous.

This chapter was written to point out some of the problems with alternatives to a processed food supply. It should be obvious by now that one can be nutritionally adequate with our food supply if the proper choices are made. Legislation can help create a safe food supply, but we can only choose the food ourselves. Nutrition is a lot more than the Basic Four, but food guides such as the Basic Four Food Plan are useful in choosing foods. Food processing is a lot different from home canning and pickling, as we will see in the next few chapters. The first half of this book has given you the stimulus to achieve better health and you have learned how food is a direct factor in your nutritional health. It is now important for us to learn about how to keep foods so that they are both safe and have the highest nutritional value.

Multiple Choice Study Questions

1. All vegetables are organic because
   A. they are composed of carbon, hydrogen, oxygen, and nitrogen
   B. they grow in soil that is organic
   C. they have organic minerals in them
   D. they are high in protein.

2. Which is not a vegetarian diet regimen?
   A. Zen macrobiotic
   B. lacto-ovo-vegan
   C. pure vegan
   D. ovo-vegan
   E. Atkins

3. The quality of foods found in a health store is ___ the quality of the foods in a supermarket.

    A. greater than

    B. less than

    C. about the same as

4. Many organic foods

    A. contain pesticide residues

    B. are less appealing than pesticide-controlled foods

    C. are more expensive than supermarket foods

    D. contain fewer additives than supermarket foods

    E. all of the above

Essay Study Questions

1. Define natural and organic foods. Why do some people prefer them?

2. Based on previous information, what foods should vegetarians substitute for the meat group of the Basic Four food groups?

3. What problems can occur with the Zen macrobiotic diet?

4. What kinds of foods are found in health-food stores?

5. Is there any value in using "organic" fertilizer?

6. What are the advantages or disadvantages of a vegetarian diet to one's own health? To the world food situation?

7. Should we feel reassured about the average American diet?

8. Summarize the general changes that have occurred in the U.S. diet over the last few decades.

Things to Do

1. Visit several organic health food stores. What kinds of products are being sold? Compare their prices to similar products in a supermarket, discount store, and pharmacy (e.g., compare equivalent dosages of vitamin C, iron, vitamin E).

2. Visit a natural foods cooperative. Discuss with the owner where they get their foods and the difficulties involved. How does the quality compare with your supermarket?

3. Plan a vegetarian or natural foods diet, using the Basic Four guide. Calculate the nutrient value.

4. Visit a regular supermarket and make a list of what we would consider to be a tailored nutrition food.

Chapter 13. Answers to Multiple-Choice Study Questions: 1, A; 2, E; 3, C; 4, E.

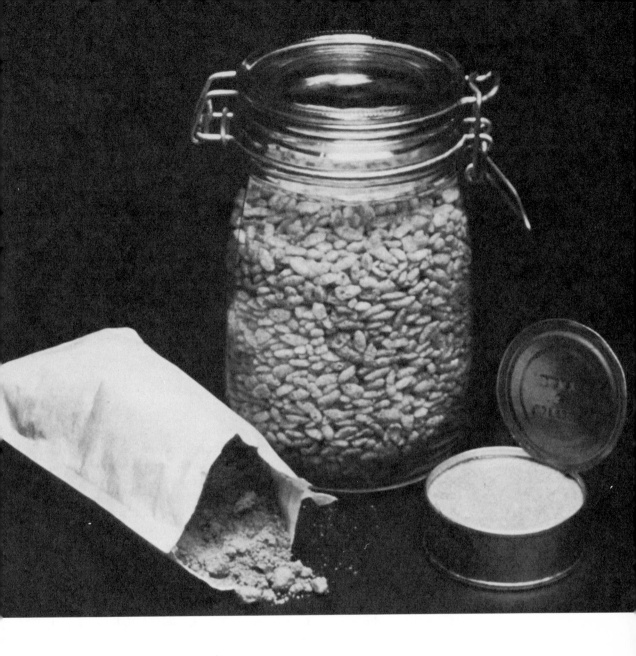

THE BASIS OF
FOOD PRESERVATION

14

THE FOOD DETERIORATION PROBLEM

Foods, whether grown on trees, in the ground as plants, or as animals above the ground, do not last forever. Fish begins to deteriorate in quality soon after it is caught. Fruits, vegetables, and cereal grains also begin to deteriorate once they are harvested. Prior to harvesting, plants are subject to attack by pests including insects, birds, and ground animals. Weeds compete with plants for nutrients. Plants and animals are also susceptible to disease that slows growth or that may eventually kill them.

In this modern society most of us do not live in a climate or on farms where we can obtain fresh food daily, so after harvest or slaughter we must use some means of preservation to insure an adequate food supply. The basis of the agricultural and food-processing industry is to assure an adequate food supply through proper care both before and after harvesting and slaughter. In addition, these preservation practices can be used to handle food and distribute it around the world to those who are needy in times of drought or starvation.

TYPES OF FOOD LOSS PROBLEMS

Pre-Harvest Deterioration

Food deterioration can be separated into many different categories. Prior to harvest, fruits, vegetables, and grains are subject to many forms of biological decay that can completely destroy a crop or reduce yield. It is estimated that in the United States these factors result in almost 10–20% loss of valuable food. For example, over 2,000 weed varieties can starve plants of their needed nutrients. In addition, food plants are subject to more than 1,500 different diseases caused by microorganisms and viruses. Some of these may destroy the plant, while others, such as molds, may grow on the plant and produce chemicals that are toxic to humans or animals and can be fatal if ingested. Genetically superior plants that resist disease are continuously being developed. Chemical sprays called herbicides, which destroy weeds, are another means of combating these losses by the modern farmer. In addition, certain chemical sprays can be used to combat plant diseases. Careful application and control are needed, however, to prevent any harmful residues of the chemical from being present on the plant after harvest. In the United States the Environmental Protection Agency (EPA) is responsible for regulating the use of these chemicals on the human food supply. In addition to chemicals, farmers may use soil nutrients to maximize the growth rate of the crop. Careful selection and application of the chemical is needed. Of even greater importance is one of the most essential substances, water. Since many weeds are more drought-resistant than the food crop, various forms of sprinkling and irrigation are needed to bring water to the plant. In the 1980s new methods including use of trickle irrigation are being pioneered because of the growing problem of lack of ground water in the United States. Of even more interest is the use of hydroponics. In this process, fruits or vegetables are grown in an enclosed green-house in which their roots are in a rock bed through which water carrying the desired nutrients is passed. The greenhouse also has an air lock to prevent pests from entering. Unfortunately this is an expensive means of producing food.

Insects can also seriously affect plants by causing decay or by eating the plant before we can harvest it. It is estimated that there are over 10,000 kinds of insects that must be controlled for maximum crop production. The Mediterranean fruit fly problem that occurred in California in 1981 is a good example of how devastating insect damage can be. Sprays such as Malthion and DDT (which was banned in the United States) can be used to combat these pests. Other insects that will eat the harmful ones can be introduced into an area, as long as the overall ecological balance is not upset. Male insects sterilized by radiation can also be introduced to the area. They mate with the female insects who then cannot produce any offspring. This was tried in the Medfly 1981 incident but the males were not properly sterilized, which resulted in an even greater problem. Unfortunately, as some new methods are developed, the insects develop resistances to the new methods. Thus research must be constantly finding ways to prevent crop destruction by insects.

Rodents and other pests such as birds will cause further losses by eating the food before it can be harvested. You may be able to put a scarecrow in your own garden but try to put scarecrows on a 1,000-acre wheat farm. It just does not work. Use of sonic devices, chemicals, rodenticides, and other means can reduce losses but we still have over 10% of crops being eaten by these pests.

Animals that we eat are subject to preslaughter stress and disease that can kill them or render them inedible. The United States Department of Agriculture, which controls meat slaughter and pro-cessing, bans the use for human foods of any dead, diseased, dying (a temperature over 106°F), or downed (crippled) animals. Ranchers must take adequate care of their animals, provide proper nutrition, and in some instances give them drugs to treat any disease. The use of these drugs is under strict control by the United States Food and Drug Administration (FDA).

Rinderpest and hoof and mouth disease are caused by viruses that ravage the cattle population all over the world. Careful control and quarantine have prevented these diseases from occurring in the United States. Recently the United States has developed a new vaccine for hoof and mouth disease that may help to eradicate it from the earth. The sleeping sickness caused by the tsetse fly prevents productive grazing by cattle in many fertile parts of Africa. Dairy cows can develop udder infections from bacteria, decreasing milk production. Chickens raised in large facilities with 100,000 or more birds are subject to a wide variety of contagious bacterial diseases. The use of proper sanitary facilities, the addition of antibiotics to animal feed, development of genetically more resistant animal breeds, and segregation of diseased animals decreases losses. Other animals also cause food livestock losses. In some states, wild dogs destroy thousands of beef and dairy cattle a year. Despite all these problems, the United States has one of the best agricultural productivity rates in the world and is able to export many of its cereal grain crops to needy parts of the world.

Post-Harvest Problems

Over 75% of our population lives in suburban and metropolitan areas, while the rest live in rural or widely separated areas. Less than 2% of the population in the United States is directly involved in food production on the farm. This can be contrasted to the more than 60% of the population living on subsistence farming in India and the 10–15% farmer population in Europe. The distance between the farmer and the consumer can be a great one. Food must be transported over these distances, and during this period it can be subjected to many hazardous conditions that must be controlled or prevented. Prevention of decay can be handled in such a way that the food is kept as close to the natural state as possible, thus leaving it only with a short shelf life. On the other hand, more elaborate preservation methods, some used as early as 4000 B.C., can extend the shelf life of the food over many weeks or months.

The modes of food loss and decay during post-harvest time can be classified into areas similar to those that occur under pre-harvest conditions: pest contamination and consumption of the food; senescence, which is the natural biochemical aging once harvested or slaughtered; chemical breakdown; physical decay processes that lead to food losses; and, most important, growth of microorganisms in the food, which spoils it or produces toxins harmful to humans.

Pests

Rodents and other pests, such as birds and insects, can cause major losses of harvested food crops. A rat can eat about 20 to 30 grams of food a day, voids 70 droppings per day, excretes almost an ounce of urine, and sheds many hairs. Droppings carry disease bacteria that are potential public health hazards. By eating food that humans could eat, or by contaminating the food so that we cannot eat it, rodents are responsible for a large portion of the food loss that occurs. The World Health Organization estimates that the loss of food due to rodents is over 30 million tons a year or 5% of the world's crop production. This loss is enough to feed 130 million people per year. According to the Food and Drug Administration, the United States' estimated losses can amount to over 10% of the grain crop. This is based on a population of over 100 million rats in the United States, almost one-half of the human population. These exceedingly high estimates indicate a very serious problem. Contamination of foods by rats during storage is considerable in foreign countries. For example, some foreign maize (corn) contains 25 rodent hairs as well as over 20,000 insect fragments per ounce. In the United States, flour with several rodent hairs and insect fragments per pound is subject to seizure and subsequent destruction by the FDA. This contamination is technically called filth and the FDA sets tolerances or action levels above which the food is unfit to eat. Obviously, adequate protection in the grain elevator, during transportation, and in storage areas is necessary. Rodenticides and buildings with controlled openings are two of the protective measures used to handle rodents. Warfarin, a very effective rodenticide, is an example of a chemical used to control these pests. Most food-storage warehouses and food-processing facilities have careful quality-control procedures to minimize this problem, including the hiring of licensed (through EPA) pesticide applicators who routinely inspect and use chemical control procedures.

Senescence

Once harvested or slaughtered, all foods are still living organisms to some degree. Plants such as fruits and vegetables are respiring, that is, they are consuming their starch stores to form ATP, carbon dioxide, and water. This ATP is used to keep the life processes going, controlled by the various enzyme reactions. During this time, ripening may occur if it has not already done so before harvest. Many fruits are picked before they ripen so that by the time they reach the consumer they are not yet at the ideal state of maturity. Otherwise they would become overripe and would begin to decay before purchase.

Eventually, the harvested plant can no longer effectively maintain its integrity because there are no nutrients being supplied by the roots from which it was separated. At this point, tissues begin to be deteriorated by the acids and the alcohols formed from the incomplete breakdown of the carbohydrate stores. The harvested plant can soften, darken in color, and rot. This process is called senescence. A similar process occurs in fish and meats after slaughter, and because muscle has very few energy stores, the decay takes place more rapidly. To some degree this is desirable in meat because the process of aging gives a better flavor and softer texture. To prevent or slow down decay from senescence, food usually is refrigerated. Refrigeration which lowers the temperature of foods enough to slow down these metabolic processes, is one means of preservation.

Another method is to lower or control the oxygen level around the food. For example, increased levels of carbon dioxide (CO_2) can be introduced into the storage area or injected into the bag in which the food is stored. The CO_2 slows down senescence and thus can increase the shelf life of many fruits and vegetables. Some producers transport lettuce from California in sealed boxcars or trucks with this type of controlled atmospheric (CA) process.

Microbiological Decay

One of the major decay mechanisms that destroys food is microbial growth. Microbes are tiny organisms sometimes called germs that can grow on the food causing it to spoil rapidly. This will be discussed in more detail in the next chapter. An example of microbiological decay is slime formation on fresh meat and fresh fish. This growth of bacteria does not make the food harmful if consumed, but the taste, smell, and texture make it inedible. Another example is the growth of mold on bread or cheese.

A second type of microbial decay is that in which toxic substances are produced by the microbes as they grow. This could cause harm if the food were ingested by animals or humans. An example is the growth of *Aspergillus flavus* on moist grain and peanuts. *Aspergillus flavus* is a mold that produces a toxic substance, aflatoxin, that can cause liver cancer and death. The Food and Drug Administration (FDA), which is responsible for the safety of the food supply (except meats, which are under USDA), expects that processors will inspect their cereal grain ingredients for contamination by this mold. Unfortunately, in the late 1970s and early 1980s wet harvesting seasons led to major contamination problems of cereal crops. This caused the destruction of much grain since no permissible procedures are known that can eliminate the toxin. In some cases, the FDA has allowed the contaminated cereal crop to be used in animal feed as long as the feed was used only in meat-producing animals and the level of use was such that no residue would show up in the meat.

A third type of microbiological destruction is the growth of infectious organisms in food. If ingested these microbes, usually bacteria, cause another type of food poisoning in humans called a food infection. This poisoning is associated with vomiting, diarrhea, and fever and can be fatal to infants and the elderly. In many cases the source of contamination is humans who carry the disease, have poor personal hygiene, and mishandle food being prepared for someone. Both the toxin formers and the infectious microorganisms are called pathogens.

Food processing is designed with three factors in mind: (1) to prevent contact of the food with the undesirable organisms; (2) to destroy any decay or pathogenic organisms present in the food so that no growth occurs in storage; and (3) to alter the food in such a manner that the organisms cannot grow if they come in contact with the food. Refrigeration is one example of controlling the growth of these organisms. At refrigeration temperature (0 to 5°C), most pathogenic organisms cannot grow. However, some decay bacteria can still grow on meat, fish, and milk at these temperatures, so shelf life is not very long. The following chapters illustrate other preservation methods. It should be noted that from a regulatory standpoint, the primary basis of food preservation is the prevention and control of pathogens. This is because foods are made in such volume that one incident of mishandling at the processing level could cause harm to thousands or millions of people.

Chemical Deterioration

The deterioration of foods discussed above was the result of living organisms degrading or growing on the food and the natural biochemical breakdown of the food itself. Some of the enzyme-related reactions have a direct effect on the quality of the food before the food may physically look unacceptable. For example, keeping corn at room temperature causes the sugar to be converted to starch as a result of enzyme reactions related to senescence. The corn still looks good, may still be crisp, but it has lost all its desirable sweetness. Senescence also reduces the vitamin content with vitamin C being the most susceptible.

Once a fruit, vegetable, or animal product is mechanically handled in some way such as peeling, slicing, or depitting, the tissues of the food get damaged. This damage releases the enzymes from their previously controlled environment and they can then catalyze decay reactions that would not have occurred previously. Examples of this are the rapid enzymatic browning that occurs when an apple or banana is bitten into or when an eggplant is sliced. In meats after cutting, released enzymes can contact fats and cause them to oxidize or split into fatty acids. Because these enzymatic processes, not normally associated with senescence, are usually rapid and result in significant deterioration, food processors use procedures to minimize the reactions such as denaturing the enzymes so that they cannot act. Blanching by heating the food is a method of enzyme denaturation.

Handling food also allows the natural chemicals present in the food to contact each other. This can result in further deterioration if the chemicals are reactive. This is important in engineered foods where various ingredients are combined. Usually these chemical reactions are much slower than the enzymatically catalyzed ones, but they can still result in similar undesirable end products. Rancidity is an example of a chemical deteriorative reaction that occurs in potato chips. In rancidity, oxygen reacts with the unsaturated fats to produce off-flavors and unacceptable odors. This same reaction occurs much more rapidly in frozen vegetables if they are not heat treated (blanched) first to destroy the responsible enzyme. A nonenzymatic reaction between certain sugars and amino acids or proteins can result in off-flavors, odors, and brown discoloration. This reaction is very slow at room temperature compared to enzymatic browning (remember a banana browns almost as soon as you bite into it) but is accelerated at high temperatures. Some vitamins, such as vitamins A and C, are also slowly destroyed by oxygen during processing and storage of foods by mechanisms other than those catalyzed by enzymes.

Processing is designed to minimize or prevent these deteriorative changes by control of the composition of the food, through process modifications, and by packaging. Some of these factors will be discussed in later chapters. It is important to note here that control of chemical deteriorative reactions also has a priority from a toxicological standpoint. There is evidence, for example, that some of the products of the oxidation of fats may be involved in promoting or causing both cancer and heart disease. For example, recent research has shown that the problem with cholesterol may not be cholesterol itself but rather the result of oxidation products of cholesterol that form during processing or storage of the food. Similarly, certain processing conditions may cause amino acids to react with sugars to produce potential toxic substances. This is called nonenzymatic browning. Minimizing these reactions during processing and storage is another priority of preservation technology.

Physical Decay

Physical decay is another type of food deterioration with economic consequences. For example, physical abuse of fresh fruits damages tissue cells that then release enzymes leading to browning or blackening at the point of abuse. These products are considered unacceptable by the consumer. Tomatoes at the bottom of a package may become squashed or broken. This makes them susceptible to infection and attack by molds and bacteria. Once this occurs the whole package may become infected with the organisms.

Meats and fish can lose water during frozen storage, which makes them tougher when thawed and cooked. Fresh vegetables can also lose water when refrigerated. This is very obvious in celery and carrots that lose their crispness during storage after losing only about 3% of their weight in water. The water loss occurs because the water evaporates in the lower humidity of the refrigerator. A plastic package slows this down considerably.

On the other hand, dry foods such as potato chips or crackers can gain water in a humid environment. They become soft and they are unpleasant to eat. Most crisp foods will become soft when exposed to humidities exceeding about 45–50% relative humidity. Higher humidities (generally >50%) make salt and sugar stick together so they will not pour. The changes in water content leading to unacceptability can be prevented by proper packaging to prevent moisture gain and storage at low humidities after processing.

Another example of physical deterioration is stale bread. It is obvious to everyone that during storage bread will get harder and tougher. This is not due to water loss entirely but rather to the crystallization of starch molecules during storage, a different physical change. This is an unusual reaction in that it proceeds faster at refrigeration temperatures. From a physical standpoint, bread keeps longer at room temperature or if frozen; however, at room temperature it may grow moldy in seven to ten days.

A final example of physical decay is the melting of chocolates. We have all experienced putting a chocolate candy bar in our pocket or purse and keeping it there for too long on a warm day. Refrigeration would have prevented the mess but we cannot carry a refrigerator around with us. Processors can modify the fat in the chocolate to prevent this but it does not always have the same flavor or texture when eaten.

There are many physical modes of deterioration that processing or proper storage must prevent or control. It is important for the processor as well as for the consumer to control these methods of deterioration in order to prevent or minimize food waste.

Naturally Occurring Toxicants

In an earlier chapter we noted that natural foods are not perfect. Many foods contain chemical substances harmful to humans that are produced by the normal metabolic pathways in the food. One, for example, is the raw soybean, which contains factors that can interfere with protein digestion, factors that adversely affect organs such as the pancreas, and factors that disrupt red blood cells. Another important priority of food preservation is to identify these factors and eliminate them either by removal or destruction. With the soybean, steam heating destroys the harmful natural chemicals. Other natural food toxicants are discussed in Chapter 26. Another classification of food toxicants are those harmful chemicals introduced into the environment that eventually get into the foods we harvest. Although not natural, they cannot be avoided or easily removed. Examples include the mercury that is found in fish, PCBs found in many foods, and DDT left from prior use. The FDA has set tolerances and actions levels for many of these chemicals based on their safety in the diet. Above these levels the foods are considered adulterated and illegal to sell.

Processors must constantly test their raw materials to be sure that any illegal chemical is not present in excess of the prescribed limit. Much research is being done to try to lower the level of these toxicants. It should be noted that pesticides in processed foods are not considered as pesticides but are treated as food additives. However, the FDA establishes the tolerance in the processed food at the same level as that allowed by the EPA on the raw agricultural commodity when ready to eat. The tolerances for pesticides are published in 21 CFR 193. This stands for the Code of Federal Regulations (CFR) Title 21, which refers to the regulations published by the FDA. Part 193 is the section that lists the tolerance levels for pesticides in processed foods. We will refer to other parts of 21 CFR in the rest of this book. Most university and city libraries carry the various titles of the CFRs.

Summary of Modes of Deterioration of Foods

Foods are subject to many decay mechanisms, before as well as after harvest or slaughter. These include biological attack by pests, disease, or decay microorganisms, senescence, chemical reactions, and physical changes. The objective of the producer and processor is to prevent or minimize these reactions as well as to eliminate human-introduced and natural toxins. Some typical processing methods will be discussed in the next several chapters. However, before we go on, let us look into the history of processing as well as review the basic principles of processing.

HISTORICAL ASPECTS OF FOOD PROCESSING

Although food processing techniques such as refrigeration, freezing, and canning are the result of the relatively new science of food technology, processing food products is actually an ancient practice. Some 2,000 to 3,000 years ago, central community bakeries were started to free individual families from having to bake bread daily. Some of the earliest guilds or unions were formed by bakers for the purpose of sustaining their trade and improving this very important staple.

The drying, salting, and sugaring of foods dates back 5,000 to 6,000 years. Drying was probably discovered by accident, such as by leaving a carcass out in the sun or by holding meat close to a fire. Cave dwellers may have quickly learned that the meat lasted much longer when dried in these ways. Of course they did not know that the process killed or inhibited microorganism growth. The origins of salting and sugaring techniques to preserve food are also lost in antiquity.

Fermenting of foods, a chemical preservation method, is also an ancient practice. Cheese was probably discovered while people journeyed across the desert carrying their milk in pouches made of animal stomachs. The milk was acted on by the enzymes from the animal stomach wall, and the right kind of bacteria growing in the milk in the warm sun produced a desirable flavor and texture. It also became obvious to them that in this form the food lasted much longer.

Unfortunately, war has been one of the most significant influences on the development of new food-processing techniques. The development and encouragement of the canning of foods during the early 1800s was due in part to Napoleon's need for a safe and varied food supply for his armies. Similarly, the method for making margarine, a substitute for butter, was also developed during that time. Canned foods, because they could be stored for long times, became a significant part of the diet in less than 50 years. During the Vietnam War, research by the military led to the development of foods canned in flexible pouches (the retort pouch). This was easier to carry than metal cans and the pouch was very light. This type of product began to be introduced to the U.S. public in the early 1980s and will probably replace the can in 50 years.

Drying of foods was usually confined to sun drying meat or fish and the making of raisins from grapes. The wet autumns in the U.S. from 1918 to 1920, which ruined the raisin crop, stimulated the advent of mechanical driers, but the use of these products by consumers was minimal. However, during World War II the United States troops in Europe needed food that could be stored easily and prepared quickly in the field. Methods for preparing dehydrated instant potatoes, vegetables, and eggs resulted. More people were exposed to the advantages of these easily stored and available foods. World War II also encouraged the frozen-food industry. This was because the U.S. government conscripted a major portion of the canned and dried foods for the military, leaving frozen foods as the only available long shelf-life products in the market. By the middle 1950s frozen foods became a much more common part of the diet.

The Vietnam War fostered the development of the process of freeze-drying. The United States Army Ranger Patrols needed food supplies that could be carried in the field for long periods of time. They also wanted a food supply that was nutritious, lightweight so as to be easy to carry, and easy to prepare. Freeze-dried complete dinners packaged in flexible film pouches resulted. Actually, without freeze-drying we might have lost more troops in World War II. Freeze-drying was used to dry preparations of penicillin since drying of the drug by other means caused the penicillin to be destroyed. Using flexible film-packaged dehydrated foods instead of canned foods greatly improved the mobility of troops. These innovations were also used in the United States' space program and are now available to homemakers and campers.

SOCIOLOGICAL ASPECTS OF FOOD PROCESSING

One important aspect of food processing is the consumer's desire for more convenient food in order to reduce the time required for meal preparation. We have seen many innovations in the food industry, including instant coffee and instant milk, frozen bread, cake mixes, instant puddings, frozen boil-in-the-bag vegetables, and complete meal replacements such as the breakfast bar. Is the consumer really the originator of this convenience mania, or are the food companies responsible? This is not an easy question to answer. The food industry is marketing many products at higher prices than the raw materials would cost the homemaker. This gives the company a profit that allows them to stay in business. With the availability of processed foods, the average consumer needs to shop less than once a week rather than every day or two because of the preservation techniques that have been used to prolong food shelf life and make many products available. This conserves gasoline. The shelf life of bread, for instance, has been greatly increased by the addition of mold inhibitors that allow a loaf of bread to be successfully stored at room temperature for over a week. Microwave-designed foods and boil-in-the-bag meals have resulted in considerably shortened meal-preparation time, leaving more leisure time for the homemaker.

The consumer has also gained an increased variety of foods because of these new innovations in processing and technology. The average supermarket has approximately 8,000 kinds of food items versus the 40 to 50 kinds in rural stores 20 years ago. The consumer is able to have exotic or foreign foods without the time and effort required to prepare them from the original ingredients. In fact, many of the ingredients would not be available without some form of processing. Consumers can also enjoy entirely new foods, such as special frozen deserts, turkey hot dogs, potato chips of uniform size and shape, instant breakfasts, and controlled-calorie meals, that have been engineered by the food industry.

Many foods are consistently eaten because they have an acceptable odor, taste, texture, and color. The criteria for judging these characteristics are largely personal and/or cultural. Food processing is designed to achieve and/or maintain these desirable characteristics. To some people Limburger cheese is highly desirable and to others it is totally unacceptable. Because of cultural practices some people readily eat horsemeat, while others cannot tolerate it. Religious practice also determines some food preferences. The processor can meet these needs for many people who cannot prepare the foods on their own or could not grow these foods where they live. Of course the food must be packaged and handled so the product remains at the highest quality when it reaches the consumer, whether the purchase is culturally, personally, or religiously oriented. In addition, as consumers may want their favorite foods all year round, processing must maintain the desired quality attributes during transportation and storage. It should be remembered that year-round availability also contributes to nutritional adequacy since a wider choice of products is available. When the pilgrims came to America they had a dangerous period from late winter to early spring called the "six-week want." During this time they had run out of all their fruits and vegetables, and certain diseases such as scurvy appeared.

In attempting to meet the goals described above, the food industry tries to use processing techniques that maintain high quality and impart long shelf life to foods without the danger of food pathogens and chemical toxins. Important criteria of quality are flavor, odor, color, texture, and nutritional value. New techniques and better control of processing have greatly improved these quality factors. To achieve part of the improved quality, processors sometimes may have to add certain chemicals (additives) to foods. The addition of these chemicals is a source of great social controversy at the present time. This is especially true if the additive is felt to be purely cosmetic, such as the addition of an artificial color. Pressure by political and social groups can change the use of approved additives very quickly. The controversy over the use of nitrite in cured meat and the use of saccharin as an artificial sweetener are two examples that will be discussed in Chapter 26.

The nutritional quality of food has become a major factor since the middle 1970s. Processors are conducting research and are making advances in developing methods that can preserve maximum nutritional value during processing while keeping the food safe. New methods of harvesting and freezing vegetables give frozen products better flavor and higher nutritional quality than can be obtained from fresh produce that is improperly stored. Although quality is important, it should be emphasized that all processing has as its rationale first, the prevention and control of disease-causing organisms; second, the control of decay microorganisms; and third, the elimination insofar as possible of chemical toxins. Many consumers are unaware of these priorities and unjustly accuse the processor of destroying the quality factors in their quest to provide convenience foods with long shelf life and to make a profit.

THE BASIC FOOD PRESERVATION METHODS

Principles and Priorities

Many microorganisms can grow in food and cause spoilage. Since microorganisms multiply so rapidly, microbial growth is the foremost cause of most food losses unless the food is processed. Some microorganisms can also cause disease and are called pathogens. Prevention of growth of microorganisms that are potential food pathogens and prevention of decay are primary priorities in the design of a food process.

Some of the processes will be described in detail in the following chapters. However, before we begin, let us list the various methods of food processing and mention how each process insures a longer shelf life with respect to deterioration. In looking at these methods it is important to remember that besides destruction and prevention of growth of microbes, the other priorities of food processing are: (a) to eliminate and control both natural and added chemical toxins; (b) to maintain nutrition quality; (c) to maintain quality in terms of flavor, odor, appearance, and texture; (d) to make a variety of foods available all year round so as to prevent nutritional imbalance; (e) to make foods convenient to use; (f) to provide a variety of foods for cultural reasons. Using these priorities we end up with three types of food systems.

1. *Perishable Foods.* Foods that are not processed at all or are only minimally processed (their shelf life is not more than 30–60 days after harvest or slaughter) usually decay by senescence or microbial growth, and generally are refrigerated. This category includes fresh meat, most vegetables, most bakery products, some fruits, and some dairy products.

2. *Semi-Perishable Foods.* Foods that are given a further process or special packaging so that they last from 60 days to six months include ice cream, many cheeses, some frozen foods such as fish, dry snack foods such as potato chips, and some refrigerated fruits and vegetables.

3. *Shelf-Stable Foods.* Foods that are given significant processing (their shelf life is generally very long, from six months to as much as three years) include all canned foods and most frozen and dry foods including pasta. Some fruits, such as apples, if properly held under the right gas conditions, can last almost one year. The same is true for potatoes.

Preservation by Application of Heat

The primary purpose of food processing is to prevent the growth of decay-causing and pathogenic microorganisms. This can be done by reducing their number, or killing them, and then packaging the food in such a way that the organisms do not recontaminate the food and grow. There are several ways to accomplish this. Heating foods generally destroys many harmful and decay organisms. Sterilization involves completely destroying all organisms present (such as the sterilization used for medical instruments). Canning, technically called commercial sterilization, is based upon the principle of sterilization except that not all organisms are killed since complete sterilization as used for medical products would result in significant loss of food quality. The commercially sterilized food is put into a package (can, jar, etc.) that prevents any further contamination from the environment during distribution.

Pasteurization, another form of heating, uses less heat or lower temperature. Pasteurization reduces the number of organisms present to a safe level but not to as low a level as in commercial sterilization. This reduction in numbers lengthens the shelf life of the food product and eliminates any pathogens present. Blanching, a third method of heat processing, usually does not eliminate microorganisms because even less heat is used. It denaturates undesirable enzymes, drives air out of the food, and softens it so it can be put into a package (like a can).

Heating is also used in other methods of preservation such as concentration, drying, baking, and extrusion (the process used to make many cereal products). Heat treatment can be used for other purposes, for example to effect a phase change such as to remove water during drying. This application does not result in elimination of many microorganisms.

Radiation Processing

Radiation is another pastuerization and sterilization technique that can be used to process foods. Three methods of irradiation are possible: (1) with gamma rays from a decaying radionucleotide such as Colbalt-60 or Cesium-137; (2) with high-energy electrons from an electron accelerator; (3) with ultraviolet light from a UV-light source. The irradiation beam hits the undesirable microbe and injures or kills it. Radiation can also cause an increase in chemical reactions, thus careful control must be used to maintain quality while treating the food.

In the United States, mainly because of the fear generated by the atomic bomb, radiation is classified as a food additive under the Food, Drug and Cosmetic Act although it is a process. Each irradiated food must be tested as if it were a food additive. Because of this, irradiation has only been approved for a few things such as insect deinfestation of wheat grain, inhibition of sprouting potatoes by surface treatment, and continuous sterilization of liquids and food contact surfaces by UV-light. Irradiation, however, is used in other countries, such as in Israel and The Netherlands, in low-surface doses for treatment of mushrooms and strawberries. This kills the surface molds and increases refrigerated shelf life for up to two to three months. In the early 1980s the United States government has begun reconsideration of the legal status of irradiation and may begin to approve the process for other foods. For example, in 1983 approval for treatment of spices was given. However with the Three Mile Island incident and the Diablo Canyon protests over nuclear power plants, it may take a long time to get consumer acceptance of sterilized irradiated foods, especially if they have to be labeled as being radiated.

Separation Methods

Separation by filtration using a special filter with very fine pores is a method of processing that can be used to remove undesirable microbes from liquid foods. It is employed in the production of some vinegars, juices, wines, and beers. Filtering is especially desirable for use in these products because it does not destroy or change flavors as heating does. Unfortunately, there are no methods available by which microbes can be filtered from solid foods.

Most separation processes for foods do not involve removing microorganisms. Instead they are used to disassemble a native food or a food process waste ingredient into its various constituents thereby creating a new food, a utilizable food, or a useful ingredient. The cutting of a carcass of beef into various portions like steaks and roasts is the simplest example of a separation process; rarely would we cook the whole carcass. At the other extreme of complexity is the use of separation to create new food ingredients. For example, special filters that allow only certain molecules to flow through a membrane are used to separate lactose and whey protein from the waste discharge of a cheese plant. These ingredients can then be used separately in other foods. The filtration method used is called ultrafiltration, which means the pores are so fine that they can differentiate between the size of the molecules. Another example is the creation of potable (drinkable) water from seawater by reverse osmosis. In this case a high pressure is created across a membrane and water is passed through the pores while the salts are retained on one side.

Complex separation techniques are also used for solid foods. The milling of wheat to create flour for baking purposes involves removing the hull, the bran layer, and the germ and then size-reducing the grain into a fine flour. This process, in fact, was begun before 2000 B.C. By 250 A.D. the process was so advanced that the Romans had a cereal grain mill in Barbegal, France (then "Provence"), that produced enough flour for 80,000 people per day. When the Normans conquered Saxony (England) in 1066 they acquired more than 6,000 grain mills in their new land. Interestingly, the Saxon word for "aristocrat" was "lord," meaning loaf giver. Of course, one can make a more nutritious bread from the whole grain, a particularly popular practice returning since the 1970s. The problem is that the finished product is coarse because the flour does not have the desired functionality with the other components present, especially the fiber. Thus consumers must learn to balance their desires between improved quality and impaired nutrition. Newer milling techniques are being researched so that the consumer can have the quality desired along with the needed nutrition and fiber content of baked products.

A second example is the manufacture of oil and protein from soybeans. The bean is cooked and treated with a solvent that removes the oil. The extracted oil is further treated to yield either a liquid salad oil, a margarine spread, or a solid cooking fat. The spent soy meal is then treated with heat, acid, or alkali to convert the protein into a dry textured product. This protein can then be made into imitation meat like bacon, into an imitation mozzarella cheese, or incorporated into ground hamburger to extend it and have a lower fat product.

Other separation processes include extracting coffee from beans to make instant coffee, extracting sugar from sugar cane or beets, and separating the butterfat from milk. The latter also produces a lower fat content milk. In the above examples, although the separation is the desired outcome, the procedures used are designed to insure that microbial contamination or growth does not occur and that any toxicants present are removed or destroyed.

Temperature Control As a Means of Preservation

Environmental factors that do not destroy organisms but prevent their growth are also important in food processing. One of the most important of these controlling factors is temperature. Refrigeration and freezing of foods lowers the environmental temperature of the food to levels that do not allow the growth of many destructive organisms. At the same time the reduction in temperature slows enzymatic and chemical reactions that could lead to deterioration. This increases their shelf life significantly. In many cases refrigeration is used as a complementary means to preserve foods that have only been minimally processed, such as pasteurized milk. These methods will be discussed in more detail in Chapter 18.

Holding foods at very high temperatures (greater than 140°F) also prevents the growth of most spoilage organisms and all pathogens. But holding foods at high temperatures creates a problem. Foods kept for a long time on a steam table at high temperature lose their desirable color and flavor as well as many important nutrients. Some vending machines serve hot canned foods by keeping them constantly above 150°F. If kept too long their quality is poor. Placement of microwave ovens in vending areas can eliminate the need to keep the canned foods hot.

Gas Environmental Control

Controlling oxygen levels around a food is another environmental control method that can be used to extend shelf life. For example, in home production of jam and jellies, the application of a layer of paraffin wax to the top of the jam in the jar prevents oxygen from contacting the surface and prevents growth of molds. On a commercial basis, a vacuum pump is used to remove the oxygen from the jar. However, in some foods, certain bacteria can grow in the absence of oxygen. We will evaluate this problem later in the book with respect to canning procedures, where oxygen is removed to prevent chemical decay. Oxygen is also removed to prevent reactions from occurring during storage of many dry foods that are susceptible to rancidity because of the oxidation of unsaturated fats. The process involves putting the product in a flexible film pouch, usually with a layer of foil in the film, pulling a vacuum, and then sealing the pouch. A good seal as well as integrity of the foil is necessary to maintain the low oxygen level. Another method involves flushing the pouch with nitrogen to drive out the oxygen. This is used when pulling the vacuum causes the pouch to collapse and crush the food such as would occur with potato chips.

A second method is the controlled atmospheric (CA) storage techniques mentioned earlier. Here both O_2 and CO_2 levels are controlled to maximize shelf life of fresh produce. The process is used extensively for storage of apples in warehouses. It is becoming more popular for transport and storage of other foods such as lettuce, meat, fish, and poultry.

Processing by Control of Water Content

Controlling the water content of a food is an important environmental factor that can be used in preservation. Freezing foods transforms liquid water into a solid form, ice. Microbes cannot grow in the solid form of water and thus the food is preserved. Two benefits of freezing are: (1) lowering the temperature of foods, which slows the rates of microbial, enzymatic, and chemical reactions and (2) freezing water into ice, which makes it unavailable to organisms and reactions. The principle here is that almost all microbial, enzymatic, or chemical reactions that cause deterioration of foods require a water phase to take place in. If the water is removed, as in freezing it into a solid, the reaction is stopped. Unfortunately not all the water in a food freezes when the food is frozen so they do not have an infinite shelf life.

Drying is another method in which the water content of a food is controlled or changed. Whereas freezing makes water unavailable for reactions and growth of microbes by converting the liquid water into a solid state, drying renders water unavailable by directly removing it from the food in a vapor state.

As will be seen in Chapter 19, the extent to which water is removed determines the shelf life of a dried food from a nutritional, microbiological, and chemical standpoint. Some of the processes that can be classified under drying include: concentration, where only part of the water is removed; baking; deepfat frying, where oil replaces the water; extrusion; and smoking of foods such as sausage, hams, and fish.

Another means of controlling water content is the addition of chemical agents or food ingredients that bind the water. This bound water is then no longer available for the chemical and microbial actions that could spoil the food. This is one of the most ancient methods of food preservation. Ancient man found that adding large quantities of sugar or salt to a food would prevent it from spoiling. They did not understand that the reason was the water-binding ability of the sugar and salt. In fact, in climates where lack of cool temperatures did not allow for refrigeration, such as Japan, many foods preserved by these "humectants" (water-binders) were developed. Other humectants include glycerol, fructose, propylene glycol, sorbitol, and glucose. However one does not need to add just these specific chemicals. Mixing a dry ingredient such as starch or protein with a wet one will cause a redistribution of the water so that the water is bound. However larger quantities of the dry ingredient are needed making the food less palatable. Humectants allow less dry ingredient to be used, with the advantage of a soft moist texture and better palatability.

The semi-moist hamburger-type dog food products, such as the Ken-L-Ration Burger® or Gaines Burger®, are products made this way. They are stable from a microbial standpoint at room temperature. In these products meat, cereal, and soy are combined with enough salt, sugar, and glycol to bind the water. This prevents the growth of deleterious and food-poisoning organisms and gives good shelf life.   In addition, the dog can eat the food directly as it has a soft moist texture.   History reveals the use of this principle by the American Indians.   During their travels and during the long winters they ate *pemmican,* which they made by mixing berries, a source of sugar and acid, with semi-dried buffalo meat, and dry nuts.   The binding action effected by the sugar and the dry nuts and the acid of the berries produced a very stable product.   Thus, the American Indians developed the process that is the basis of the new pet-food product that has come into existence during the 1960s.   In 1981 the Swiss government bought almost $20 million worth of a pemmican-type product from the Nestle Company to be put in disaster shelters for their population.   The same principle of water binding is used in jams, jellies, fruitcake, and some of the shelf-stable breakfast toaster tarts and meal bars.

Fermentation Processing

Fermentation is a natural method used to preserve foods by changing the chemical environment of the food.   Natural organisms or prepared cultures of desired organisms are added to the food.   The food is then held at the right conditions, allowing growth of the microorganisms to take place.   During growth these microbes produce chemical byproducts such as acids or alcohols.   These chemicals in turn prevent growth of harmful microbes or other decay microbes.   This is the basis of making wine, beer, cheese, bread, and vinegar, as well as many other foods such as olives and pickles.   The chemicals produced by the desirable organism prevent the decay organisms from taking over through a change in pH (acid level), increase in alcohol content, or by direct inhibition.   To get the desired organism to grow, however, initially we may have to use some heat to kill the undesirable ones present or we may need to add sugar or salt, which binds water and thereby prevents growth of the undesirables.   Thus we are using a combination of processes.   Fermentation can also be used to create a new food product out of some food component.   The fermentation of flour with other ingredients in making bread is one example as is the making of beer from cereal grains.   These two fermentation processes as well as the making of cheese from milk are ancient practices that were performed well before we had any knowledge of microorganisms.

Preservation by Addition of Chemicals

The addition of chemicals can be included as an environmental method of food preservation.   It may be used to change the internal environment of the food in such a way as to prevent the growth of or kill undesirable microorganisms.   In addition, other chemicals may prevent or inhibit chemical and enzymatic reactions. The lowering of the pH of a food by adding some acid such as citric acid or vinegar can inhibit the growth of many organisms, especially pathogens. This method is used to preserve many foods such as pimentos, mayonnaise, salad dressing, jams, jellies, and relishes. In many cases no other preservation is needed as long as the package is unopened. It is important to reduce the pH below 4.6, since below that level pathogens generally do not grow.

Some foods such as citrus products are naturally preserved to some degree because of their natural acid content. The acid foods are generally those with a pH of less than 3.5 and include many citrus products. Acidified foods (those to which acid is intentionally added) have a pH generally less than 4.6. A low-acid food is one with a pH greater than 4.6 but less than 6.8 and includes most vegetables, cereals, meat, and fish. These foods need some means of preservation because of senescence and rapid microbial growth. Very few foods have a pH above 6.8. These include eggs, tortillas, and soda crackers. In the fermenting of non-acid foods (such as milk to cheese) we use an organism that "naturally" produces the desired inhibiting chemicals. This "natural" definition, however, is really semantics, since one could achieve the same effect by adding a chemical. The difference, however, is that as the organism grows it produces other compounds that impart the "natural" flavor to make the food into something different and acceptable.

Certain chemicals added to foods can directly prevent the metabolic processes of microbes from occurring by damaging or killing the cell. This constitutes another environmental factor for controlling deleterious organisms. Antibiotics function by this principle. In the production of some beers, certain antibiotic inhibitors can be used to extend shelf life instead of using filtration or pasteurization methods, both of which destroy flavor. Thus a shelf-stable draft beer can be produced.

Other chemicals used to inhibit microbes include nitrite, sorbate, and benzoate. One of the most common metabolic inhibitors found in foods is the calcium propionate that is listed on the label of many bakery products. In the making of Swiss cheese, the fermentation organisms produce gas to make the characteristic holes, but they also produce propionic acid, which retards the molding of the cheese and gives it the desired flavor. When intentionally added to bakery products, propionic acid prevents the spoilage molds from growing on the surface and prevents certain bacteria from growing and producing a ropey texture in the interior of the crumb. Thus, the use of propionate extends shelf life for several days. This allows the bread to be used rather than thrown out, illustrating the usefulness of chemical inhibitors. These chemicals prevent the waste of the energy that went into making the product and the waste of the commodity itself.

The use of humectants such as sugar and salt, which bind the water to make it unavailable, is another form of controlling the growth of microbes. The method can be classified as both a water control and chemical process because many of the humectants also specifically inhibit the growth of spoilage and pathogenic microbes. A good example is propylene glycol. Smoking foods over a fire is an old process that uses the same principles. Smoke from wood or charcoal coats the food with some chemicals that are highly inhibitory to bacterial growth on the surface of the food. At the same time the smoking process dries out the surface, thereby using water control as a preservation principle. The heat from the fire also kills some organisms. Besides these three preservation principles, smoked cured meats also contain sugar and salt that act as humectants. Sodium nitrite is also added and acts as another metabolic inhibitor. Thus, one can take a highly perishable food such as pork and make it into a semi-perishable one by a combination of several methods that act synergistically.

Certain heavily smoked foods have been shown to contain specific chemicals on the surface that may be carcinogenic, that is, they might cause cancer in humans. Most food companies today use a liquid smoke instead of smoking the food directly over wood the "natural" way. The liquid smoke has been treated with an extraction process to remove the carcinogenic agents. The fact is that although charcoal-grilled foods are very desirable to most of us because of the taste, they may involve some risk because the smoke and burning of the fat as it drips into the fire produces carcinogenic chemicals. This brings up the risk/benefit ratio with respect to additives that we shall discuss in detail later. The individual consumer must decide whether or not to eat foods that could involve a certain risk to health. The question is whether we should take the risk, no matter how small, in light of the high degree of acceptability of the food. The possible carcinogenic effects of many chemicals are under investigation. The FDA has the authority to investigate these risks and either eliminate them through banning the chemical (or process) or, if the risk is small, informing the consumer, especially when the risk involves chemicals that are used solely to enhance or preserve color, texture, or flavor rather than act as preventors of pathogenic growth. This risk/benefit approach by education has led to some controversies between the government, the food industry, and consumer groups and will be mentioned in a later chapter.

Packaging

Packaging is also important to the preservation of foods because it controls the environment inside the package so as to maintain shelf life and protects the food from being contaminated by spoilage microbes, pathogenic organisms, external chemicals, or pests such as rodents, birds, and insects. For example, the can or glass jar used for heat-processed food serves these purposes.

Unripe bananas emit a hormone (ethylene) into the gas space surrounding themselves. This hormone controls the ripening process. Packaging unripe bananas in polyethylene bags traps this gas that speeds the rate of ripening. If the right package is used that traps just the right amount of ethylene, the bananas will reach the desired degree of ripeness by the time they are ready for sale.

Another function of the package is to prevent the transport of moisture and oxygen across the barrier. Dried foods are sometimes packaged in foil to keep these gases from coming through, thereby preventing both browning reactions and rancidity. Opaque packages also prevent light from reaching the food. The ultraviolet part of light can accelerate lipid oxidation and destroy both riboflavin and vitamin A. Studies at the University of Minnesota have shown that the pasta viewable through the window of a box has lost over 50% of its riboflavin compared to the pasta in the dark corners of the box.

Other functions of the package include: entrapment and prevention of loss of desirable odors; encasement to prevent physical damage; use as a means of handling the food; and use as a medium for advertising and education about the food as well as containing the required legal information (see Chapter 24).

SUMMARY

The basic goals of food processing are to eliminate any potential microbiological harm to the consumer while maintaining quality and nutritional value from the time of harvest to the time of consumption. Many factors can cause loss of foods prior to harvest and slaughter; they may account for almost 20% loss of foods produced in this country. Pesticides, insecticides, herbicides, and animal drugs help keep these pre-harvest losses at lower levels than occurs elsewhere in the world. After harvest or slaughter, foods are still subject to decay and loss of quality. With fruits and vegetables senescence occurs, which leads to overripening and a decreased resistance to microbial attack. Microbial attack is the biggest problem after harvest because the food loses its natural protection. Two types of microbial deterioration can then occur—one causes quality loss and one can cause human disease. The main purpose of processing is to prevent these types of microbial deterioration. Other post-harvest food deterioration mechanisms include chemical, enzymatic, and physical decay. From a historical standpoint, the need to feed troops in wars between nations has led to the development of food-processing techniques that provide a better food supply. Other goals of food processing are to increase shelf life so as to provide foods all year round and to provide foods in more convenient forms. Finally, it must be emphasized that the basic principle in all food processing is to make the foods safe so that the consumer does not get food poisoning from dangerous microbes or naturally occurring toxins. Heat can be used to destroy the organisms, and cold can be used to prevent their growth. Other environmental factors such as addition of chemicals and control of water and oxygen level can also be used to help preserve foods.

The first priority of food preservation is the control of or prevention of contact with pathogenic microbes, that is, "food safety." Secondly, the process is designed to help slow down or prevent the deteriorating chemical and microbial reactions that can eventually make a food unacceptable. Also, processing can remove any naturally occurring toxicants if they reach an undesirable level. The process used depends on the food itself, the type of quality and convenience desired, the effect on nutritional losses, and, of course, the safety of the food when consumed. Today processors must also design the process to minimize the amount of energy used and minimize environmental pollution. It should be noted that processing accounts for only 30% of the total energy involved in the food chain. Agricultural production uses 20% and distribution and marketing about 17%. The most energy used, 33%, is involved in home storage and preparation of foods. Of total energy used in this country the food chain accounts for only 16–17% whereas energy used for comfort control such as home heating or air conditioning totals 30%. Finally, we should point out that processed foods do not last forever. Table 14.1 gives the expected shelf life for some common foods under optimum conditions. The table also includes the typical mode of deterioration and the type of open dating information that should be included on the label to help the consumer be aware of the shelf-life limits. Open dating will be covered in more detail in the chapter on food labeling.

TABLE 14.1 Major modes of deterioration, critical environmental factors, shelf life, and suggested type of open dating for typical food products

Food product	Mode of deterioration (assuming an intact package)	Critical environmental factors	Shelf life (average)	Date most suitable for product	Suggested additional information on label
Perishables					
Fluid milk and products	bacterial growth, oxidized flavor, hydrolytic rancidity	oxygen, temperature	7–14 days at refrigerated temperature	sell by	length of time product can be stored at home
Fresh bakery products	staling, microbial growth, moisture loss causing hardening, oxidative rancidity	oxygen, temperature, moisture	2 days (bread) 7 days (cake)	sell by	
Fresh red meat	bacterial activity, oxidation	oxygen, temperature, light	3–4 days at refrigerated temperature	pack or sell by [a]	
Fresh poultry	pathogen growth, *microbial decay*	oxygen, temperature, light	2–7 days at refrigerated temperature	sell by [a]	length of time product can be stored in home either frozen or refrigerated
Fresh fish	bacterial growth	temperature	14 days when stored on ice (marine fish)	pack (catch date) [a]	
Fresh fruits and vegetables	microbial decay, nutrient loss, wilting, bruising	temperature, light, oxygen, relative humidity, soil & water physical handling	[b]	pack [a]	
Semiperishables and perishables					
Fried snack foods	rancidity, loss of crispness	oxygen, light, temperature, moisture	4–6 weeks	sell by or best-if-used-by	home storage information such as "store in a cool, dry place"
Cheese	rancidity, browning, lactose crystallization	temperature	processed cheese 4–24 months, natural cheese 4–12 months	best-if-used-by	
Ice cream	graininess caused by ice and *lactose crystalization* loss of solubilization (caking) lysine loss	fluctuating temperature (below freezing)	1–4 months	sell by or best-if-used-by	recommended home storage temperature
Long shelf-life foods					
Dehydrated foods	browning, rancidity, loss of pigment, loss of texture, loss of nutrients	moisture, temperature, light, oxygen	dehydrated vegetables 3–15 months, dehydrated meat 1–6 months, dried fruit 1–24 months	sell by or best-if-used-by	estimate of shelf life beyond sell by date; store in cool, dry place

TABLE 14.1 Major Modes of deterioration, critical environmental factors, shelf life, and suggested type of open dating for typical food products *(Continued)*

Food product	Mode of deterioration (assuming an intact package)	Critical environmental factors	Shelf life (average)	Date most suitable for product	Suggested additional information on label
Long shelf-life foods (Continued)					
Nonfat dry milk	*flavor deterioration*, loss of solubilization (caking), lysine loss	moisture, temperature	12 months	best-if-used-by	
Breakfast cereals	rancidity, loss of crispness, vitamin loss, particle breakage	moisture, temperature, rough handling	6–18 months	best-if-used-by or sell by	recommended storage conditions
Pasta	texture changes, *staling*, vitamin and protein loss	too high or low moisture, temperature	pasta with egg solids 9–36 months, macaroni and spaghetti 24–48 months	best-if-used-by	
Frozen concentrated juices	loss of turbidity or cloudiness, yeast growth, loss of vitamins, loss of color or flavor	temperature	18–30 months	sell by or best-if-used-by	months of high quality left for home storage
Frozen fruits and vegetables	loss of nutrients; loss of texture, *flavor*, color; and formation of package ice	temperature	6–24 months	best-if-used-by	recommended storage conditions
Frozen meats, poultry, and fish	*rancidity*, protein denaturation, color change, desiccation	temperature	beef 6–12 months, veal 4–14 months, pork 4–12 months, fish 2–8 months, lamb 6–16 months	best-if-used-by	recommended storage conditions
Frozen convenience foods	rancidity in meat portions, weeping and curdling of sauces, loss of flavor, loss of color	oxygen, temperature	6–12 months	best-if-used-by	recommended storage conditions
Canned fruits and vegetables	*loss of flavor*, texture, color, nutrients	temperature	12–36 months	best-if-used-by	
Coffee	*rancidity*, loss of flavor and odor	oxygen	ground, roasted, vacuum-packed, 9 months; instant coffee 18–36 months	best-if-used-by	
Tea	*loss of flavor*, absorption of foreign odors	moisture	18 months	best-if-used-by	

[a] This date applies only if the product is packaged prior to sale. If unpacked or sold in bulk prior to sale, this product is exempt from an open date.

[b] Depends on the specific commodity. Sweet corn has a shelf life of 4 to 8 days, and apples range from 3 to 8 months at proper temperature. For this specific information, see Theodore Labuza, *Shelf Life of Foods*, (Westport, CN: Food and Nutrition Press, 1982.)

NOTE: When known, the primary mode of deterioration is in bold italic type.

*Multiple
Choice
Study
Questions*

1. In food processing, the primary concern should be

A. the nutritional content of the food
B. food additives
C. prevention of growth of decay organisms
D. safety from pathogens

2. Senescence is the process whereby fruits

A. are sprayed with various scents
B. age after picking thereby shortening shelf life
C. are put in plastic bags to prevent water loss
D. produce odor compounds while they grow, to give a better flavor

3. The major principle of blanching is to

A. destroy microbes
B. inhibit chemical reactions
C. destroy enzymes that cause adverse biochemical reactions
D. cook food
E. prevent rancidity

4. Which process does not control growth of decay organisms through direct chemical means?

A. smoking
B. fermentation
C. sugaring
D. pasteurization

5. Which method does not preserve foods by killing organisms?

A. canning
B. smoking
C. pasteurization
D. filtration

6. Layering wax on the surface of jams and jellies prevents growth of

A. bacteria
B. yeast
C. molds
D. viruses
E. staph aureus

7. From an energy standpoint the area that consumes as much energy as industrial food processing is

A. agricultural growing practices
B. home storage and preparation
C. food wholesaling and retailing
D. transportation of foods

Use the following list to answer questions 8 through 11.
    A. growth of decay organisms
    B. growth of microbial pathogens
    C. biochemical reactions
    D. rancidity
    E. non-enzymatic browning

8. From the standard of food safety which of the above is the most important to prevent?

9. Which process applies to the aging of fruits and vegetables?

10. Which applies to the oxidation of fatty acids during storage of dry food?

11. Which best explains green mold appearing on bread?

Essay Study Questions

1. Why preserve foods at all?

2. List the basic methods by which foods deteriorate both pre- and post-harvest.

3. What is senescence? Give examples of useful and harmful outcomes of senescence.

4. Indicate some examples of food deterioration by physical and chemical means.

5. Discuss some food preservation techniques that were developed as the result of wars.

6. List the various processes used to preserve foods and indicate how they control or prevent microbiological problems.

7. What are humectants? Name some foods in which they are used.

8. Discuss the principles of food preservation.

9. Discuss the consequences of water gain or loss from foods.

10. List the major methods of food processing and describe briefly how they work.

Things to Do

1. Make a list of foods found in the home or at the supermarket. Try to list them under the various categories of how they are preserved.

2. Prepare a saturated solution of sodium chloride and place it in the bottom of a small fish tank (one gallon or less) with a cover on it. Place crackers and potato chips above the solution on a platform. Determine how fast they become soft (the equilibrium relative humidity in the chamber is 75%). Similarly place carrots or celery in the chamber and measure how long it takes for them to lose crispness.

3. Place two batches of mushrooms (or lettuce) in the refrigerator, one in a plastic bag and another in the open. Determine how long it takes before they go moldy.

4. Obtain a copy of Science Experiments You Can Eat by Vicki Cobb, J.B. Lippincott Co., New York ($2.50). This book gives about 38 different experiments on food preservation methods that can be done at home or in the classroom. This is an excellent book for use with this chapter. Several other applicable experiments will be referred to in the following chapters.

5. Obtain a copy of "Food of Our Fathers" put out by the Institute of Food Technologists, 221 N. LaSalle St., Chicago, IL 60601 ($1.00), and read about the preservation and nutritional practices of the pioneers. Discuss their problems in class and how they were eventually solved.

6. Read the regulations and laws on pesticides and give examples of how a pesticide is controlled in the environment.

Chapter 14. Answers to Multiple-Choice Study Questions: 1, D; 2, B; 3, C; 4, D; 5, D; 6, C; 7, B; 8, B; 9, E; 10, D; 11, A.

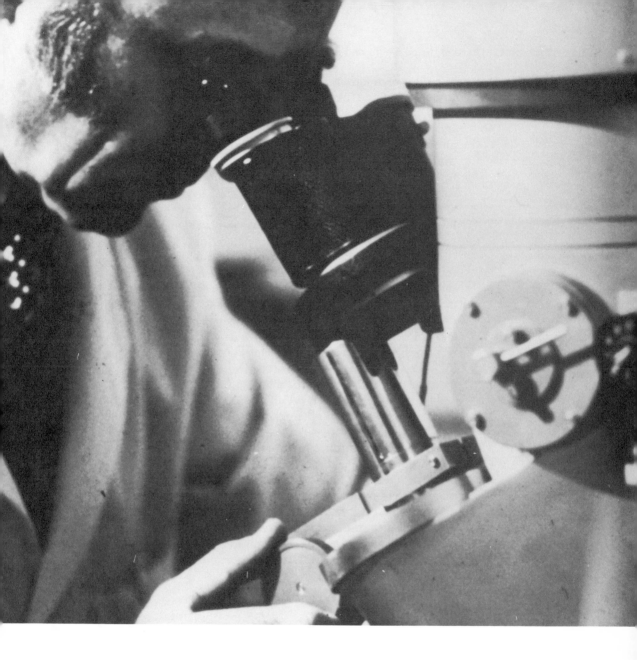

MICROORGANISMS IN FOODS: GOOD GERMS AND BAD ONES

15

THE TYPES OF MICROBES IN FOODS

Microbes or microorganisms are tiny living beings, usually invisible to the naked eye. Anton van Leeuwenhoek was the first to describe these "animalcules" in 1680 when looking into his crude microscope. Their nature and significance was not understood, however, and most scientists believed that the spoilage occurring in foods was the result of life being created through "spontaneous generation." An Italian scientist, Lazzaro Spallanzani, did experiments to disprove this theory in 1750, but his ideas were not accepted. It was not until 1876, through the work of Louis Pasteur who was helping the French wine and beer industry, that the relationship of microorganisms or "germs" as he called them, to spoilage became accepted. Pasteur also explained the cause of some human and animal diseases through his germ theory. He showed that it was these invisible microorganisms that could grow on foods and either spoil them, that is, ferment them or create a new product such as wine, which was desirable. In the past 100 years, this science has expanded dramatically to help us understand spoilage as well as the beneficial use of microbes. The genetic engineering revolution of the 1980s is creating a new era in which microorganisms will be used to solve many food, health, and medical problems.

Before looking at the types of microbes in food it should be noted that they are classified as fungi, generally do not contain chlorophyll as plants do, and are so diverse in metabolic pathways that the biochemistry and nutrient requirements we learned for humans in the earlier chapters sometimes do not apply. They can just about grow on anything, including cement and asphalt roads! In general, microbes important to foods are classified as (1) bacteria, (2) yeasts, or (3) molds, each of which has many diverse forms and many environmental and nutrient requirements. Their characteristics, shapes, and environmental and nutrient requirements are used to identify and classify particular microbes.

Bacteria

Unicellular bacteria are some of the most primitive of the living species on earth. Of importance is the fact that they do not have a cell nucleus as we do. The nucleus is the location of our genes. In bacteria, however, the genetic material is either floating around freely inside the cell or is attached in strands to the cell wall. This classifies them as prokaryotes. This is very important to the field of genetic engineering because it becomes easier to manipulate and change the genes.

Bacteria are generally the fastest growing of all microbes. They produce by division in which a cell divides in half to produce two daughter cells. Then after the same period of time, called the generation time, the two daughter cells divide (multiply) and each produces two more cells and so on (see Figure 15.1). In this process the genetic material is duplicated and split into the two daughter cells so they carry the same traits as the parents. They are sometimes called clones. Sometimes along the way the genes are affected by environmental or chemical factors and a mutation arises creating a daughter cell with different characteristics. This can have both positive or negative effects in processing, as will be seen in Chapter 20.

Generation times for some bacteria in foods can be as short as seven minutes. Thus, if all the nutrients were available, in six hours a population starting with one cell would exceed one million billions, a number too astronomical to understand. Fortunately, since the growing condition may be less than perfect and nutrients not all that available, populations rarely exceed 10^{12} per gram of food, that is one million millions or 1,000,000,000,000, which is still a rather large number. The reason for the limitation may, in part, be due to the fact that the waste products the organisms produce may be poisonous to them and either slow down growth or even kill the organisms. A typical curve is illustrated in Figure 15.2 showing the various periods of growth, including the initial lag or slow phase, the log or rapid growth phase, the stationary phase with no more population increase, and finally death due to lack of nutrients or self pollution from metabolic wastes. The growth of the world's human population has followed the form of this graph in the lag and log phases. One may speculate on whether the increase in world pollution or lack of nutrients, that is the world food problem, will cause us to enter the last two phases. On the other hand we may, if the environment continues to be limiting, enter the stationary phase

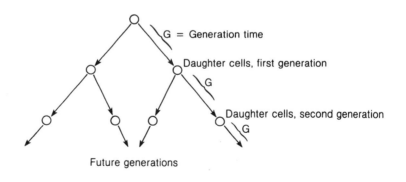

FIGURE 15.1 Duplication process for bacteria

by using birth control methods to allow individuals to reach their full potential.

Some bacteria can take two biological forms, a vegetative state and a dormant or spore state. In the vegetative state, which is shown in Figure 15.2 the bacteria are actively metabolizing the nutrients in their surroundings and producing waste products. The growth rate and type of end products produced are dependent on many environmental factors and on the nutrients available. This will be discussed later. In general, the types of products produced may be gases like hydrogen sulfide (the odor of rotten eggs) or it may be small molecular weight compounds such as aldehydes, ketones, acids, or alcohols that cause off-flavors and odors such as those in soured milk. The product may also be a slime, like that formed on the surface of meat or fish.

Not all end products are undesirable. Some cheeses produced from milk are fermented with bacteria to achieve desirable flavors. The type of bacteria used will determine the end product. Thus we have yogurt, sour cream, buttermilk, cottage cheese, cheddar cheese, Swiss cheese, and so on, each fermented with a particular strain of bacteria. Sauerkraut is another example. In this case, three different bacteria work together to produce the desired acids and flavors through fermentation of cabbage. Unfortunately, as noted in Chap-

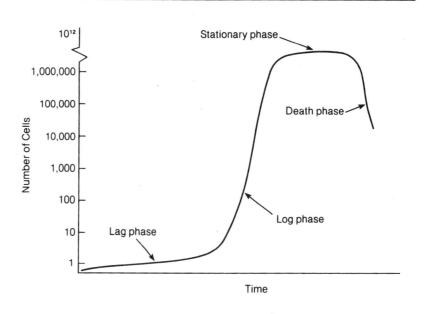

FIGURE 15.2 Growth curve of a microorganism

ter 14, some bacteria may also produce a chemical that is toxic to humans or, if we ingest them, they may grow on the nutrients in our digestive tract and cause an infection in our body. The important ones will be discussed in the next chapter.

Bacteria have two general shapes. Circular bacteria are called cocci. The cocci may be singular or may bunch up into long chains, cubes, or even grape-like clusters. Other bacteria take the general shape of a rod, which also may be irregular, short and stubby, curved, or long and narrow. Some of these rods may also have tiny projections called flagella, as shown in Figure 15.3, which vibrate and can cause the organism to move along in different directions. Although the coccus and the rod are the general shapes, other forms can also be found in nature.

Certain rod-shaped bacteria can form a spore during their growth process and eventually die while they eject the spore into the environment. This is a way of surviving adverse environments. Spore formation is not really reproduction since the bacteria does not divide. In sporulation, all the genetic material of the cell gets put into the spore to maintain it through stress. It is like suspended animation. This spore is usually extremely resistant to heat and other adverse environmental conditions compared to the vegetative state of the same organism. For example, some bacteria in the vegetative state can be killed by a few minutes of heating in solution at only 70°C but require heating for 20 minutes at 120°C to be killed when it is in the spore state. The spore is dormant and therefore does not metabolize and use nutrients. It can survive being dried and thus can be borne on the wind and spread throughout the environment. When the spore finally finds a favorable medium (environment) again, it somehow senses it and the genetic material becomes active. The spore then germinates, which is a process in which it forms a new vegetative cell (like being born again from the dead). Microbiologists are actively studying this whole process of spore formation and germination because it is poorly understood but is important to the safety and quality of foods.

The canning process is based on the heat treatment required to kill the spores of a pathogenic bacteria called *Clostridium botulinum*. If the spores are not destroyed, they can germinate and change back

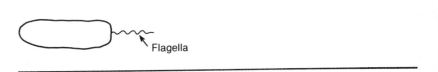

Flagella

FIGURE 15.3 Bacteria with a flagella which imparts mobility

into vegetative cells inside a can of food. There they can grow rapidly in an oxygen-free environment and can produce a chemical that is highly toxic to humans.

Removal of oxygen does not prevent all bacteria from growing and multiplying as it would do to humans. Some bacteria are called anaerobes because they cannot grow in the presence of oxygen. These organisms use a somewhat different metabolic process to produce energy than the one we described earlier for humans. Those that grow in air are called aerobes. Facultative anaerobes is the name given to microorganisms that can grow either with or without oxygen by being able to change their metabolic pathways.

Bacteria can also be separated on the basis of their optimum temperature for growth. Psycrophiles are those that grow best at low temperatures (0 to 10°C); mesophiles grow best from 15 to 40°C; and thermophiles can only grow above 40°C. Although some organisms can grow in several ranges, the classification describes their optimum temperature range for growth. Most bacterial pathogens cannot multiply or produce toxin below 5°C. Thus, quickly refrigerating warm foods is one way to prevent food poisoning.

The recent clamor about genetic engineering concerns the multiplication step we illustrated earlier. Since some genes of a bacteria may float freely in the cell as a circular particle called a plasmid, the plasmid is fairly easy to remove from the cell. One can then split the plasmid and insert a new gene into it from some other organism. This new plasmid containing a new gene is then reinserted into a cell of the first type and the new trait will be carried in the division process so the daughter cells take on new traits. Thus, if one inserts a human gene that controls the production of pancreatic insulin into a bacteria plasmid and reinserts this into the bacteria, the bacteria, if given the proper nutrients, may then be able to produce insulin very cheaply. Of course, this is easier to say than to do, but that is what makes the technique so fascinating. Recent research has shown that the fermentation ability of some useful dairy fermentation bacteria is due to the presence of transferable genetic material in a plasmid in the bacteria. It is quite possible to insert more of the fermenting genes into this plasmid and make a "super" bug, one that can ferment the milk very rapidly. In fact, genetic engineering has already been done to create a bacteria for control of oil spills. The genes necessary to ferment or utilize the various fractions of crude oil were inserted into certain types of bacteria and we now have a "super pollution bug" that can be used to eat up the oil spill.

Yeasts

Yeasts are another type of microorganism associated with foods. They are larger than most bacteria and contain their genetic material in a nucleus, that is a cell organelle that has a membrane around the genes. This means they are more highly advanced and are called eukaryotes. Yeast multiply by several different means. Some produce multiple ascospores, much like the bacteria spore, and release the spores into the environment. However, since several spores are produced per cell, the population can increase dramatically unlike bacteria spores. Others divide by fission, much like the bacterial division in which the genetic material is duplicated and split into the two cells. Most yeast reproduce by a process called budding, as illustrated in Figure 15.4. In this process they produce a growth on the cell wall like a new leaf or stem forming on a plant. This eventually takes shape and then cleaves off the original cell to form a new one.

Yeast can usually grow under more adverse conditions than can bacteria. Thus they can withstand a lower water content or higher sugar and salt content and can grow under somewhat reduced oxygen conditions. However, yeast are easily killed by heat during pasteurization.

Although many yeast produce undesirable fermentations that cause food decay, we usually associate them with useful products. Fermented yeast foods include apple cider, vinegar, wine, beer, and bread. There are at present no known poisons produced by yeast.

Molds

The molds are the hardiest of the microorganisms that can grow on foods and form diverse shapes that are too numerous to classify. Molds contain a nucleus and are thus eukaryotes or more highly advanced microorganisms. Rather than being unicellular they can form multicellular plants. They produce more slowly by growing first in a mycelial mat. This is seen as the fine hairy filaments that may occur on the surface of moldy bread. Thus, molds are visible to us at advanced stages of growth. The mold then may produce spores at the ends of these filaments. In some cases these spores are

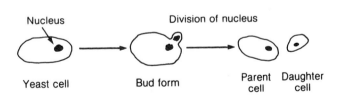

FIGURE 15.4 Budding process for reproduction in yeast

highly colored, from red to green to blue to black. The spore is a dormant stage, just like the bacterial spore, and can be carried by air currents to be deposited in another place where it might grow. Mold spores are extremely resistant to heat in the dormant stage. However, their resistance is usually much less than that of bacteria spores.

Molds generally need oxygen to grow and thus are usually seen only on the surface of foods. Waxing the top of homemade jams is a way to prevent mold growth. Molds are the microorganisms most resistant to reduced water content and can grow in conditions of high salt or sugar content.

Some molds produce toxic substances that can have a great effect on the food processor as well as on the consumer. These will be discussed in the next chapter. It should be noted, however, that many molds are used by the pharmaceutical industry to produce drugs, nutrients, and chemicals such as antibiotics, some vitamins, and citric acid. It may be that with the techniques of genetic engineering, the abilities of molds to produce these products or other new ones can be dramatically increased.

Viruses

Viruses are not living organisms in themselves but carry genetic material in a capsule surrounded by protein. In nature the particle is dormant. The virus must first invade a living cell. Many of the mechanisms by which this occurs are not well understood. But when viruses see the right cell its metabolism somehow turns on, much like a spore germinating. After attachment to a living cell, the virus then ejects its own genetic information into the cell. These genes take over the metabolic process of the cell and eventually produce more viruses as well as destroy the cell. The virus particles are then released and can attack other living cells. If this happens in human or animal tissue it can result in disease or death. Polio in humans and hoof and mouth disease in cattle are two diseases caused by viruses. Vaccines against these diseases either destroy the virus in the blood or prevent it from attaching to a cell. Viruses may also be one mechanism in causing cancer. It is felt that the attacked cell literally goes wild, reproducing and growing into a malignant tumor, all controlled by the viruses' DNA. One virus (hepatitis) is transmitted in a human/food vector, that is, it is carried by humans. The poor sanitary habits of these people result in the contamination of foods with fecal matter. This inoculates the food with the virus particles. When we eat the food, the virus enters the body and starts its disease cycle.

**PROCESS
CONTROL**

Microorganisms or germs can be beneficial or harmful to food or humans because of their metabolism of food components and production of waste products. In processing we are concerned with the prevention of the undesirable effects such as slime formation, tissue breakdown, production of off-odors or flavors, as well as growth of pathogens or production of toxins. Some laws, in fact, have been passed that limit the number of microorganisms allowed in a food product. For example, Oregon at one time set standards for the total number of bacteria that could be present in meat. Most states have similar standards for milk. To achieve these standards, controls must be used during processing and storage. The ingredients and the process are analyzed by the hazard analysis critical control point procedure (HACCP). The food from the field or slaughterhouse must initially have as low a microbial content as possible so that we start out low on the growth curve. Then each step is examined on the basis of what environmental or metabolic factors present would result in the prevention of growth or in the death of the undesirable organism. A procedure is then established whereby some readily measurable controlling factor is continuously monitored; for example, if the pH or temperature is kept within a certain range the food will be safe. The rest of this chapter reviews those important environmental factors that can be used to control the growth of microorganisms.

A more detailed outline of a HACCP analysis follows. The FDA uses a HACCP analysis when they inspect food plants and they have published regulations (21 CFR Part 110) called Current Good Manufacturers Procedures (CGMPs) that outline how a plant should operate to produce safe foods. In the analysis we have tried to show how HACCP can be applied to quality factors as well, that is, not just to microbial growth.

**HAZARD
ANALYSIS
OF FOOD
PROCESSING**

The concept of HACCP is best described as a system of classification that uses the basis of identifying and controlling any potential health hazard or quality loss hazard during food processing. The food process HACCP classification consists of three major hazard categories.

Hazard 1. The product contains a "sensitive" ingredient or ingredients, that is it may contain pathogens or it has a sensitive flavor, color, or nutrient in it.

Hazard 2. The manufacturing process does not contain a controlled processing step that effectively destroys harmful bacteria, prevents their contamination, or stops or controls a particular reaction leading to quality loss.

The processing step referred to here can be heat or chemical processing or the engineering of a food system that, by its chemical or physical composition, destroys or prevents growth of harmful microorganisms or denatures a deteriorative enzyme, for example, by reduction of the water content of the food.

Hazard 3. There is a substantial potential for storage abuse in distribution or in consumer handling that could render the product either harmful or of unacceptable quality when consumed.

The principle judgment criterion for abuse potential is whether the food product is a good medium for chemical reaction or microbial growth in the state in which it is distributed or as normally prepared by the consumer. Consideration must be given to low levels of microbial contamination that have escaped control screening or processing designed to prevent contamination by harmful bacteria.

The critical control points (CCPs) can be divided into microbiological and quality factors.

The microbiological control point (MCCP) concept is used to describe those locations in a food-processing operation and the rapid microbiological laboratory tests or other important criteria (such as time/temperature or pH recording) that can be used with good assurance and in a reasonable time to assess the potential for either pathogenic or other microbial growth that would render the product unacceptable or harmful.

The quality control point concept (QCCP) is used to describe the locations in a food-processing operation and the rapid laboratory tests or other important criteria that can be used with good assurance to assess the potential for loss of eating or nutrient quality of the final product.

Figure 15.5 shows a general process diagram with the critical control points identified.

ENVIRONMENTAL FACTORS CONTROLLING THE GROWTH OF MICRO-ORGANISMS

Temperature

Each microorganism has an optimum temperature range for growth. Above or below this range growth cannot occur. For pathogens, temperatures below 45°F and above 145°F are adequate to prevent their growth. Thus, any process with temperatures within these limits has a potential hazard to health. To prevent food poisoning the food processor must make sure that the numbers of microbial pathogens are low in the ingredients entering the process line, must

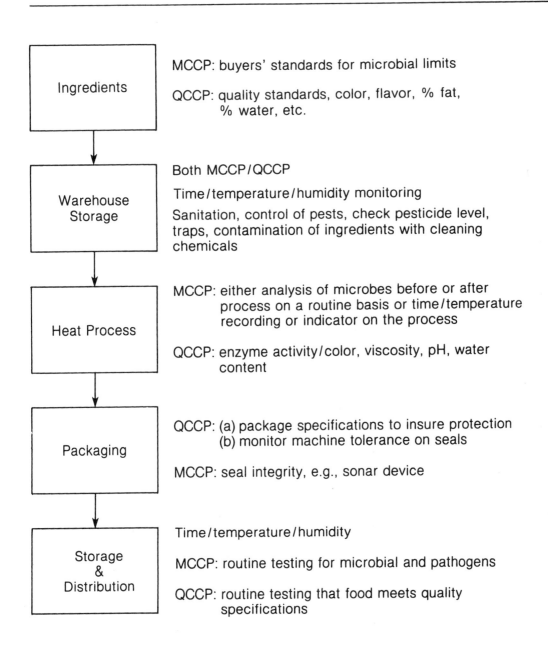

FIGURE 15.5 Critical control points

monitor the process time as well as control it to cause death or prevent multiplication, and must sanitize the equipment on a regular basis so the organism numbers do not increase. If possible, the processor could also add a heating step that raises the temperature high enough for a long enough time to destroy any pathogens or the toxins they produced.

Oxygen Level

As with temperature, each microorganism has a particular requirement for oxygen. Some require O_2 while others are killed or inhibited in its presence. *Clostridium botulinum*, a potent pathogen, can grow and produce toxin in an oxygen-free environment, for example, in a can of food. We could eliminate this problem by allowing air to remain in the can, but the food would then spoil rapidly by other means. Thus, oxygen per se is not used to control this organism. Instead we heat treat the food at high temperature to kill the organism. With jams and jellies, however, control of oxygen levels is very important at the surface of the foods. Jams and jellies are very susceptible to mold growth on the surface. The processor must nitrogen flush or vacuum pack the jar to insure long shelf life. Once opened, however, the protection is lost and we are instructed to keep the product refrigerated as molds do not grow very well at low temperatures.

pH

Most organisms can grow only in a specific pH range just as most have a specific temperature range; pH control can be used to prevent or slow down decay in many foods. We usually separate foods into four acidity ranges:

1. Nonacid foods: pH greater than 6.8. Examples are eggs and soda crackers.

2. Low-acid foods: pH from 4.6 to 6.8. This includes foods such as meat, fish, milk, poultry, and most vegetables.

3. Acid foods: pH 3.5 to 4.5. This is the pH range of many fruits such as apples and grapes, some vegetables, and tomatoes.

4. High-acid foods: pH less than 3.5. Most citrus fruits and sauerkraut fall in this range as do many carbonated beverages such as colas.

Sauerkraut is a good example of a food that is preserved by the production of natural acids during fermentation. Sauerkraut is produced as the result of fermentation by organisms found naturally on the cabbage. In fact, this fermentation is an example of ecological balances. One type of bacteria grows first, producing some acid, which lowers the pH. This acid eventually kills the first bacteria, and then a second type of bacteria, which has a lower optimum pH, takes over and produces additional acid. Finally, as the pH decreases further, the second type of bacteria dies and, a third species begins to grow, producing acid as well as certain flavoring compounds that are characteristic of sauerkraut. The acid also ruptures the cabbage cells to change the texture. All three species of bacteria are naturally present. They start growing when the cabbage is first mixed with salt and shredded. The salt inhibits other organisms present from growing and spoiling the food during fermentation. The shredding releases the nutrients from the cells so the microbes can start to grow. Molds, however, can also grow on the cabbage in the vat in which the process is carried out, so the cabbage shreds must be covered with enough salt solution to exclude oxygen at the surface.

As pH is lowered in food the amount of heat necessary to thermally process (can) foods to make them safe decreases. Thus peas at pH 5.6 must be heat processed in a pressure cooker at 115°C for 40 minutes while tomatoes of pH 4.0 only require 30 minutes in a boiling water bath (100°C). Lastly, most pathogenic bacteria cannot grow in acid conditions (pH less than 4.6), so acid conditions can be used to prevent foods from causing food poisoning. Of course we cannot add acid to all foods because of the flavor problem. In a food process in which pH is important, measurement of it would be one of the critical control points described earlier.

Water Availability

Removing water can control microbial growth. Different organisms have different resistances to water removal. The availability of the water in a food to the environment or to an organism is called water activity or equilibrium relative humidity (ERH). The water activity scale (a_w scale) goes from 0 to 1. Multiplying by 100 converts it to the equilibrium relative humidity scale (% ERH). As an example, let us imagine a food that has an equilibrium relative humidity of 50%. This is the case for many cookies and pasta products. If a cookie was held in a room at 50% relative humidity, it would neither gain nor lose water. In other words, the water in the food is not available to the environment. If the room had a higher percent ERH the food would gain water until it equilibrated to the new moisture content and the new percent ERH. A room with a lower humidity would cause the food to dry out until it reached the new equilibrium

ERH at a lower water content. This relationship is known as the water sorption property of a food.

Microorganisms are also controlled by the a_w or % ERH of their environment. When most tissue foods are harvested or slaughtered, they usually have an a_w close to 1.0 or are near 100% ERH. At this level most food spoilage bacteria can grow very rapidly. By drying the food out or adding humectants, we can lower the % ERH. This is the basis of drying as well as sugar and salt addition to foods. Drying food drives off the water. The use of humectants such as sugar and salt is based on the fact that the chemicals bind the water and lower the % ERH. As this happens, growth of microorganisms slows down or ceases since the water availability is decreased.

Bacteria have the least resistance to lowering the water activity. Most stop growing above 92–93% ERH. But a very important bacteria, *Staphylococcus aureus,* can grown down to at least 84–85%. This bacteria is important since it is a pathogen and can produce toxins harmful to humans and animals. It is resistant to moderate levels of salt or sugar. The semi-moist or intermediate moisture dog foods like the Ken-L-Ration Burger ® (Quaker Oats) are processed according to the water-activity principle. Sugars, glycol, and salt are added to lower the ERH of the meat to below 85%. Thus bacteria cannot grow or spoil the food. Some of the breakfast toaster tarts are made in the same way by adding sugar to lower the ERH to 60–65%. The sugars present in table syrups, jams, and honey have the same effect.

Yeasts are more resistant than most bacteria and can grow down to 86–88% ERH. Some, however, can grow much below that level but are rare in foods. As noted before, molds are the hardiest microorganisms. Many can grow in foods in which the water activity or ERH has been lowered to 70–75%. Thus, the dog food mentioned above must be heat-treated, which destroys the mold spores, since the a_w is lowered to only 0.85. In addition, acid may be added (pH control) to prevent growth of molds that may contaminate the product before packaging, and a mold inhibitor, such as propylene glycol or potassium sorbate, may also be added. Usually, processors combine all four process techniques. In fact, the combination has a synergistic effect such that the processor can go to higher a_w's by using less salt or sugar and still get the desired protection. This allows the food to have a higher water content and thus a more pleasant soft, moist texture. A synergistic effect is one in which total protection is greater than the sum of the protections afforded by each technique when used alone.

From the standpoint of microbial growth, all foods below an a_w of 0.6 or 60% ERH are safe. Thus, when we dry foods we try to remove enough water to be below this level. Since chemical deterioration can still occur at this level, however, processors usually dry foods to below 30–40% ERH where deterioration is extremely slow.

Nutrients

The availability of nutrients also controls microbial growth. A microorganism that requires protein will not grow in soda pop or cornstarch. We can use the food composition to help predict which organisms will not grow. For example, many food poisoning organisms grow better in high-protein foods. In the hazard analysis of a food process, one can recognize a potential problem by looking for those ingredients that supply the needed nutrients for harmful bacteria. One may not always be able to eliminate the ingredient but critical control procedures could be set up to monitor and regulate any potential problems.

Those microbes that are important to spoilage of foods generally require some carbon source such as carbohydrate or protein, they may require some vitamins although many make all they need, and they require certain minerals, for example, potassium, phosphorus, iodine, sulfur, iron, and calcium. The ability of a microbe to grow on a certain test medium is another means by which organisms can be classified, for example, those that can grow on lactose versus those that cannot. This fact has also been used to develop a test to determine whether certain chemicals can cause a mutation and thus might be a carcinogen. Organisms that require a certain nutrient, such as an amino acid, are treated with the test chemical during their rapid growth (log) stage (Figure 15.1). If the chemical affects the cell DNA and causes a certain mutation, the cell may no longer require the nutrient. Thus, treated daughter cells put on a medium without the amino acid can now grow, while untreated ones will not grow and multiply.

Inhibitors

The last general method of controlling the growth of microorganisms is through the use of chemicals that can have a direct toxic effect on the metabolism of the cell. Several possible mechanisms by which they act include:

1. Preventing absorption of nutrients across the cell wall, as sorbic acid does.

2. Stopping protein synthesis by interrupting the RNA/DNA mechanisms for gene expression. Some antibiotics may do this.

3. Preventing spore outgrowth. Nitrite may act in this way on *Clostridium botulinum* spores.

4. Preventing certain metabolic pathways by irreversibly binding with important enzymes.

5. Preventing DNA replication and thus preventing the multiplication of the cell. Again many antibiotics work by this method.

Not only are these agents used in some foods themselves, but many types of inhibitors are used as sanitizing agents on food contact surfaces. This is another way to reduce contamination. A common sanitizing agent used at home for medical purposes is ethanol. However in this case the mechanism works by binding water, causing an osmotic shock that kills the cell.

SUMMARY

Microorganisms that are present in all foods after slaughter or harvest can cause decay or food poisoning. The organisms may also be introduced into the food from the environment. Microbes can be divided into three types: bacteria, yeast, and molds. Some are useful and can be used to produce fermented foods such as bread, wine, and cheese. Others must be destroyed or inhibited because they result in disease or in the loss of the food. To prevent growth or to destroy the microbes, several environmental factors can be used as controls in processing of foods: temperature, oxygen level, acidity, availability of water, nutrients, and chemical inhibitors. Food processors use these factors individually or in combination to preserve foods by a method of controlling critical points in the process.

There are many different ways to control the growth of microorganisms in foods. It must be stressed that the basis of processing is prevention of the growth of pathogenic organisms since food safety comes first. The next chapter discusses some food-safety problems caused by microbes.

Multiple Choice Study Questions

1. All bacteria are
  A. harmful
  B. useful
  C. molds
  D. generally useful or harmful
  E. multi cellular

2. Which of the following has no direct chemical antimicrobial effect?
  A. sugar
  B. propionate
  C. salt
  D. sorbate
  E. nitrate

3. The optimum range of growth temperatures for thermophilic bacteria is

    A. 210–312°C
    B. 35–90°F
    C. 110–150°F
    D. 6,000–8,000°F
    E. −20 to −40°F

4. Which of the conditions below would be best for prevention of mold growth?

    A. a refrigerator at 55°F
    B. a refrigerator at 40°F
    C. room temperature
    D. 100°F
    E. a freezer

5. The mircoorganism that can grow to the lowest water activity (a_w or % ERH) is

    A. mold
    B. bacteria
    C. staphylococcus
    D. yeast
    E. clostridia

6. Jams and jellies are stable food products because

    A. heating prevents mold contamination
    B. the enzymes present destroy the bacteria
    C. the % ERH is low enough to prevent bacteria from growing
    D. the % ERH is low enough to prevent bacteria and yeast growth
    E. the % ERH is low enough to prevent bacteria and mold growth

Essay Study Questions

1. What are the types of germs found in foods?

2. What are the specific differences between bacteria, molds, and yeasts?

3. How are bacteria classified?

4. What is the difference between the vegetative and spore state of a bacteria?

5. List the specific environmental factors used to control microbial growth.

6. Define and discuss the effect of water availability on microbial growth.

7. Discuss the various acidity classifications for foods.

8. How are semi-moist pet foods preserved?

9. In what foods are yeasts used for desirable effects?

Things to Do

1. Do the experiments on yeast in Section 8 of the *Science Experiments You Can Eat* book. See Chapter 14 for reference.

2. Obtain some nutrient agar from a laboratory supply house (or make it by preparing plain gelatin with about 5 g. of dextrose and a crushed vitamin pill added to one quart liquid). Pour it into a flask or glass beaker covered at the top with a cotton plug. Cook it in a boiling water bath for at least two hours to sterilize it and then pour it into sterile short jars or petri dishes (sterilize in boiling water also).

   A. Make cultures of your hands, mouth, nose, a healing wound, the air (leave standing out), and the surface of various foods. To do this swab the surface with sterile gauze, then touch the surface of the growth medium. Store the jars or dishes covered at room temperature and examine the formed colonies to determine what they are (a microscope is useful) and how much grows.

   B. When preparing the medium, add vinegar to it to get pHs of 6, 5, 4, and 3 (use litmus paper to check pH). Spread some mold spores (from moldy bread) on each plate and store at room temperature. Examine the effect of the acid on growth.

   C. Do an experiment similar to (b) but add 10, 20, 30, 40, and 50 cc. of ethanol (use twice that amount of 100-proof vodka) before sterilizing. Examine the effect of ethanol on growth of the molds (you can also do it with other microbes).

   D. Do an experiment similar to (b) but add 10, 20, 30, 40, 50, 60, 70, 80, 90, and 100 g. of sucrose before sterilizing. Examine the effect of sucrose (i.e., reduced a_w) on the growth of molds or other organisms.

3. Get fresh apple cider (unprocessed with no additives). Pour similar quantities into a small heat-resistant jar (about one-half pint) and heat the cider in a water bath at 60°C for 2, 4, 6, 8, 10, 12, etc., to 20 minutes. Determine the time needed to preserve it. Higher heating temperatures can also be used but the heating time segments should be decreased.

4. Prepare saturated salt slurries of the following salts (obtained from a pharmacy or science lab):

	% ERH	a_W
$Mg(NO_3)_2 \cdot 6H_2O$	55	0.55
NaCl	75	0.75
Li_2SO_4	85	0.85
NA_2HPO_4	95	0.95

Place the slurries in the bottom of individual small (one-gallon) fish tanks and put a platform (plastic strawberry basket) above the solution. Cover the tanks with glass or plastic. Take fresh white bread (one homemade without preservatives and one with calcium propionate) and put a small piece (about ¼ slice with no crust) of each into each tank. After two to three days spread some mold spores on each slice. Determine how long it takes for the mold to grow at room temperature.

5. Obtain a copy of the article, "Hazard Analysis of Home Recipe Methods" by Dr. E. Zottola and I. Wolf (*Journal of Food Protection,* vol. 44, p. 560, 1981). Discuss the use of this for typical meals you prepare or are served in the school/office cafeteria.

6. Read the Food and Drug Administration's regulations on Good Manufacturing Practices in 21 CFR Part 110. Try to figure out which factors they consider most important in a process. Then visit a food plant and try to identify the critical control points.

7. Obtain the September 1981 issue of *Scientific American.* The whole issue deals with genetic engineering. Read it and try to project which factors will be most important to both nutrition and food processing.

Chapter 15. Answers to Multiple-Choice Study Questions: 1, D; 2, E; 3, C; 4, E; 5, A; 6, D.

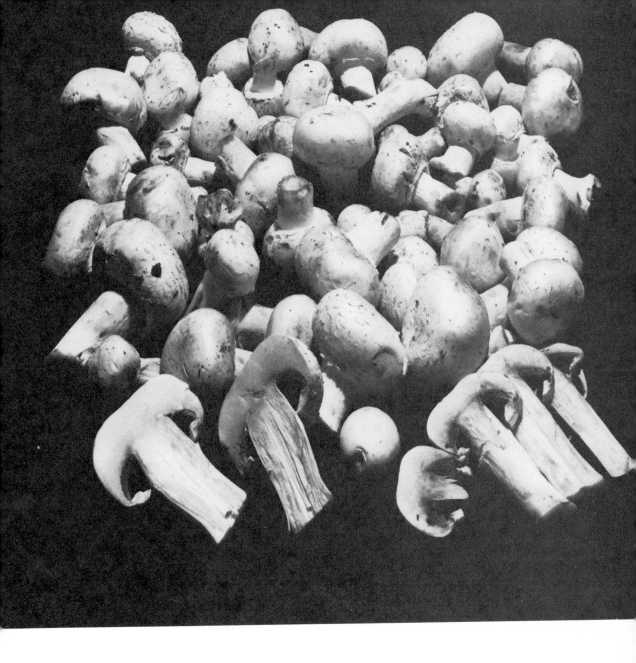

16

FOOD-BORNE DISEASE:
THE HARMFUL GERMS

The diseases discussed in this chapter are those that occur as the result of consumption of foods that carry toxic materials produced by microbes or from microbes themselves that cause infection. As should be obvious by now, sanitation and proper processing and proper preparation and handling of the finished food should prevent disease. However, food-borne diseases still occur because many people do not follow sanitary practices. The Center for Disease Control (CDC) of the United States Public Health Service estimates that over 94% of the incidents of food poisoning occur because people in the home or in the food service establishment do not follow or are unaware of good sanitation and health practices. Less than 6% of food poisoning incidents are caused by unsanitary conditions during food processing. This is a small percentage. It shows that where the right food-processing procedures are carried out, such as HACCPs, health protection can be maintained. However, the major efforts of the Food and Drug Administration (FDA) to prevent food-borne disease are still based on control at the industrial processing level through regulations and inspections. This is because the industry produces large batches of foods. Thus, one incident of an unsanitary practice has the potential to result in disease for thousands of people.

It should be emphasized that food poisoning is really a variety of illnesses caused by foods. The expression "ptomaine poisoning" is a misnomer. Foods high in protein that become spoiled could smell very bad and cause vomiting if someone tried to eat them. The compounds formed in the breakdown of protein were generally called ptomaines, from which we get the inaccurate label "ptomaine poisoning." But foods containing food poisoning organisms may carry few or almost no off-flavors or odors. The poisoned food may look and taste all right but still could cause an illness. One cannot use odor or flavor to determine that a food can cause a disease or illness.

FOOD INTOXICATIONS

Food intoxications are caused by organisms that grow on foods and produce harmful or lethal chemicals called toxins. *Clostridium botulinum, Staphylococcus aureus,* and some molds produce harmful toxins that can cause diarrhea and even death in humans. Other intoxications can occur from foods being contaminated with harmful chemicals such as arsenic, mercury, PCBs (polychlorinated-biphenyls), or vinyl chloride monomers, although these intoxications are not the result of microbial growth.

Mold Intoxications

Human poisoning from molds that produce toxins in foods is uncommon in the United States but has occurred repeatedly in other parts of the world. In the Orient, cooked rice that is allowed to remain at room temperature for several days is susceptible to the growth of a very lethal mold. This green mold, *Aspergillus flavus,* produces a toxin—aflatoxin—that kills ducks or turkeys when present in their feed even in small doses. The toxin is suspected of causing death in many young children in the Orient, especially in Thailand and Laos. The toxin can also cause liver cancer if consumed in low doses over a long period of time. Foods containing this toxin in the United States can be impounded and destroyed by the FDA. Contamination can occur when cottonseed, cereal grains, and peanuts are not dried long enough before being held in silos or grain elevators, especially when there is a lot of rain around harvest time. If the percent ERH of the grain is above 80%, the mold can grow and produce the toxin. The toxin can be discovered by using a black light because the chemical, if present, will fluoresce. The FDA has set a maximum of 20 µg/kg. of food or 20 parts per billion (ppb) for the toxin. This means that in one billion pounds of food there cannot be more than 20 pounds of the toxin distributed evenly throughout it. Based on animal studies, the FDA feels that this amount will cause no harm to humans. Any food with greater than this level is considered to be adulterated and subject to seizure and destruction. Mixing a batch of cereal grains of high levels with one of low level to achieve less than 20 ppb in the final batch is also illegal. Because it is consumed by infants and children, milk has a lower action level, 0.5 ppb. To insure that processed foods are free from aflatoxin, HACCP procedure demands constant testing of potentially hazardous ingredients and maintenance of low humidity storage conditions for susceptible foods.

Another potent toxin, ergotamine, is produced from the mold *Calviceps purpurea.* Many thousands of Russians died during World War II when they consumed rye and wheat contaminated with this mold. The cereals were left in the field during the winter and were not harvested until the following spring when the soldiers had returned from the battlefront. The mold grew and produced the toxin on the grain, since the ERH was high under the snow. One should never eat cereal products that have a purple mold growing on them, since it could be this organism. The chemical is similar to LSD but will cause death if a high enough dose is ingested. A major incident occurred in 1953 in Pont Esprit, France, from contaminated rye. Recent meteorological and anthropological evidence also suggests that the Salem Witch trials may have had their origins in the population eating rye contaminated with ergotamine.

The way to prevent intoxication from molds is to handle peanuts, grains, and cereals properly by controlling the percent ERH or by heat treating to kill the spores before they germinate. Methods to detect the toxin must also be found, and the contaminated food should be destroyed. However, in the future, when food is less available to the world, we may have to find a method to get rid of the toxin once present in the food. Current food laws and regulations do not allow us to do this in the United States.

Patulin, a toxin produced by many common mold species that grow on cheese and bread, has only recently been identified. How dangerous it is to humans is not known. The best precaution is to not eat moldy bread and to cut off the area of cheese where a mold contaminant may have grown. This means that certain cheeses that rely on mold fermentation, such as Brie, Camembert, and Roquefort, have a potential for risk from toxins. This is a good example of the risk/benefit decision mentioned earlier. Since we do not really know the risk, the aesthetic benefit of consuming these cheeses, especially with a good wine, may far outweigh the risk. With the advent of sophisticated analytical techniques that can find chemicals at the ppb and even ppt level (i.e., one part in a trillion), one can expect the identification of many more toxicants from molds that grow on the foods we eat. The important issue will be how we classify these risks and how the Food and Drug Administration will regulate them.

Bacterial Food Intoxication

Bacteria are probably the biggest cause of food intoxication diseases for humans. Some of the important organisms will be discussed individually.

Botulism. *Clostridium botulinum* is an anaerobic spore-forming bacteria that can grow in low-acid foods. Its spores are ubiquitous and can be found in the ground that vegetables grow in. The biggest potential for the outgrowth of the spore is in a canned food which by the nature of the process has an anaerobic environment. If the food is underprocessed, that is, it is not given a long enough heat treatment, the spores may not have been completely killed. *Clostridium botulinum* spores have one of the highest resistances to heat of all bacteria spores. Since the oxygen has been completely removed from the can, the spores if present can germinate, and the cells can grow at room temperature. A toxin is produced by the growing cells that is very deadly. It is a protein and is one of the most toxic chemicals known to humans. An amount equal to about one-half pound is enough to kill everyone in the United States. The disease is called botulism.

Botulism poisoning symptoms can occur from about one to seven days after the ingestion of the toxin. Botulism poisoning used to be about 50% fatal, but because of the use of anti-toxins and early recognition of symptoms, this has dropped to less than 20%. Symptoms, which are similar to those of a stroke, include double vision and muscular paralysis. Death occurs because nerve transmission fails, resulting in respiratory arrest (an inability to breathe). The simple procedure of boiling low-acid canned foods for ten minutes prior to consumption would prevent the poisoning. Since the toxin is heat-sensitive it would be destroyed. This suggests that the common practice of eating from a can of food before heating is not a good idea. It also suggests that canned foods (low-acid type) that are not typically heated before eating, such as sardines, tuna, or mushrooms may present a greater safety hazard. Some canned foods such as tomatoes, citrus juices, and pickled produce are safe because the organism cannot grow in acid conditions (a pH less than 4.6). To avoid contracting this disease, one should not eat food from smelly, damaged, or bulging cans although the toxin can be present without any off-odors. Technically all low-acid canned foods should be cooked before consumption. The amount of botulism that occurs in the United States is small, however, because of the controls industry and the FDA requires. The outbreaks are mainly due to consuming home-canned foods that have been underprocessed and fermented foods that are not acid enough. Alaska has the highest incidence of botulism in the United States, mainly from improperly preserved home foods such as smoked salmon.

In 1980 a botulism incident occurred when people ate potato salad in a restaurant. After careful sleuthing, the FDA found that the cook had baked potatoes in their skins covered with foil for a banquet. There were some leftover potatoes. Unfortunately, the unused baked potatoes were not refrigerated but kept at room temperature in the foil. The next day the cook removed the foil, cut open the potatoes, and used them to make a potato salad. Subsequent consumption of the salad made many people ill. Unknown to the cook, the baking of the potatoes set up the incident. Baking is not hot enough to kill botulinum spores but it killed all the bacteria competitors. The heat also drove out the air, setting up anaerobic conditions on the skin. Potato skins that touch the dirt underground are a good source of the spores. Thus we had a sensitive ingredient (Hazard Class I), and an incomplete process (Hazard Class II). The next culprit was the mishandling by the cook (Hazard Class III) in letting the potatoes stay at room temperature, which is in the optimal growth range for the organism. The spores germinated, produced toxin, and then the toxin became part of the salad. How many times do we have close calls like this at home without knowing it? Botulism has also been associated with the death of infants given honey since the honey is a good source of the spores. The infant does not have a very acid stomach, so the spores can outgrow there. Then the cells produce toxin in the intestine in the infants that leads to rapid death.

Staphylococcus Food Poisoning.   One of the most common types of food poisoning in the United States is the result of foods containing the toxin formed by *Staphylococcus aureus*. In 1978 this toxin accounted for about 30% of all individual cases of food poisoning. Symptoms occur within two to four hours after consumption of the contaminated food. The symptoms include explosive diarrhea, vomiting, dehydration, and abdominal cramps. The disease lasts about 24 hours. It is so violent that those who get it often wish they were dead. Unfortunately, the very old and the very young react much more violently to the intoxication.

This intoxication is most commonly associated with cream-filled pastries, salted meats and sausage, and with tuna salad, chicken salad, and similar mixtures, especially when made for picnics. The myth that mayonnaise causes this food poisoning is common but untrue. The actual cause is dilution of the acid of the mayonnaise with sensitive (Hazard Class I) food ingredients coupled with unsanitary food preparation (Hazard Class III). The organisms can grow in the system if the addition of food raises the pH above 4.6 (Hazard Class II). The organisms, however, can enter the food only if there is unsanitary food preparation or use of a contaminated ingredient. *S. aureus* can be present in all parts of the human body, especially in small cuts, in boils and around the mouth and nose. People often do not clean their hands before making salad mixtures by hand. They also do not follow good sanitary practices of not scratching various parts of the face while making the food.

Usually salt, sugar, or acid, such as that found in mayonnaise, is added to the foods associated with this intoxication. Since the organism is resistant to moderate concentrations of these water binders and chemical inhibitors, conditions are set up that allow growth of the *Staphylococcus aureus* but that prevent growth of other competing bacteria. Rapid growth occurs if the food is left unrefrigerated. If quickly cooled to below 45°F the food presents no hazard. Thus sanitary habits and refrigeration are important for preventing the growth of *S. aureus*. Cooking the finished food does no good since the toxin, once produced, is heat resistant and cooking does not destroy it. Refrigeration is imperative because the organism is a mesophile and cannot grow below 45°F. All foods should be rapidly chilled.

One of the most famous cases of staphylococcus food poisoning occurred in 1975 when an airline had improperly prepared (Hazard Class III) a ham and egg omelette mixture for a breakfast on a large charter plane. The cook had a cut on his hand that was infected. The pus from it must have contaminated the omelette during preparation. The organisms grew on the ham/egg interface since he left the mixture at room temperature and the reduced water activity and higher salt content of the ham favored the growth of the *S.*

aureus. The meals were placed on the plane the next morning as it came in for refueling in Anchorage, Alaska, on the way from Japan. After take-off the meal was heated and served. Remember that cooking does not destroy the toxin. Several hours later, on the way to Copenhagen, out over the Arctic, over 150 people became violently ill. The plane had no place to put down so they had to go on. One can imagine the scene with very few restrooms and 150 people with violent diarrhea, cramps, and vomiting. Fortunately, everyone recovered, but the head chef of the airline was so upset that he later committed suicide. The latest data available in the United States is for 1978 and indicates that there were three confirmed deaths from *S. aureus* intoxication that year. These could have been prevented.

Clostridium perfringens. Food poisoning from the bacteria *Clostridium perfringens* is another one of the most common forms of food poisoning. Because it is rarely recognized it accounts for only 8% of confirmed outbreaks. The disease can be classified both as an intoxication and as an infection. Symptoms of this food poisoning are mild cramps and diarrhea occurring about 4–22 hours after eating, similar to the symptoms for the 24-hour flu. This food poisoning is usually contracted from meats, eggs, gravies, and other protein foods. The organism is a rod-shaped spore-former with high heat resistance. The spore is usually present on all foods including meats when tested (Hazard Class I).

The way the toxin is produced is unusual. For example, cooking roast beef in an oven will kill the growing cells, which are normally present, but it does not kill all the spores since they are much more heat resistant. If the roast is immediately cooled, there is no problem. Similarly, if it is held for at least 15 minutes at >60°C and then cooled it will be safe. Holding the meat, however, for a long time at serving temperature (<140°F) as is done in many homes and restaurants, especially under infra-red warming lamps, will activate the spores to the growing vegetative state. We then eat the food. Once the live cells are inside the intestine, the adverse conditions cause spores to form again. In the process a toxin is produced. If a large enough number of organisms are ingested and a great enough amount of toxin is formed the disease results. Sanitation, such as using clean utensils, is only slightly important in the prevention of this disease. More important is good handling through the rapid cooling of meats and gravies if they have to be held for any length of time. If the food must be served warm, it should be held above 65°C (150°F) to prevent growth of the *Clostridium perfringens* microorganism. Unfortunately, holding at the higher temperature also destroys nutrients and causes loss of eating quality (no rare roast beef) so keeping it cold after rapid cooling is preferred. When needed it should then be warmed. This illness is especially prevalent because of the improper practice of keeping meats and gravies warm in food service places such as restaurants. A common home practice is also responsible—the practice of letting hot meat cool down slowly before refrigeration. Most meats and gravies should be refrigerated as soon as possible after serving or cooking. The problem with this disease is that it is so mild it is not recognized as food poisoning; we confuse it with a 24-hour flu.

Others.   There are many new food intoxications from other organisms, such as *Bacillus cereus*, that microbiologists are discovering. Their significance to human disease has not yet been established so it is not known whether we should worry about them. In any case, if we follow the HACCP principles we should be able to prevent problems.

Chemical Food Intoxication

There are many foods in their natural state that contain toxins. Manioca (tapioca) and soybeans contain toxins that are destroyed through processing. Many species of mushrooms, such as the Amanita species, as well as some species of fish , contain deadly poisons. It is important to know which foods are poisonous. Some of these will be discussed in Chapter 26. It should be noted that many plants contain various chemicals that are extracted for use as drugs. If taken in large doses, death could occur from some of these chemicals, but if used cautiously they provide a benefit.

There are also intoxications from eating food that has become contaminated with an industrial chemical. Accidental spills of chemicals, such as PCBs or dioxin, on feed grain have caused the death of many animals. Some people have also eaten seed grain that was treated with a mercury fungicide. It caused death and deformities. Unfortunately, they had not read the label to see that there was a warning against eating the seeds. The fungicide was to prevent mold from growing so the seeds could be used for planting without rotting.

Under the Food, Drug and Cosmetic Act all foods that contain poisonous and deleterious substances are considered adulterated and subject to seizure. The law does however, recognize the problem that even foods in the natural state contain some poisonous substances, so these foods are exempted if the level of the toxin is low enough to "not render the food injurious to health." The problem is that there are many synthetic and other chemicals that have increased in the environment, thereby contaminating raw foods, including banned pesticides, PCBs, PBBs, mercury, etc. The courts recognized that they might have to ban all foods if the law was carried out to the letter. Thus, the FDA has set tolerances and action levels in foods for these poisonous or deleterious substances. An action level is based on the fact that new technology may come about to help reduce the level in the environment and/or the food in the near future while the tolerance level is based on the fact that there does not exist a known potential way to reduce the level. Action levels are generally set near the level at which the chemical can be detected in the food. Tolerances and action levels have been set for PCBs, the banned pesticides Aldrin, Dieldrin, and DDT, lead, mercury, and many other substances. THe FDA can prevent a company from selling foods that are above the action level for a substance. The list of levels can be obtained from: Food and Drug Administration, Industry Program Branch, Bureau of Foods HFF–326, 200 C St. S.W., Washington, D.C. 20204

FOOD INFECTIONS

Food infections are caused by bacteria that grow rapidly in the intestinal tract of humans causing diarrhea, vomiting, and other unpleasant symptoms. The bacteria enter the body on food we eat that is contaminated. *Salmonella* species are common infectious types of bacteria that can grow in food as a result of improper processing or handling (Hazard Class II or III). When consumed, these bacteria subsequently cause a serious food infection in our intestinal tract. The reasons that they contaminate foods will be discussed below along with the methods of prevention. Other food infection organisms include *Vibrio parahemolyticus* present in shellfish, *Escherichia coli,* which sometimes causes Montezuma's Revenge, and various cholera species. Other food infections include viral hepatitis and parasites transmitted from animals, such as trichinosis from pork and toxoplasmosis from beef.

The Center for Disease Control (CDC) in Atlanta, Georgia, run by the United States Public Health Service, attempts to collect data on food poisoning throughout the United States. Since 1973 there have been approximately 14,000 cases of food poisoning reported to them every year. Those cases occurred in about 300–350 outbreaks per year. An outbreak is an incident whereas the case is an individual. On the average an outbreak is responsible for making 40 people ill. It is estimated however that over 200 million cases of food poisonings occur every year. These cases are not reported either because the disease is not recognized as food poisoning or because not enough evidence is collected to verify it as such. Many states just don't have the facilities to investigate.

Salmonella

Reporting of confirmed outbreaks of Salmonellosis was on the decline in the early 1970s but increased again in 1975. Salmonellosis still accounted for about 25% of all confirmed outbreaks of food poisoning. The major symptoms of salmonellosis are vomiting, diarrhea, and fever, similar to other food poisonings. One type of salmonella poisoning organism is transmitted in water contaminated by sewage. If we drink the water we could get typhoid fever.

The salmonella organisms normally inhabit the large intestines of humans and animals. The species that causes food poisoning may get into the food supply by contamination from fecal matter because of improper toilet habits or from poor sanitation (Hazard Class III). If the food is high in protein (Hazard Class I) growth will occur when the temperature is kept at 80–100°F (about 25–37°C). Over 70% of all salmonellosis cases are the result of eating contaminated meats and poultry.

The food-related organism is *Salmonella typhimurium*. It has been associated with meat and poultry processed under unsanitary conditions in some slaughterhouses. Under poor sanitary process conditions, fecal matter from the intestines of diseased animals contaminates the edible meat or poultry (Hazard Class II). If the meat is held warm, the organism can multiply. Once ingested the organisms grow rapidly in the intestine of humans and cause severe reactions. Symptoms are usually not evident until about 7 to 72 hours after eating and can last for about 48 hours causing severe dehydration. Young children and elderly people, having less resistance, are severely affected by salmonellosis. In some cases they die. In 1978 there was only one confirmed death but since then several serious incidents in nursing homes have occurred.

Good process control, personal sanitation, and adequate refrigeration are the primary methods for preventing food poisoning from *Salmonellae*. Hands should always be washed and gloves should be worn when preparing foods. Do we ever do this at home? It is not usually necessary if we eat the food rapidly after cooking since the level of contamination is low. In addition, if the food is cooked properly, the organism is killed because it cannot survive high heat. Usually what happens, however, is that a contaminated roast is first prepared on a wooden cutting board and then roasted. The board, if used again for slicing the meat after cooking, but before washing, will recontaminate the roast or other foods. The roast if then kept unrefrigerated for a long enough time serves as a good medium for growth of the bacteria. Good sanitation and good personal toilet habits are important means of prevention. It has been estimated that the real cost to the economy from salmonellosis infections alone may exceed one billion dollars.

Pet turtles have been banned from sale in the United States because they harbor this organism in their intestinal tract. Many young children have been poisoned by handling these turtles or the water in which they live. Salmonellae-free turtles have recently become available but they may still be a potential hazard.

Vibrio Parahemolyticus

This organism has been implicated in food infections only since 1970. In 1978 there was one confirmed outbreak affecting 82 people. It is an organism associated with seafood because it can grow in salt water. The symptoms are like those of other food poisonings. About four to eight hours after consumption of the food, vomiting, cramps, and diarrhea occur. A fever that lasts one to two days may occur. The organism is easily destroyed by cooking, but eating raw oysters and clams can be a hazard. Good sanitation and rinsing the shellfish in clean chlorinated water are good precautionary measures.

Parasite Infections

There are probably many parasite infections transmitted to humans by animals, but very little is known about them. Amoebic dysentery is caused by a parasite common to many parts of the world. At the present time it is very difficult to kill this parasite once it is in the body, so it is possible for humans to carry it around for many years. It infects those who eat fresh produce such as fruits and vegetables that have been contaminated as a result of the use of fecal matter (night soil) for fertilizer. In many parts of the world people must wash their fruits and vegetables with a chlorine solution before eating them. This destroys the organisms but makes the food taste terrible.

Schistosomiasis. Schistosomiasis, another infection is one of the most prevalent diseases in the world, although it is not common in the United States and is not a disease transmitted by food itself. This disease, which is caused by a parasite transmitted by snails, afflicts people who work in rice paddies or other aqua culture. The snails bite the humans, allowing the parasite to enter the body. The afflicted person develops a wasting anemia-type disease because the parasite feeds on the blood cells and destroys them. Life expectancy after infection is about two to three years unless treated. Unfortunately the best medicine for combatting this disease has also been shown to cause mutations in rats. The advisability of using the medicine is under dispute since it could possibly cause human mutations; however, no other drug has been found to be as effective.

Trichinella.   Trichinella is a parasite carried in pork as well as in other animals. The disease trichinosis can result in liver and brain damage and eventually death if contaminated pork is eaten.

In most cases severe reactions are rare. There has been little evidence of this parasite in USDA-inspected meat over the last 40 years but the disease still occurs in areas where people consume meat that has not been inspected. The meat is either game meat, such as bear, or from pigs fed unsterilized garbage. In 1978 there were six outbreaks affecting 12 people while in 1981 the CDC reported 206 cases, 70% of which were from pork. The animals came mostly from small farms in the northeast. One way in which food animals such as pigs can get the infection is from wild animal droppings. Thorough cooking or freezing of pork for several weeks can kill these parasites. This is still recommended today, since the USDA does not inspect for trichinella. Instead they rely on consumer education to encourage people to properly cook the meat. Because of the increased incidence of trichinosis, the USDA is considering putting cooking information on the package label for pork products.

An internal temperature of 140°F (60°C) is more than enough to kill the parasite. One must be careful with microwaves; since the food heats up so fast longer cooking times are needed. Pork or pork products are responsible for about 80% of the outbreaks of trichinosis, ground beef for 8%, and bear meat for 5%. Cattle do not carry the parasite, but beef gets contaminated when it is ground in a meat grinder that has not been washed after it was used for pork.

SUMMARY

The most common food poisonings in this country are due to the presence and growth of harmful microorganisms in food, although chemicals have also been implicated as causes. Those microbes from food that grow directly in the human body and affect it are called infections and are much like an infection in a wound. Other microorganisms produce chemicals that are toxic to humans causing a disease called a food intoxication. Molds are common sources of toxic materials especially *Aspergillus flavus* which produces aflatoxin in peanuts and cereal grains. Control of the equilibrium relative humidity (ERH) of the grain is the best method of prevention. Many bacteria also produce toxins. The two most important are *Clostridium botulinum,* which is involved in underprocessed canned foods, and *Staphylococcus aureus,* which is involved in high sugar and salt

TABLE 16.1 United States statistics: food-borne disease

Disease	1969 [a] Outbreak	1969 Cases	1970 [a] Outbreak	1970 Cases	1972 Outbreak	1972 Cases	1973 Outbreak	1973 Cases	1978 Outbreak	1978 Cases
Staphylococcal	55(39) [b]	2,809	42(60)	2,881	34	1,948	20	1,272	25	1,493
Salmonellosis [a]	40(9)	1,770	44(4)	4,699	36	1,880	33	2,462	50	1,883
Colstridium perfringens	36(29)	16,825	14(40)	2,574	9	973	9	1,424	9	617
Botulism	9(1)	15	6(1)	13	4	24	10	31	12	58
Bacillus cereus	3	14	2(1)	46	–	–	1	2	6	248
Shigellosis [a]	10	1,444	8	1,668	3	86	8	1,388	3	163
Streptococcal pharyngitis										
Enterococcal gastroenteritis	2(2)	32	(1)		1	35	1	250	–	–
Vibrio parahemolyticus	(2)		(2)		1	50	–		1	58
E. Coli	2(3)	276	4(3)	240	6	701	1	2	1	82
Giardia lamblia infections	1	19			1	39	–	–	1	35
Trichinosis	11	35	9	41	8	20	10	59	–	–
Viral hepatitis	9	116	4	107	5	90	5	425	6	12
Mushroom poisonings	2(2)	6			9	21	9	41	4	267
Other toxic plants	1				1	–	–		1	7
Toxic fish and shellfish poisonings	4		(1)		9	82	14	333	30	96
Heavy metal poisonings	4		3	15	3	8			1	41
Other chemical poisonings	16(5)	125	3(13)	24	6	35	5	18	5	19
Unknown or unconfirmed	166	5,077	227	11,140	165	8,567	181	4,735	300	8,611
Total	371	28,563	366	23,448	301	14,559	307	12,442	457	13,709

[a] Includes water-borne outbreaks

[b] Numbers in parentheses refer to unconfirmed outbreaks

Center for Disease Control U.S. Dept. of Public Health. 1978 is the latest data available.

content foods. Another food intoxication, caused by *Clostridium perfringens*, is so mild that very few people recognize it as such. However, it is the result of the common practice of not cooling meats rapidly enough. Of the organisms that cause food infection the *Salmonella* species is the most important. As with other food infections, good sanitary practices, rapid cooling, and refrigeration are the most important preventive measures. Food poisoning, a serious threat to the people of this country, could be prevented by understanding these principles. It is estimated that the average cost per person for food poisoning is over $400, including the medical expenses and lost time on the job. This amounts to a cost close to $100 billion per year. Table 16.1 lists the number of cases of various food-borne diseases investigated and reported by the CDC from 1969 to 1978, the last year for which data have been compiled. This should give the reader some idea of the tip of the iceberg, since most cases are not reported. Also listed in Table 16.1 are some food-borne diseases that we have not discussed but are important as well.

Multiple Choice Study Questions

1. Most food-related diseases in the U.S. are found

A. at McDonald's
B. in food produced by the food industry
C. in homes and food service establishments
D. at General Mills
E. at the Bon Vivant Company

2. Which of the following does not cause a food intoxication?

A. *Clostridium botulinum*
B. *Aspergillus flavus*
C. *Caviceps purpurea*
D. *Staphylococcus aureus*
E. *Salmonellae typhimurium*

3. It has been reported that the hysteria of the Salem Witch Trials may have been the result of

A. consumption of cheese that had been contaminated by patulin
B. consuming raw milk
C. consuming rye grain that had ergot
D. consuming too much alcohol
E. consuming aflatoxin

4. Which of the following conditions is the most likely to permit growth of *Clostridium botulinum?*

    A. acid foods in anaerobic package
    B. low-acid foods in aerobic package
    C. refrigerated milk
    D. dried green beans in an anaerobic package
    E. low-acid foods in an anaerobic package

5. Which one of the following organisms causes a food infection?

    A. *Clostridium botulinum*
    B. *Staphylococcus aureus*
    C. *Saccharomyces cerevisiae*
    D. *Salmonellae typhimurium*

6. Which food poisoning usually shows up the fastest?

    A. botulism
    B. perfringens
    C. staphylococcus
    D. salmonellosis

The following is a list of food poisoning organisms. Use it to answer questions 7 through 16.

    A. *Clostridium perfringens*
    B. *Salmonella*
    C. *Staphylococcus aureus*
    D. *Clostridium botulinum*
    E. *Trichinosis*

7. Which organism is associated with the "mayonnaise" disease?

8. Which one is the suspected cause of the "Roast Beef" disease?

9. Which organism causes death from paralysis, with the first symptom being double vision?

10. Which organism produces explosive diarrhea in two to four hours after eating the contaminated food?

11. Which organism is associated with fecal matter?

12. Which organism is the basis for preservation in canning?

13. Which organism produces a very mild disease like 24-hour flu?

14. Which organism is associated with boils and cuts?

15. Which organism produces a toxin that is stable to heating?

16. Which organism is associated with disease from wild game, especially bear meat?

Essay Study Questions

1. Define food infection and food intoxication.

2. What problems occur with the growth of *Aspergillus flavus* in foods? How can they be controlled?

3. Discuss the problem of botulism poisoning.

4. Describe the process by which *Staphylococcus aureus* can contaminate foods. Indicate the symptoms of the disease and what the hazard analysis would show.

5. Why is *Clostridium perfringens* intoxication so common? How can it be prevented?

6. Discuss the importance of *Salmonella* food infections and how they can be prevented.

7. What is the significance of parasite infection diseases in the United States?

8. How great is the overall problem of food poisoning in the United States?

Things to Do

1. Visit the local public health authorities. Obtain information from them on cases of food-borne disease occurring in your area. Discuss the incidents in class.

2. Try to find people who have had a case of food poisoning. Interview them to try to determine which disease it was and the food that caused it.

3. Visit a local food-processing plant. Discuss with the manager the steps they take to prevent food-borne illnesses. Identify the critical control points.

4. Watch the sanitary habits of your family in food preparation. Try to list the good and bad points. Explain to them why they should change, if necessary.

Chapter 16. Answers to Multiple-Choice Study Questions: 1, C; 2, E; 3, C; 4, E; 5, D; 6, C; 7, C; 8, A; 9, A; 10, C; 11, B; 12, D; 13, A; 14, C; 15, C; 16, E.

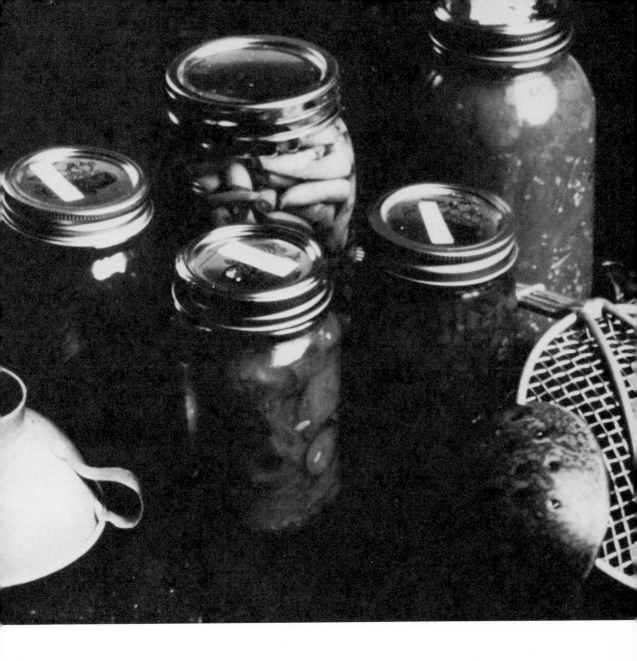

HEAT PRESERVATION
OF FOODS: CANNING

17

HISTORY OF HEAT PROCESSING

Napoleon was partly responsible for stimulating the development of canning foods. Around 1780 he needed a means of supplying meats, fruits, and milk to his troops during lengthy campaigns away from home. He set up a Society for the Encouragement of Industry that offered prizes for methods that would help industry.

By this time a Frenchman, Nicholas Appert, had already devised a heat preservation process. It was referred to as "Appertizing." His process involved placing food in glass bottles wrapped in burlap. The top was left open so that the air inside could escape when the bottles filled with the food were heated in a boiling water bath. After boiling for a given length of time, Appert put waxed corks in the bottle opening and wired the bottle shut. The bottles were then allowed to remain in the boiling water for a further period of time, after which he held them at room temperature for a two-month period. During this storage, some of the bottles exploded; from this he deduced that the products had not been processed long enough. He then experimented with longer cooking times to find the time that gave a stable food. For some foods, such as meat or vegetables, he found that four to six hours of boiling were needed. Appert sold his products in his shop in Paris. In 1809, a French newspaper wrote, "At his hand, spring, summer, and autumn live in a bottle." In 1809 the Society for the Encouragement of Industry offered Appert a prize of 12,000 francs if he would publish his method, which he did in 1810 as a patent.

Durand, an Englishman, secured the rights to the French patent with the addition of enclosing the food in vessels other than bottles. He sold this patent to three Englishmen for 1,000£ in 1811. By 1813 they began production of foods in "tin cannisters," the origin of our "tin can." The tin cans had a small hole in the top. The hole was soldered shut after heating the food for the required time. These cans were hard to make (10 per worker per day) and also had to be opened with a hammer and chisel. However, the idea caught on and their shop supplied the Royal Navy, Admiral Ross on his Arctic expeditions, and consumers. The concept was brought to the United States by William Underwood (of Deviled Ham fame) who set up shop in 1820 in Boston canning seafood. New methods were eventually developed to make cans more easily but there were still problems.

The "Appertizing" or canning process was based on the belief that when the food was heated, the oxygen was forced out of the container so it couldn't react with the food. In this manner the food was preserved from spoiling since it was felt that without air, spontaneous generation or spoilage could not occur. Joseph Louis Gay-Lussac, a French chemist, strongly supported this idea. He had a method of testing for the presence of oxygen and found that food that was Appertized did not contain oxygen.

During the years from 1820 to 1880, some owners of food-canning factories played the roles of magicians. Some of them would enter their plants during the canning process wearing magicians' costumes. They would mumble mystical incantations over the boiling water baths and throw handfuls of a mysterious white powder into each vat. By adding the special powders, they found they could reduce the process time needed for canning foods, in some instances from four hours down to only two hours. Many guilds developed that used these techniques. The basis of the effect, the addition of salts such as sodium chloride or calcium chloride, was that it raised the boiling point of the water in which the foods were being preserved. Instead of heating at 212°F (100°C), which is the normal boiling point of water, the foods were being processed at temperatures of up to 240°F (115°C). This reduced the needed process time but processors did not really understand why.

By 1875 retorts or autoclaves were devised. These are large pressure cookers that achieved a higher temperature. Interestingly, the commercial retorts of this period sometimes exploded after six or seven months' use; because of the lack of adequate metal technology and high-quality steel, they couldn't operate under such high temperatures. This inhibited the canning industry for some time but stimulated the iron industry to search for methods to produce stronger steel. Today the industry uses retorts that can process foods at temperatures as high as 280°F (138°C).

Prior to 1860 most scientists believed that food spoiled as a result of spontaneous generation, the creation of living organisms from nonliving matter in the presence of air or oxygen. This theory was well supported by some scientists and philosophers. The discovery of oxygen helped to further promulgate the concept. During the late 1860s, however, Pasteur discovered that microbes were the main cause of food spoilage. Taking this idea in the late 1880s, a professor of biology at the Massachusetts Institute of Technology, Samuel Cate Prescott, and Mr. Underwood whom we mentioned earlier, began a study of the microbiology of the canning process. They, along with W. Russel at the University of Wisconsin who was doing similar research, conclusively proved that the basis of canning was the thermal destruction of very heat-resistant spores. Thus they did for the canned-food industry what Pasteur did for the beer and wine industry. Eventually the work showed that the process had to be based on killing the most heat-resistant pathogen, *Clostridium botulinum*, in order to make the food safe. By 1920 C. Olin Ball of Rutgers University published equations by which processors today still calculate the safe process time based on the can size and temperature used. To be safe, however, processors verify the correct heating time by inoculating cans with test microorganisms and then determining if any are left after the heat treatment. Because of the safety factors needed, the calculated process sometimes leads to overprocessing of food from a nutritional standpoint. Newer techniques of heat processing are being investigated to help maximize nutritional value while maintaining safety. Since 1979 all processors who process foods with a pH greater than 4.6 and a water activity greater than 0.85 (85% EHR) in hermetically sealed containers (cans, bottles, pouches, etc.) must register their process with the FDA according to 21 CFR 113, which are the CGMPs for canning low acid foods. This means that the company must provide information that the sterilization process is adequate before the food can be put into interstate commerce. In addition, one of the plant personnel directly responsible for the retorting operation (heating in the pressure vessel) must have attended a special school on thermal processing that gives instructions in HACCP (Hazard Analysis and Critical Control Point) methods that insure safety. The regulations also require keeping track of the process time and the temperature of the retort for every batch. This is an excellent example of a microbiological critical control point based on a Class II Hazard (process control) that was discussed earlier.

THE SAFETY OF CANNED FOODS

The safety of canned foods is based on following 21 CFR 113, which insures that a properly processed product will not have any pathogenic organisms present in it. As Prescott and Underwood realized, the process should be oriented toward the pathogenic organism that would be most likely to pose the biggest problem in a given product. Since the canning process removes all the oxygen, those pathogenic organisms that grow in the absence of oxygen should be the most important. Thus *Clostridium botulinum,* which grows in the absence of air under low-acid conditions and has spores that are more resistant to heat treatment than most other microorganisms, became the basis for the evaluation of the safety of the canning process. The overall heat-processing time, however, is based on other microorganisms as well, which are even more heat resistant than *Clostridium botulinum.* This is done to provide an added safety factor, and because many of these more resistant spores are naturally present in food and could germinate and spoil the food during storage.

To understand how the process is calculated, let us examine the microbiology and heat transfer of the process. From a microbial standpoint, a drop of liquid can be packed with over one trillion tiny microorganisms of various types. A drop of food in the natural state can contain from 100 to several million of these organisms prior to processing. The different organisms are affected differently by heat, that is, they are destroyed at different rates. The rate of kill for each organism is also dependent on the temperature used, as illustrated in Figure 17.1. An equation for predicting how many organisms would die in the canning process can be formulated using this information if the temperature history of the food during processing is known. In order for the organisms to be destroyed, heat must penetrate into the interior, through the can and then the food. The slowest heating point in the can must be found because that is where the least amount of thermal destruction would occur. The processing time is then calculated, based on the amount of heat necessary to reduce the number of organisms to a level that their presence in any one can has a very low probability. If the organisms are destroyed to such a low probability at the slowest heating point, it can be assumed that the probability of destruction at all other places within the can is greater. In the case of solid-pack foods, such as ham or hash, the center of the can is the slowest heating point, whereas with liquid foods it is further down the central axis. Therefore, the temperature at that point, as a function of time, is used to determine the probability of kill. This is what Dr. Ball did in his mathematical evaluation of the process.

In order to insure safety of canned foods, all process calculations are based on the destruction of about one thousand billion spores (one trillion) of *Clostridium botulinum* at the slowest heating point. Since in general there are only about 100 organisms present at the slowest heating point, the food would end up being processed for a

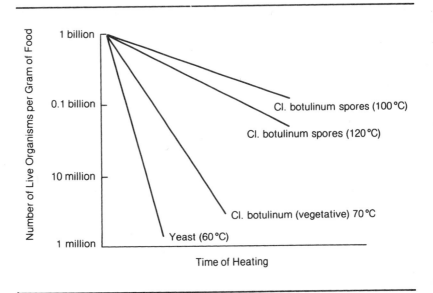

FIGURE 17.1 Effect of temperature on the number of microbial deaths as a function of time

time such that there is only about one chance in about 10 billion that one organism could survive in a can, grow, and produce toxin. Since the process used is longer to destroy potential storage organisms the probability in fact may be so infinitesimally small as to be meaningless.

Theoretically the higher the temperature of the process, the shorter the time needed to achieve the required safety factor. All canning processes for low-acid food theoretically operate with this safety factor. Hypothetically, if a canning plant were large enough to manufacture 10 billion cans of a food product from one batch at one time and it was given the minimum time required for botulism safety, one can should be unsafe. However, there are no canning plants in operation that have the facilities to process this number of cans in a single batch.

Some factor over and above the required botulinum kill is used by all processors because of the presence of more heat-resistant nonpathogenic mesophilic organisms. These organisms could grow at room temperature and spoil the food if not destroyed.

The reasons some commercially processed canned foods spoil are: (a) inadequate processes based on improper process times (too short for spoilage organisms); (b) improper sealing or damage to cans with subsequent recontamination by spores or bacteria; (c) growth of nontoxic, much more heat-resistant microbes (thermophiles) during storage, when held at high temperature. If the food were processed to completely destroy these latter thermophilic organisms, it would be too overcooked and would lose much of its quality and nutritional value.

High-acid (pH less than 4.6) foods do not have to be processed for botulinum because the organism cannot grow under acid conditions. For acid foods a process equivalent to a heating value needed to destroy a minimum of 100,000 spores is used. Because of this, a shorter time and lower temperature can be used. Thus a boiling water cooker is used; a retort is not needed. One problem, of course, is in mixing a low-acid food with a high-acid food such as meatballs with spaghetti sauce. Since the acid may not penetrate the meat, the more stringent process time must be used.

In fact, canned meat products do not come under the jurisdiction of the FDA. They are covered, rather, by the USDA whose regulations appear in 9 CFR 318.11 (Title 9 applies to meat food products). The regulations are not as stringently written as are the FDA's. However, meat is processed under continuous inspection, and samples of each retort batch have to be held at 95°F for 10 days prior to shipping the batch. This incubation should be enough to allow the botulinum spores to outgrow if present, produce gas, and swell the can. The USDA is, however, considering adopting the FDA requirements.

**HOME
CANNING**

Home-canned food has been responsible for over 90% of the outbreaks of botulism in this country over the past 70 years. In the last 20 years, home canning has probably resulted in an average of five deaths a year because of improper home-canning procedures. In 1970 there were six reported outbreaks of botulism poisoning affecting 13 people, five of whom died. All the cases were from home-canned food. In 1971 there were 24 outbreaks of food poisoning from botulism, resulting in four deaths, again from home-canned foods. In 1973 there were only 10 incidents, with one death; but in 1974 there were 20 outbreaks, which affected 30 people. Only one involved commercially processed food. Fifteen outbreaks, which resulted in six deaths, were traced directly to home canning. The rest were from sources other than canned food. In 1978 there were 12 outbreaks affecting 58 people with three deaths occurring. The biggest outbreak occurred at a Michigan restaurant where home-processed chili peppers were served. The chili peppers were only processed in a boiling water bath. The restaurant owner had never read anything about canning. As food prices rise and more people decide to grow and process their own foods, these incidents may increase. Unfortunately, many home canners do not read the instructions, and some use outdated procedures or equipment.

The failure of the home canner to check the operation of the pressure gauge on the pressure cooker is one of the chief errors resulting in the spoiling of home-canned foods. This results in a lower degree of heating and the chance that all the spores may not be destroyed. Another problem is improper seals on the jar lids. In addition, many people think they can process all foods safely in boiling water or even in an oven. The boiling water method should only be used for acid foods. Even there, some people make the error of mixing a high-acid and low-acid product (like meat in spaghetti sauce) and then assume they can use a boiling water bath. A dry oven should never be used for processing; there is a great danger the jars will explode. There have also been reports of tomatoes causing botulism. This should not occur as most tomato varieties have a pH of less than 4.6 as was recently confirmed by a University of Minnesota study. However, if people use damaged or rotten tomatoes containing a high degree of spoilage organisms, the pH may be changed enough to allow botulinum growth. The solution is to always use high-quality foods for home processing.

The sampling of home-canned foods prior to meal preparation is another cause of death by food poisoning. In 1972 a woman opened a jar of home-canned green beans, tasted the beans, heated them, and served them to her family. The family lived; she died. This shows how sensitive the toxin is to heat. Ten minutes of cooking at moderate to high heat is usually enough to destroy it completely.

NUTRIENT DESTRUCTION IN CANNED FOODS

The destruction of nutrients is the primary drawback in the canning process. The processing procedure used for destroying the spores of the organism *Clostridium botulinum* also results in the destruction of some sensitive nutrients, such as vitamin C. The heating that occurs can destroy up to 30% of vitamin C. Preparation for canning fruits and vegetables also requires washing, sorting, peeling, cutting, and blanching (scalding the vegetables or fruits in hot water or steam). Some nutrients such as vitamins and minerals are lost in the peeling, cutting, and washing steps. Blanching of the food is a mild heat treatment of two to three minutes in steam or boiling water, done prior to filling the jar or can. Blanching destroys the enzymes in the fruits or vegetables that could cause the production of off-odors, off-flavors, and off-colors during storage. The use of hot water for blanching can cause a loss of up to 25% of vitamin C as well as the leaching out of some minerals. Steam blanching results in only a 5–10% loss. When vegetables are reheated at home in preparation for the meal, the possibility exists for the destruction of an additional 25% of vitamin C. This can result in a total loss of vitamin C in canned foods as high as 75%.

Other vitamins that are affected by heat treatment are thiamin and vitamin A. In a product such as canned soup containing meat, approximately 10–20% of the thiamin is lost during canning. Vitamin A losses are 15–20% for the same type of product. These losses could be reduced if we could find faster ways to heat process food. Home-canning procedures are designed to insure maximum safety, because people are not as careful as they are in an industrial setting. Therefore, nutrient destruction for home-canned food is usually much greater than for commercially canned foods.

Nutrition labeling of certain foods, according to the Food and Drug Administration, has created an impetus to investigate the effect of heat processing on nutrients in foods. In the past, the food industry has been selling foods primarily on the basis of flavor and texture acceptability. These criteria had been the most important considerations to the consumer. A 1974 survey of 50,000 homemakers over the United States revealed that only 20% of those surveyed placed nutrition as the principal criterion for selection of foods. However, this has changed slowly, as the consumer became more aware of nutrition and food processing. This increased nutritional and food awareness has led the food industry (including the canning industry) to find methods to improve the nutritive value of processed canned foods. Shelf-life studies of canned foods are also being conducted. It is known that they may have a shelf life of up to three years because there is no oxygen in the can. Some companies label their products with a best-if-used-by date. The various chemical reactions causing quality loss and nutrient loss rates are one of the areas of research. Some information on shelf-life of canned foods will be presented in Chapter 22.

COMMERCIAL CANNING

Since 1925 commercial canning operations have produced close to a trillion cans of food products, the magic number we talked about, but of course not in one batch. In over 40 years there have been only five confirmed deaths in the U.S. and 2 in Belgium due to botulism from commercially canned foods produced in the U.S., as shown in Table 17.1. The reasons seven deaths have occurred since 1940 were that the retort operators failed to make certain that the cans were processed at the required time and temperature, that the can was not sealed properly and became recontaminated with the bacteria, or that the machinery caused a pinhole in the metal through which the organism entered. This latter cause resulted in a massive financial loss for the Alaskan salmon canneries. The problem was that the older sealing machines were not adjusted for the newer, lighter weight metal cans and rough handling caused pinholes to form.

Under most circumstances *Clostridium botulinum* produces off-odors and gas when it grows. A swollen can or off-odors when the can is opened are good indications that the food is contaminated and dangerous but, unfortunately, this does not always occur. Death can be avoided by cooking canned foods at home prior to serving, since the toxin is not resistant to heat. As seen in Table 17.1, most of the commercial foods that caused death were foods that could be eaten without heating such as tunafish, cold potato soup, or salmon.

The steps in a commercial process are varied but follow some basic principles. These will be described here and are outlined in Figure 17.2 using canned string beans as an example. The process begins in the field in which the product is checked constantly so that it can be picked at optimum maturity. For string beans, both sweetness and texture would be important to check. After harvest

TABLE 17.1 Deaths due to botulism from commercially canned low-acid foods

Year	Number of deaths	Implicated Food
1941	1	Mushrooms
1963	2	Tunafish
1971	1	Vischyssoise
1974	1	Beef Stew
1982	2	Salmon *

Center for Disease Control, Dept. HHS.
* Deaths in Belgium, salmon made in Alaska.

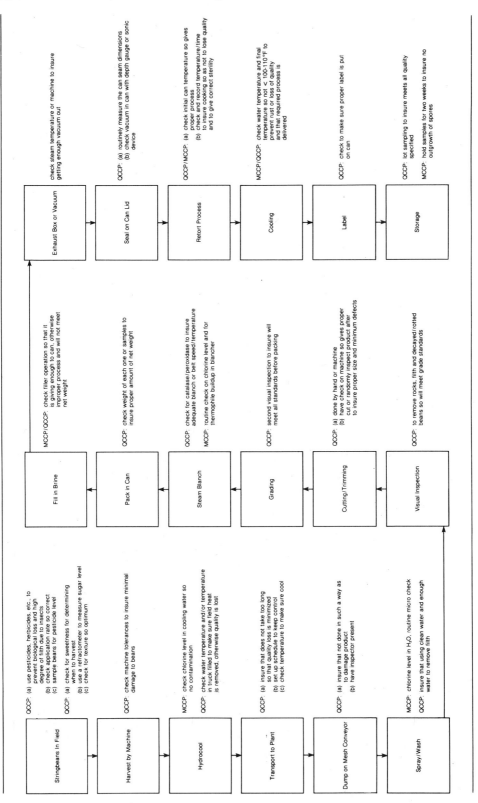

FIGURE 17.2 A process outline for canned string beans showing the typical QCCPs and MCCPs

the product must be cooled in the field unless it can be delivered and processed rapidly. One needs to remove the field heat, otherwise quality would be rapidly lost. After delivery the beans are washed and trimmed with several visual inspections to make sure both filth and undesirable decayed material will not get into the can. The beans are then blanched, packed into the can with brine, evacuated, the lid is sealed on, and the can is retort processed. Figure 17.2 illustrates several of the MCCPs and QCCPs in the process.

Those who want to know more about the reasons for these steps should consult some of the food technology references listed at the end of this book. Once processed, the cans are cooled rapidly to prevent both rust and the growth of thermophiles. They are then labeled and once again thoroughly examined to make sure they meet both legal standards and company requirements. It should be obvious from our discussion that the process is severe in order to insure safety (i.e. low risk). Thus the benefit of very high quality is lost, but we do end up with the desired long shelf life. Perhaps today with the availability of supermarkets we do not need foods that can last over two years. However, we can't compromise the safety of the product. Methods to heat treat rapidly without destroying quality are being sought.

Improved Methods of Thermal Processing

It is possible to process foods by methods that are not as nutritionally destructive as the normal retort canning procedure. For example, peas are normally processed in cans at 240°F (116°C) for 35 minutes, destroying 20–50% of the vitamin C. In the process of aseptic canning, peas in brine are pumped rapidly through a tube heated on the outside by a hot liquid or steam. Because of the turbulence and the much smaller distance the heat has to travel through the pipe as compared to the can, the peas are heated rapidly in less than two minutes to 350°F (177°C). This process destroys less than 5% of the vitamin C but it destroys the same amount of botulinum spores as in a batch retort pressure cooker. This is because at the higher temperature there is a much higher rate of bacteria kill compared to the rate of destruction of nutrients. The sterile peas can then be put directly into sterile cans or flexible pouches. Peas processed this way have the taste and texture of fresh peas. The method is called aseptic processing or high temperature-short time (HTST) thermal processing. Sterile milk (UHT milk or ultra high temperature milk) is made this way in Europe and requires no refrigeration. However, it has not been accepted by the United States consumer. In 1982 some companies began to market this product as well as aseptically sterilized juices in flexible soft cartons in the U.S.

Other methods used to improve nutritional quality include agitating the cans during heat processing, processing in foil (retort) pouches, and using direct gas flames for heating cans. For products with fluid, such as peas in brine, agitating the cans in the retort increases the rate of heating. This is because the food inside the can rotates rapidly, distributing the heat evenly. Thus the slowest heating point is no longer in the center but is distributed throughout the can. This method cannot work for solid foods, however.

Solid foods can be processed in foil pouches to increase quality. Foil pouches heat faster because they are much thinner than a can containing the same amount of food. They also have a larger surface area for contact with the heating system. This method was approved for use by the FDA in 1977 and several companies are now marketing retort pouched foods in the U.S. This method is used extensively in Japan and Europe.

The use of a gas flame results in faster heating rates, than can be obtained with steam. With steam in a retort, because of the danger and cost of creating high pressure and temperature, the maximum temperature that can be used is about 200°C. Gas flames can heat at 1100°C (2000°F). If the can is rotated very rapidly in the flame, the contents, if liquid, can heat quickly without burning. Solid foods cannot be done this way. Several food companies are now using this process after it was approved by the FDA in 1978. The original problem was to insure that each can met the required process schedule per 21 CFR 113. Some companies have even advertised that their product is Dragon Fired to bring out the natural flavor. At the very high temperature the time needed to kill the spores is so short that the nutrient and quality changes are minimal. All the above processes, it should be noted, would still need all the pre-retort and post-retort steps listed in Figure 17.2.

Bacteria Resistant to Processing

Canned foods are not completely sterile but are considered to be commercially sterile. Bacteria spores that are much more heat resistant than *Clostridium botulinum* can survive the process. They usually do not grow at normal room temperature nor do they produce any toxin. These bacteria are known as thermophiles, and can grow only at high temperatures. If a shipment of canned food travels by truck or railroad car across a desert and is allowed to become very warm (about 45 to 50°C), it would be possible for these spores to germinate and the cells to start to grow within the cans. The same is possible in a warm warehouse. This could turn the food product sour and/or cause the formation of gas, subsequently causing the cans to explode. It is unlikely that canned foods are subjected to such conditions. However, with the energy crunch in recent years some warehouses have reduced the amount of air conditioning they use so it is possible for this to occur. The consumer should not use swollen cans but should save them and call the local Food and Drug Administration so they can check the contents.

Pasteurization

Some foods are given heat treatments that do not kill all microorganisms. Pasteurized foods are heated to destroy some pathogens and reduce the microbial load thereby extending shelf life. Longer heating or high temperature would induce undesirable color and flavor changes in the food, making it unacceptable. Pasteurization was first applied to destroy those pathogens in raw milk that were responsible for tuberculosis and brucellosis. Today pasteurization is used for beers, wine, many dairy products, and other refrigerated foods. Usually a pasteurized food is further processed, for example, by refrigeration. As with canning, rapid high temperature-short time (HTST) procedures have been developed for pasteurization. In the United States, most milk is pasteurized at 71°C (160°F) for 15 seconds whereas it used to be heated for 30 to 40 minutes at 60°C (140°F). In Europe, a sterile milk packed in foil-lined cardboard pouches is sold that is processed for a very short time at ultra-high temperatures (over 300°F). The milk is stable for six months at room temperature. This process has not met with success in the United States because of its slightly cooked flavor but in 1982 some companies introduced fruit juices made this way.

SUMMARY

The canning process was discovered by Nicholas Appert in the early 1800s. However, it was not until the early 1900s that the reasons behind the method were understood. Heat processing of low-acid foods is based on the destruction of the spores of the pathogen *Clostridium botulinum* in the slowest heating point in the container being heated. The process is such that there is a chance of much less than one can in 10 billion having any botulinum spores left. Since other more heat-resistant microbes can be present, heat-processed foods are processed for an even longer time. Thus food poisoning from botulism is rare from commercially canned products. It does occur, more frequently in home processing, however, because less care is taken to insure safety and because of ignorance of the problems.

Because of the long heating time required to insure safety, significant destruction of some nutrients such as vitamin C, thiamin, and vitamin A can occur. Newer methods of heat processing are being designed to reduce these nutritional losses. Generally, one can say that commercially processed canned foods are extremely safe to use but do have a poorer quality and lower nutritional value than other processed or unprocessed foods.

Multiple Choice Study Questions

1. The method of canning preservation was discovered by
   A. alchemists
   B. Louis Pasteur
   C. Gay-Lussac
   D. Samuel Prescott
   E. Nicholas Appert

2. The principal pathogen on which the canning process is based is
   A. *Clostridium perfringens*
   B. *Clostridium botulinum*
   C. *Staphylococcus aureus*
   D. *Costridium salmonella*

3. Canned foods
   A. can never spoil because they are sterile
   B. will spoil if held at 110–120°F because of yeasts
   C. will spoil if held at 110–120°F because of spores that are thermophiles
   D. need a longer process time if they are acid (pH less than 4.5)

4. Commercially canned foods
   A. are absolutely sterile
   B. still contain organisms that eventually spoil the food if held for one or two years
   C. contain spores that can grow at higher than normal temperatures
   D. *Contain Clostridium botulinum*
   E. have lost over 90% of the nutritional value

5. Puffy cans of food usually indicate that
   A. the product was processed at too high a temperature, causing gas to be produced
   B. storage was at an improper temperature causing yeast to grow and produce gas
   C. they were underprocessed
   D. it should be sold at a lower price than was marked
   E. underprocessing or seal damage occurred

6. The chance of getting botulism from commercially canned foods is
   A. very high
   B. moderately low
   C. one chance in a thousand
   D. one chance in a billion
   E. much less than one chance in 10 billion

7. Which processed canned food would have the lowest potential for causing death due to botulism because of the way it is consumed?
   A. tunafish
   B. potato soup
   C. mushrooms
   D. cream-style corn
   E. salmon

8. In developing the time-temperature sequence for safely processing canned foods, an important factor is
   A. the location of the fastest heating point
   B. the location of the slowest heating point
   C. the amount of yeast present in the food
   D. the amount of carbohydrates present
   E. the nutrient destruction

9. Which food could be preserved in the shortest time by boiling the can in water (212°F)?
   A. sauerkraut
   B. carrots
   C. meat
   D. red cabbage
   E. peas

10. HTST stands for:
    A. high treatment for celsius temperatures
    B. histological–teratogen–short treatment
    C. highly toxic–substance testing
    D. high temperature–short time
    E. heavy–tensile steel treatment

Essay Study Questions

1. Find a copy of the translation of Appert's books and analyze the experiments that led to the development of canned foods.

2. How is the process time established for a canned food?

3. How safe is canning (both home and industrially prepared products)?

4. Indicate the amount of nutrient destruction that occurs in canning operations. Why does it occur?

5. What types of heat processing methods are used to maintain nutritional and quality values of canned foods?

6. What is commercial sterility?

7. What dangers are there in home-canned foods?

8. What is the difference between pasteurization and canning?

Things
to Do

1. Prepare home-canned fruits and vegetables. Use either the USDA guidebook (USDA Pub. # 8) or your local state experiment station canning booklet. The Institute of Food Technologists (221 No. LaSalle St., Chicago, IL 60601) has an excellent pamphlet on the problems of home canning. It costs about 25¢. Describe your success.

2. Find friends who have canned foods. Try to determine whether they used safe guidelines.

3. Look for foods preserved by the newer methods of heat preservation. Bring some to class. Since September, 1977, retort pouches, flame-sterilized foods, and aseptically filled pouches (juices and puddings) have appeared.

4. Obtain a copy of 21 CFR 113 and the original Federal Register notice that describes why the regulation was written. It appeared in Volume 44 of the official Federal Register beginning on page 16204 (the March 16, 1979 issue). Examine how the FDA incorporated the HACCP principles.

5. Visit a canning plant and make a process outline like Figure 17.2 showing the various MCCPs and QCCPs.

Chapter 17. Answers to Multiple-Choice Study Questions: 1, E; 2, B; 3, C; 4, C; 5, E; 6, E; 7, D; 8, B; 9, A; 10, D.

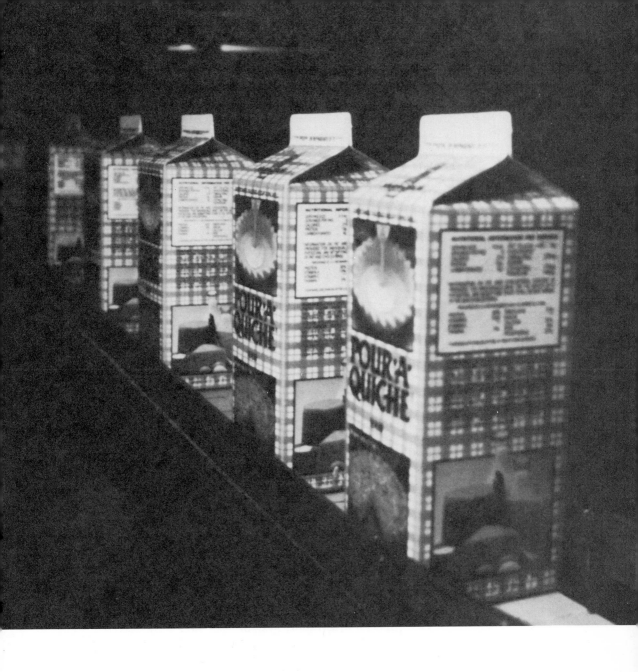

COLD PRESERVATION OF FOODS: REFRIGERATION AND FREEZING

18

THE PRINCIPLES OF REFRIGERATION AND FREEZING

The principle behind refrigeration and freezing for preservation of foods is the lowering of temperature to slow down microbial growth as well as chemical and biochemical reactions. In general, for every 10°C lowering of temperature, shelf life increases by two to five times in the refrigerated temperature range. Below 45°F (7°C) bacterial pathogens cannot grow, although some molds may produce toxin. Since water becomes a solid when frozen, it is no longer available as a phase for chemical, microbial, and enzymatic processes to take place in. This factor is the additional principle of freezing and can increase shelf life anywhere from 3 to 40 times for every 10°C lowering, much more than just refrigeration. No known pathogens can grow under frozen conditions. Almost 55% of the foods consumed at the present time in the U.S. diet are refrigerated or frozen. Another 30% of the foods consumed are preserved by canning, while only 5% are dehydrated. Refrigeration is the major process used for meat, fish, dairy products, fruits, and vegetables while freezing is used for almost every type of food because of the enhanced shelf life and superior quality.

HISTORY OF COLD PRESERVATION

Chinese poetry of 1100 B.C. described how the Chinese used to cut ice and store it until spring when it was then used to keep foods cold. The Greeks used evaporation techniques to make chilled water for drinking, as noted by Potagoras in 500 B.C. And as the old story goes, Roman emperors used to send runners up into the mountains to bring down snow for cooling some of their foods and drinks. Since not much ice or snow was available year round, this was not done to a great extent. Refrigeration in the United States before the 1800s was accomplished by using ice blocks cut from lakes in the northern states, and placing the chunks in a box with food. Ice was stored in huge ice houses for sale in the summertime as well as for keeping meat and fish cold on ocean-going ships, in many cases in vain.

A mechanical refrigeration system was first developed by John Gorrie, a medical officer stationed in Appalachicola, Florida. He was trying to cure malaria since the area was very swampy. One of his theories about the cure was that the patients needed to be kept cool. Since the ice he was buying from the north was costing him over a dollar a pound, in 1834 he invented an air expansion device to make the ice. It worked exactly the opposite of the bicycle pump that gets hot when you compress air. Although he was granted a patent for his device in 1851, a John Harrison in Australia invented a similar device at the same time. The *New York Times* said about Gorrie, "There is a crank . . . down in Appalachicola who claims he can make ice as good as God Almighty." Gorrie's idea did not catch on and he died penniless in 1855 but by this time Europeans recognized the principles and improved on them immensely. Instead of air, the new refrigeration machines used ammonia or sulfur dioxide. Unfortunately, they were bulky and also tended to explode so they were not destined for home use. The major endeavor was to produce ice blocks to replace the frozen winter lakes. This ice was used extensively by the large meat packers in Chicago to ship meat around the country as well as by vegetable growers in California to ship fresh produce to the East Coast.

In 1874, a German, Carl von Linde, improved on the crude designs and after first developing a refrigeration system to make lager beer (which must be chilled during aging), he developed and was producing 12,000 domestic refrigerators a year by 1890. The cost was high and domestic mechanical refrigerators didn't make it to the United States for 30 to 40 years. Instead, the emphasis was still on ice houses producing ice for the home ice box. It is estimated that in 1930 less than 3% of homes had a mechanical refrigerator in the U.S. However, at about that time a much better and safer refrigeration gas was invented—"freon"—and large companies like Kelvinator, Westinghouse, and General Electric began to mass produce refrigerators with small ice-making compartments.

This is about the time freezing came in. From the late 1880s, refrigeration was used on ships and trains to freeze meat and fish for transcontinental and intercontinental shipment. Clarence Birdseye of Gloucester, Massachusetts, realizing the greater quality potential began to develop a company in 1923 to sell frozen vegetables. In 1929 his idea was bought by the Postum Company, which later became General Foods, for a price of $22 million. By 1933 this company, which retained the Birdseye name, was basically freezing fruits and vegetables for sale to commercial operations, not for the consumer. By 1933 only 516 retail stores even had a frozen food cabinet. What caused the growth of frozen foods was the result of the U.S. government conscripting most of the canned and dried foods for the military during World War II. Thus, people at home got exposed to more frozen foods. In addition, new refrigerators with better freezer space became available.

**REFRIGERATOR/
FREEZER DESIGN**

Figure 18.1 shows the design of a refrigeration cycle. As the refrigerant freon comes out of the compressor it is a hot gas at high pressure (like a hand bicycle pump). It flows to the condenser, which consists of the coils on the back wall or under the refrigerator. There air (sometimes blown by a fan) removes heat from the

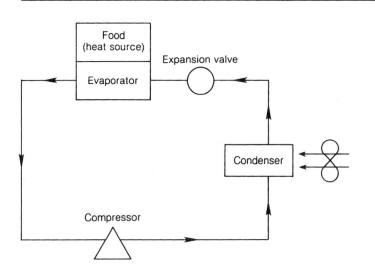

FIGURE 18.1 Design of refrigeration cycle showing direction of flow

gas changing it into a fluid. The fluid, which is still at high pressure, then goes through an expansion valve or nozzle, exiting at low pressure much like the spray from a hose or atomizer. This expansion causes it to cool rapidly to the desired refrigeration temperature. In the evaporator, which is another set of coils, the liquid boils at the same temperature much like water boiling at 100°C (212°F). The heat to boil the refrigerant comes from the air and food that enters the freezer or refrigerator compartment where the coils are placed. These coils may also be imbedded in the walls. There may be separate sets and expansion valves for both the refrigerator and freezer space. A thermostat (like on the wall of a home for the furnace) automatically opens the expansion valve and starts up the compressor. The compressor takes the evaporated gas, now at low temperature and pressure, and compresses it to start all over again. Since the evaporator coils are cool, ice builds up on them and lowers the efficiency of a refrigerator. To prevent this, automatic defrost cycles run the refrigerant cycle backwards for a short time. This melts the ice which then runs out a drain. Some freezers also have electric coils in the walls to do the same thing. It should be noted that air conditioners operate using the same cycle, but run at higher temperatures. In the air conditioner the air is cooled and dehumidified simultaneously, as the water condenses on the coils. One usually buys an air conditioner on the basis of tons, i.e., a three-fourth ton air conditioner. The term ton comes from the capacity to freeze or melt one ton of water/ice in one day.

USES OF REFRIGERATION

When we lower temperature we slow down the rates of quality loss. For fresh produce like fruits and vegetables, the rate of senescence slows down by a factor of two to three times for a 10°C drop while microbial growth slows down three to six times. Most quality changes of these refrigerated foods leading to loss of desirability are due to senescence. With meats, fish, poultry, and dairy products, on the other hand, senescence is not as important, and growth of undesirable microbes leads to slime, off-odors, and off-flavors.

Each food has an optimum temperature at which it should be refrigerated. Meats should be as cold as possible. Green bananas, however, should not be refrigerated because the ripening mechanism is impaired. Once they are ripe they should be refrigerated for maximum shelf life. Green tomatoes will also fail to ripen if refrigerated. Potatoes have an enzyme system that will turn the starch into sugars if the potatoes are kept at too low a temperature. Potatoes so stored will turn dark brown if fried or baked. On the other hand, unrefrigerated corn quickly loses its sweetness, and tomatoes can lose up to 40% of their vitamin C within three days after picking if kept at room temperature.

The best temperature for maximizing shelf life and minimizing the rate of senescence for many fruits and vegetables is 1.5°C to 5°C (35 to 41°F). Most refrigerators operate at around 7°C (45°F), which is a little too high, but lowering the temperature to 40°F (4.5°C) increases energy demand by almost 30%. As senescence proceeds, the produce becomes soft, and vitamin C content is also lowered. Eventually molds can grow on the surface and decay becomes obvious. However, some produce such as apples become damaged if the temperature drops below 5 to 8°C (41 to 47°F). This is called chill damage. With apples and limes brown spots develop because the low temperature damages internal tissues that spill out enzymes even though the produce is not frozen. These enzymes (polyphenol oxidase) cause browning. Thus many refrigerators are designed to be coldest near the bottom or top where meats are kept and warmest near the other end for storage of fruits and vegetables.

The shelf life of refrigerated fruits and vegetables can also be increased by placing them in a plastic film bag. The film slows the loss of water, thereby preventing wilting. If wilting were not stopped, the produce loses vitamin C quickly and also becomes susceptible to microbial attack. Since refrigerators take water out of the air, they are designed with a produce drawer to lower the exposure of the produce to the dry air steam.

The packaging film must be slightly permeable to oxygen for fruits and vegetables because they are still living and utilizing storage starch for energy. Usually, the higher the oxygen levels, the faster the rate of utilization of the starch and the shorter the shelf life. Therefore, packaging to keep oxygen levels low will help preserve the food for a longer time. One problem, however, is that a destruction of tissues, yielding acids and alcohol, will result if the oxygen level in the package gets too low. This is similar to the acid production in muscles during extreme exertion. When this happens, the fruit or vegetable turns mushy and is subject to microbial decay. For each fresh product, the packaging must be designed to balance the amount of water going out and the amount of oxygen coming in. This is the reason why plastic film bags for potatoes have holes in them. The waxing of fruits is an old process that also helps preserve fresh produce in much the same way as film packaging since the wax slows water loss from the surface. Apples and grapes produce their own wax to do this while maturing. Some major producers hold fresh produce under controlled atmospheric conditions in large warehouses. Here temperature, humidity, CO_2 and O_2 are all controlled to maximize shelf life. Boxcars and trucks with these units are used to distribute fresh lettuce and tomatoes nationally.

Ethylene is a gas used on fresh fruits and vegetables to induce ripening. For instance, oranges picked in Florida are not usually all in the same stage of ripening when they come from the tree. For marketing purposes, it is desirable for all of them to be at the same stage when they reach the consumer. For this reason the oranges may be placed in chambers and exposed to ethylene gas. Ethylene, although a gas, is produced by the plant itself as a growth-stimulating hormone. By spraying it over the fruit, or by using the film packaging to trap the natural ethylene produced by the fruit within the bag, the ripening process is controlled as is done with bananas. The use of film packaging can eliminate the need for external spraying with ethylene. Thus all produce will ripen at about the same time and decay will be prevented.

HOLDING FRESH FRUITS AND VEGETABLES

It is usually reasonable to assume that fresh garden fruits and vegetables picked from your own garden and quickly refrigerated at home under desirable conditions have the highest quality and nutritional value. It is not reasonable to assume that produce is as carefully handled from the time it is picked on the farms to the time it reaches the supermarkets. In fact, the opposite may be true in many cases. Although most supermarkets have produce in refrigerated cases or over ice, the farmers who pick and deliver the produce may not use refrigeration. Thus a great amount of nutritional deterioration can take place. In addition, some supermarkets inadequately refrigerate fruits and vegetables. It is hoped that future legislation on the holding of refrigerated fruits and vegetables will help upgrade the shelf life and nutritional quality of our food supply. This has certainly been the case for meats and dairy products. Table 18.1 shows the shelf life for a few fresh products at different temperatures.

FREEZING

Freezing serves much the same purpose as refrigeration. Both processes use low temperatures in order to slow the rate of decay of foods. Freezing is more effective, however, because the temperatures are much lower than they are for refrigeration. Freezing also converts liquid water into a solid, thereby making the water needed by the microbes for growth or necessary as a medium for deteriorative chemical reactions unavailable.

Although frozen foods keep much longer than refrigerated foods, they are not infinitely stable, since not all the water freezes out when the food is frozen. At $-20°F$ ($-29°C$) as much as 10% of the water can remain unfrozen in the food. Thus some chemical and enzymatic reactions can still go on in the unfrozen water, destroying food quality, although at a rate usually slower than at room temperature. However if frozen foods are held just below the freezing point, the concentration of the reactants can lead to a much faster loss of quality than at higher temperatures. In addition, as the water freezes, the salts and acid builds up in the unfrozen water. This can result in damaging physical and chemical effects on the protein structure of cell membranes, making them leaky. Chemicals that were normally separated in a cell can now come together and react.

Many frozen foods actually have a relatively shorter shelf life in comparison to canned foods, as was seen in Table 14.1. To see why this is so the various changes that occur during frozen storage will be described.

Physical Changes

Textural damage can take place in foods when they are frozen. Fruits and vegetables become mushy when frozen, losing their

TABLE 18.1 Average shelf-life of fresh foods

Commodity	Temperature		
	32–40°F	68–72°F	95–100°F
Meat	7–10 days	1 day	8 hours
Fish	2–5 days	1 day	5–6 hours
Milk	14–21 days	8 hours	4–6 hours
Leafy vegetables	3–20 days	1–7 days	1–3 days
Many fruits	1 week–1 year	1–20 days	1–7 days

natural crispness. This is because freezing can break apart the glue (pectin) that holds the cells together. The cells then slip past each other very easily when we bite into the product. This breakage is due both to the expansion of water into ice (about a 9% volume increase) and to a build up of salts in the unfrozen water which affects the pectin. In addition, as the salts concentrate in the extracellular fluid, they draw water out of the cell. In the process the cell shrinks. As some cells shrink they reach an elastic limit. At this point the cell wall breaks and the cell contents are spilled out. Upon thawing the cell does not take back all the water. An illustration of this process is the fluid that is found on the plate or in the pot when frozen food is thawed or cooked.

Meats such as pork or fatty fish such as salmon can toughen during freezing and frozen storage. This is due to salts denaturing (toughening) the protein and salt and ice causing the cell breakage that leads to a condition known as drip. Thawed meat often leaks a runny, red liquid that looks like blood but is actually the cell liquid content. Once frozen and thawed, the tissues and protein can no longer take back and hold the original amount of water that was within the cells because the cell protein and cell walls have been irreversibly affected (denatured). Besides the drip, this loss of water makes the thawed tissue foods seem dryer and tougher when eaten. However, it has relatively little effect on nutritional value.

The worst method of freezing from a quality standpoint is the one most people use at home, that is, they freeze foods in the home freezer. Because of the typical temperature and slow rate of air movement, freezing occurs very slowly. This can result in a very high loss of quality. However, from a home-processing standpoint, freezing of fruits, meats, and garden vegetables, is the safest method of preservation, and preserves more nutrients than canning or drying. It is also the simplest method since the food only needs to be blanched, put in a container, and then frozen. Fast freezing as practiced by industry results in less physical damage. However, major damaging physical effects such as drip can occur while the product is thawed slowly, for example, in a refrigerator. Faster thawing, such as on a kitchen counter, is better from a textural standpoint but can result in conditions that would allow microbial growth including growth of pathogens. This is especially true for those foods classified in the Hazard I category such as meats, poultry, eggs, and milk. To be safe, foods should be thawed rapidly under running water or in a microwave oven. If the frozen food is going to be baked, it can be put directly in the oven, as is done for pizza. This minimizes the chance for pathogens and maintains quality. It should be noted that improper handling (Hazard III) of frozen meat pies has resulted in botulism. In 1983 a woman cooked a frozen dinner, then left it on the counter for two days. The heating killed all the vegetative cells but left the more heat-resistant spores of *C. botulinum* that are always present. The heat also drove out the oxygen, thus the spores outgrew and produced the toxin. There have been four other botulinum incidents from mishandling of frozen pot pies after cooking.

Package ice is another form of physical damage caused by freezing. For example, frozen pizza may develop ice crystals within the package above the surface of the product. These ice particles are caused by the evaporation of water from the food into the air space left in the package as the product warms slightly during the freezer defrost cycle. The water crystallizes out as snow inside the package as the defrost cycle ends and the freezer drops in temperature. Although it makes the product look unacceptable, the ice itself is not damaging. However, the lost water can result in another problem. For example, dry spots can be detrimental to the appearance of frozen turkeys or chicken. In fact, the areas from which water is evaporated can darken and become tough. This area or spot is called freezer burn and is due to acceleration of certain chemical reactions taking place in that spot. With turkeys, the area can appear as a green- to brown-colored spot and may look like a mold growth, which it is not. The discoloration is the result of reactions of fats and proteins. Elimination of the air space is the best way to prevent such an ice buildup. This is done by using shrink wrap (very tight seal) or vacuum packaging to pull the film very close to the food surface. Unfortunately, with some foods like pizza tight packaging is difficult, and ice buildup is inevitable. Of greater importance is controlling temperature fluctuations during storage and defrosting, which minimizes package ice and freezer burn.

People who freeze foods at home usually do not wrap the food tightly enough in freezer wrap or foil and end up with package ice and freezer burn. Freezer burn is accelerated by the fluctuating temperatures that occur in a home freezer due to the automatic defrost cycle. As the temperature increases, water can evaporate more rapidly into the air space of the package. As the temperature decreases, the water vapor does not go back into the food; it crystallizes out as ice. If this happens repeatedly the food surface dries out and undesirable color changes occur.

Freezing also damages emulsions, causing them to separate upon thawing. This is why you don't see frozen salad dressing. An emulsion is a suspension of oil droplets in a water phase. Emulsions separate because the oil, being lighter than water, rises to the top (the cream layer in unhomogenized milk). The smaller the oil droplet the more slowly it separates; if the droplet were doubled in size it would rise four times as fast. The rate can be slowed down by homogenization that breaks the oil into as small a droplet as possible. In addition, if sugars, protein, gums, or starches are added to the water phase it becomes more viscous, i.e., thick. This also slows down the rate of creaming.

When an emulsion is frozen two things occur. First, the salts and sugars are concentrated as ice is formed. Because they compete with the proteins and starches for the remaining unfrozen water, the polymers may get chemically and physically damaged and precipitate out. Thus, when the emulsion is thawed the viscosity is less and the oil separates more easily. Second, as the ice is formed the droplets of oil are forced closer to each other, and can grow together (coalesce) and get bigger. On thawing they will separate to the top more quickly. Emulsifying agents (as noted on food labels), that have a charge on them such as lecithin, help prevent this by repelling the drops from each other.

The last physical effect that can cause quality loss in frozen foods is growth of ice into larger crystals. The crystals themselves may be damaging to the food membranes or they can impart a grainy texture if the food is eaten frozen as is the case with ice cream. Minimizing temperature fluctuations also helps slow this but with automatic defrost cycles some graininess is inevitable.

Chemical Changes

Chemical reactions that cause deterioration also occur in frozen foods because of the concentration effect in the unfrozen water and the spillage of reactants and enzymes from organelles with damaged membranes. Rancidity is one of the most rapid chemical deterioration reactions in frozen foods. Fish, beef, pork, and cured meats like ham (which contain unsaturated fats) are susceptible, especially if they are cooked before freezing. The fats break down in the presence of oxygen and a rancid flavor develops very rapidly. Rancidity is accelerated in the frozen food due to the fact that the oxygen is highly concentrated in the unfrozen water. In addition, if the food is uncooked, the lipoxidase enzyme may be released from damaged membranes and can then attack the unsaturated fats. Usually the lower the temperature the slower the rate of oxidation so that at least several months of shelf life are possible for very fatty foods. Vacuum packaging also helps slow down this reaction even more.

Browning, another chemical reaction, is a problem in frozen fruits. For example, peaches will brown in frozen storage due to certain enzyme-catalyzed reactions (polyphenol-oxidase enzymes). These enzymes cause some of the components in the fruit to react with oxygen and produce a brown color. Remember that plenty of oxygen is available and enzymes can be released from damaged cells. The brown color is disagreeable from an aesthetic standpoint and can cause bitter flavors to develop. Browning in fruits can be prevented by packing the fruits in a heavily sugared syrup prior to freezing. This serves as a barrier to oxygen. The fruits can also be blanched to destroy the enzymes, but this is not done because it softens the tissues causing loss of the desirable crisp texture. In addition, blanching causes a cooked flavor that is undesirable. Sulfur dioxide may also be used to slow the browning reaction, but it causes an off-flavor in many fruits. Sulfuring should not be done in the home because it is too difficult to control the level properly. An excess can be toxic and some individuals may be allergic to any amount of it.

Vitamin loss, especially loss of vitamin C, also occurs in frozen foods during storage. The rate of loss of vitamins is usually faster in frozen foods than in canned foods, even though the temperature is lower. This is probably because enzymes and the excess oxygen cause the destruction of some vitamins. The rate of nutritional loss in frozen foods, however, is much slower than that for fresh produce. For example, during storage, fresh green beans can lose 50% of their vitamin C in two days at 20°C (68°F), whereas, at −18°C (0°F) it takes one year for the same loss to occur.

Because of the high initial nutritional value and quality of frozen foods, the frozen food industry has been growing, particularly in the production of frozen dinners and convenience foods. The freezing process makes it possible to obtain good-quality vegetables all year round and thus helps to balance the diet, albeit at a higher processing cost.

Frozen foods are usually of a better quality than canned or fresh foods. Table 18.2 shows the length of time foods can be kept frozen and still maintain very high quality. It should be pointed out that frozen foods have a higher quality initially than canned foods because they do not receive the high temperatures that are needed in canning. This quality can be lost however, if foods are not held at a low enough temperature. The highest quality frozen foods are produced by the fastest freezing method. Liquid nitrogen (−320°F) is currently one of the best methods of freezing fruits and vegetables on a commercial basis. These foods are frozen in a matter of seconds, or minutes, in liquid nitrogen. The home freezer, on the other hand, may require more than six to ten hours to freeze a similar food, such as a frozen meal. Freezing foods at home can mean much poorer quality than can be obtained commercially unless a deep freeze, which has a lower temperature than a refrigerator/freezer, is used. Some appliance companies are developing a freezer with a fast-freeze section. It is best to remember that the smaller the portion frozen and the thinner cross section it has, the faster it will freeze.

TABLE 18.2 High-quality shelf life of frozen foods

	Home refrigerator freezer section −12°C (10°F) (months)	Home frozen food locker −18°C (0°F) (months)
Apple pie filling	9	12
Beef	2	6
Bacon	1	3
Bread [1]	6	24
Cauliflower	2	10
Chicken (raw)	7	14
Chicken (fried)	1	3
Corn on cob	4	10
Fish (fatty)	(1 wk.)	2
Green beans	3	10
Hamburger (ground)	10	20
Peaches	1	12
Peas	3	10
Pork sausage	1	4
Spinach	2	5
Strawberries	3	10

[1] Bread will toughen at a faster rate when refrigerated than if stored at room temperature.

Thawing of Frozen Foods

The process of thawing operates on the same principle as freezing, that is, faster thawing gives better quality. In fact, very slow thawing may cause significant quality loss, since many reactions are accelerated near the thawing temperature. Due to the inherent properties of ice and water, the thawing process takes three to five times longer than the freezing of food. Some of the physical and chemical damage that occurs takes place during the thawing process. The food industry has been looking at several different ways to thaw frozen foods to maintain high quality. One example is the suggestion to roast directly from the frozen state, as is recommended on the label for frozen turkeys and chickens. Another is the frozen boil-in-the-bag vegetable pouch, which insures rapid thawing without burning in the pot. Many frozen foods can also be thawed and cooked directly in microwave ovens, which are being used extensively in hospitals and restaurants and increasingly in the home. Thawing at room temperature is the least recommended thawing method because of the probability of the growth of microorganisms while the food is on the countertop. This can lead to food poisoning if pathogens are present.

One of the biggest problems is the handling of frozen foods after they leave the frozen food plant. Sometimes the truck that carries them breaks down and the food thaws out, or the frozen food cases are left on the loading dock of the supermarket too long. In many instances, clerks at supermarkets do not fill the frozen food cases quickly enough, leaving the frozen food on a cart till it thaws, or they may overfill the frozen display case. All of these factors combine to cause physical and chemical changes that decrease quality and nutritional value. Thaw indicators have been developed. Placed on the frozen food package, they reveal to the customer if a frozen food product has been subjected to improper storing or handling conditions. The use of thaw indicators raises the problem of who pays for the loss. Many consumers wrongfully blame the manufacturers for spoiled food when it is really the fault of the handler. Legislation may be needed in this area.

The refreezing of foods is not forbidden, as is sometimes believed, providing the conditions under which the foods were thawed and held did not allow the growth of poisonous microorganisms. Since most people have little knowledge of the microbial problems that can develop, they probably should not refreeze food.

SUMMARY

The basic principle in preservation through reduced temperature is the fact that lower temperatures reduce the rates of quality losses and microbial decay of foods. In addition, if the food is subjected to freezing temperatures, the liquid water becomes unavailable for reactions since it turns to ice. With fresh produce, an optimum refrigeration temperature exists for each product to give maximum shelf life. These temperatures vary with the food product. The plastic film package around fresh produce helps increase shelf life by preventing water loss and induces ripening.

With frozen foods, both slow freezing and thawing cause most of the physical and chemical changes that decrease quality. These changes include toughening, drip, browning, and rancidity. Changes also occur during storage but decrease as storage temperature is decreased. Another problem is freezer burn, which is due to evaporation of water from food into the package head space during storage. This can cause an unsightly spot called freezer burn. Undesirable package ice may also form if the storage temperature fluctuates. With respect to quality, frozen foods are better than canned, especially if held properly, but they do have a shorter shelf life.

1. Which of the following represents chill injury?

   A. package ice in a frozen food box

   B. freezer burn

   C. drip

   D. non-enzymatic browning

   E. lipid oxidation

2. Ethylene is

   A. an environmental contaminant of significant proportion

   B. a plant hormone used to stimulate ripening

   C. a toxin produced by *Aspergillus flavus*

   D. a major component of gasoline

   E. none of the above

3. Which food would be best to keep at lowest refrigeration temperature to extend shelf life?

   A. potatoes

   B. meat

   C. apples

   D. unripe bananas

4. When potatoes are kept below 50°F

   A. the sugar content increases

   B. their starch content increases

   C. more solanine is produced

   D. they turn brown very rapidly

   E. none of the above

5. Package ice is the result of

   A. improper freezing rates

   B. ice crystals getting into the package during processing

   C. water migration into the food

   D. poor packaging

   E. fluctuating temperatures

6. Which of the following combinations of meat-storage conditions would give the longest (acceptable) shelf life?

   A. fish at 25°F

   B. pork at 26°F

   C. beef at 10°F

   D. pork at 0°F

   E. beef at 0°F

7. Which food when frozen has the longest shelf life?

   A. beef

   B. pork

   C. fatty fish

D. corn

E. bread

8. The red liquid that forms when meat is thawed under normal conditions is

   A. blood that ran out of the tissues

   B. due to a very rapid thawing rate

   C. the fluid that leaked from the tissues

   D. none of the above

9. From a food quality standpoint, which would be the best way to thaw a frozen steak?

   A. put in the refrigerator overnight

   B. leave out on countertop (2–4 hours)

   C. thaw under running water

   D. microwave oven

10. Freezer burn is caused by

   A. the food touching the defrost pipe or tape in a freezer

   B. roasting from the frozen state

   C. temperature cycling in the freezer and an air space in the package

   D. packaging the roast in a tight film.

Essay Study Questions

1. What are the basic principles in cold preservation of foods?

2. Give some examples of the effect of refrigeration temperature on fresh foods.

3. How does packaging of fresh fruits and vegetables increase their shelf life?

4. What effect does ethylene gas have on fruits?

5. Why don't frozen foods last for a very long time?

6. What types of physical changes occur when a food is frozen?

7. What are the chemical reactions that deteriorate frozen foods?

8. Discuss the methods that can be used to minimize quality and nutritional losses during thawing of frozen foods.

9. What are freezer burn and package ice and how can they be prevented?

Things to Do

1. Observe the quality of some refrigerated foods during storage in the refrigerator. Compare the actual shelf life you measure to the shelf-life date on the package. Good foods to study are cottage cheese, milk, and luncheon meats. Why did they deteriorate? How much food that you consume is refrigerated food?

2. Obtain some fresh vegetables such as tomatoes, green beans, and peas. Wash, clean, and cut them. Place them in plastic bags and freeze them. Hold for one, two, and three months, thaw out, and examine their quality.

3. Visit the supermarket and compare prices of equal weights of similar foods that are fresh, canned, and frozen. (Use peas, corn, green beans, tomatoes, etc.) Why are there any differences?

4. Perform the experiments on freezing points of solutions in *Science Experiments You Can Eat.*

5. Look in the freezer for foods with package ice and freezer burn. Try to design an experiment that induces package ice.

Chapter 18. Answers to Multiple-Choice Study Questions: 1, D; 2, B; 3, B; 4, A; 5, D; 6, E; 7, E; 8, C; 9, D; 10, C.

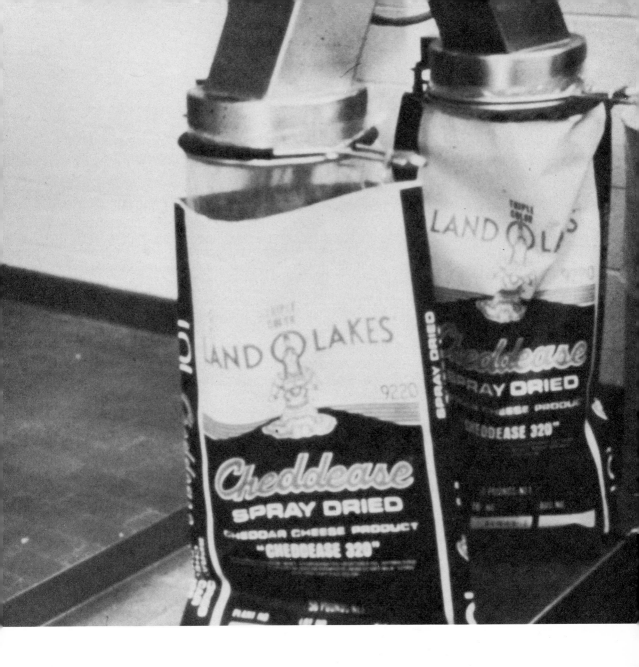

THE DRYING
OF FOODS

19

A wide variety of dehydrated food products are currently available for home use. Instant dry milk, many cereals and snacks, dry soups, spices, instant coffee (vending machines use dehydrated coffee), hamburger-type meal mix products, and many pharmaceuticals are produced by the dehydration process. This chapter will discuss some of the aspects of dehydrating foods.

There is very little recorded early history of the dehydration of foods, although sun-drying and smoking over a hot fire, which are mentioned in biblical writings, were probably the first methods used for drying foods. Drying in the sun was one of the principal methods used for meat and fish preservation for several thousand years. In addition, it was the principal method used to keep fruits during the winter. Products that are still commonly sun-dried in the United States at the present time are raisins and prunes. The major technological developments in drying took place in wartime when lightweight shelf-stable foods were needed for the military. Much of this technology has been transferred to the consumer.

PRINCIPLES OF FOOD DEHYDRATION, WATER ACTIVITY, AND STABILITY

Food preservation by drying is based on the principle that microbial growth and chemical reactions can occur only when enough water is present. By lowering the water content to a certain level, deteriorative reactions are prevented. The level necessary to preserve foods is established by the term water activity, a_w, or equilibrium relative humidity (% ERH). The ERH curve, as a function of moisture content, is shown in Figure 19.1, indicating the general a_w of various types of foods. In fresh-tissue foods, the water activity is very close to one, thus rapid growth of microbes leads to deterioration. Dry foods have a water activity of about 0.2 to 0.6. Microorganisms cannot grow below an a_w of 0.6. However, certain chemical reactions can still occur in dry foods and can reduce shelf life unless the a_w is reduced to about 0.2 to 0.3. The special moist burger-type dog foods on the market today have an a_w of 0.8 to 0.9. These foods are similar to fig newtons, cheese, and fruitcake, in that sugars are used to bind the water. In these products, the level of water availability does not allow most microbes to grow, but enough water is present so that the food is palatable and can be eaten without rehydration. However, these foods have a fairly short shelf life because many chemical reactions still occur at the higher a_w. Since molds are the least affected by lower a_w, acids and some mold inhibitors such as potassium sorbate are used to prevent their growth in these foods.

Since the a_w of a food is critical to its safety, the FDA has promulgated proposed regulations under the Good Manufacturing Practice Regulation (21 CFR 110). The regulations specify that dry foods, nuts, intermediate-moisture foods, and dry mixes must be

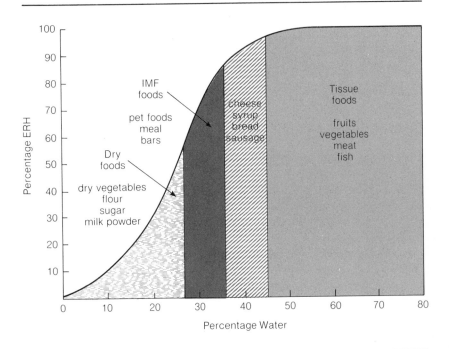

FIGURE 19.1 % ERH as a function of water content for different types of foods

maintained at a safe moisture level so that there is destruction or prevention of growth of organisms of public health significance. Once dried, the food must be packaged to prevent moisture pickup beyond the point where the food would become unsafe. That is why most dry foods are packaged in foil-laminated pouches. Of critical importance with dried foods from a HACCP standpoint are the Hazard II and Hazard III categories. If the process is not adequately controlled to eliminate pathogens, there is potential for disaster if the consumer abuses the product. This can occur during rehydration when the dried food is mixed with water and left at room temperature. The organisms may survive the drying, rehydrate, and multiply, thus producing a hazardous food. One food with this potential is dried milk or infant formula. In fact, in the past, there have been several incidents of large-scale food poisoning in children because of lack of process control and consumer abuse. Because of this the dairy industry has instituted very stringent HACCP strategies.

In addition to water pickup making the food unsafe, moisture gain can also result in sogginess, caking, and loss of crispness. This deterioration usually occurs at fairly low relative humidities, generally in the 30–50% relative humidity (RH) range. Thus, not only is a good package needed but the consumer must either consume a susceptible product rapidly after opening or reseal the food in a jar or plastic container. Foods subject to the problem of loss of crispness include crackers, potato chips, and other dry snack foods. This fact can be useful in predicting when a product is near the end point of drying, if you do home drying of foods. All one has to do is take a piece out of the dryer, let it cool, and bite it. If it is soft further drying is needed; if it is crunchy it is near the desired a_w. In industry, electronic devices that rapidly indicate a_w or moisture content are used to insure proper quality.

Foods that cake easily at low humidity are those that contain natural or added dried sugars (not the crystalline type) such as tomato powder, spice powder, some sugared cereals, and brown sugar. Crystalline salt will cake above 75% RH and table sugar (sucrose) cakes above 85% RH. At these RHs the surface of the crystal absorbs water and begins to dissolve it. If two crystals are touching, a liquid bridge containing the dissolved material forms. When the percent RH decreases, the bridge dries out and a permanent connection forms, causing the product to lose its flowability. Certain agents called "anticaking" compounds can be used to prevent this, including silicon dioxide and dextrose. At home one can put rice in a salt shaker since it binds more water than the salt and cuts down on caking.

The amount of water in a food, as measured by its availability or water activity, controls the rates of chemical deteriorative reactions. Below an a_w of 0.2 to 0.3, most dry foods are very stable. Unfortunately, since it is hard to reduce water content to this level, not all dry foods can be processed as such. In addition, if the food contains unsaturated fat, below this a_w range the fat is very susceptible to oxidation leading to rancid flavors. Because enzymes may also be active in dried foods even at low a_w's, the product is usually blanched first to denature the enzymes. This is not done with fruits because it would cause a cooked flavor, nor with onion powder and garlic powder. The latter require enzyme activity to produce the desired flavor.

It has been generally found that above an a_w of 0.3, the rate of loss of quality or nutrient value doubles or triples for each 0.1 increase in the a_w. Reactions susceptible to this include, for example, oxidative rancidity, browning, thiamin destruction, and loss of vitamin C. These will be discussed in Chapter 22. Proper packaging is important to insure minimal moisture gain during storage. This is one of the problems facing the person doing home drying since home package sealers may not do an adequate job. Lastly, it should be noted that once the food exceeds an a_w of 0.8, the rates of many chemical reactions fall because of dilution by water. This is why canned foods have such a long shelf life compared to dry foods.

ENGINEERING FACTORS

In drying a food, several factors that control the rate of moisture removal are important. Most drying operations use air. The air must be heated to evaporate the water. The humidity of the air must be low enough so that the water will want to evaporate (remember the % ERH principle). To achieve this the hot air is blown rapidly over the food so that the air humidity around the food does not build up. This is a problem in most home dryers. Since high air velocities cannot be achieved in these home devices, drying is much slower than it is industrially. The food itself also limits the rate of drying. Once the surface is dried out the water must pass through the pores that resist the flow. The longer the path for flow, the greater the resistance. Since the water is bound to the dissolved solids and the internal surfaces of the food, there is additional resistance to its removal. In addition, as the food dries out it acts as an insulator to heat; the heat energy in the hot air has a more difficult time getting into the food to evaporate the water. One way to overcome this is to go to higher temperatures, but this might scorch the surface of the food causing objectionable colors and flavors. The higher temperature also means a faster rate of loss of nutrients and quality. In addition, at high temperature case hardening may occur in which a dense dry layer is built up on the surface that resists the flow of water through it. Finally, most piece foods, when dried, shrink causing the pores to restrict the flow of water further. It is no wonder that with all these problems we do not consume many dried fruits, vegetables, meats, or fish. Industrial food drying techniques can overcome these problems and produce dried foods, such as instant coffee, that cannot be created at home.

Of additional concern is the fact that given all these engineering factors, the drying time is proportional to the thickness of the food piece squared, that is, if you double the thickness the drying time is 2^2 or 4 times longer. Thus, to insure uniform drying, control of piece size is important from both a QCCP and MCCP standpoint. It is important microbiologically since if the drying is slow and the air temperature is low (120–140°F), pathogenic microorganisms, if present, may grow and/or produce toxins in the food during drying before they reach the limiting a_w for their growth. Most organisms can survive to some degree when dry. When the food is rehydrated and if microorganisms are present in high enough numbers or enough toxin in present, food poisoning could result.

Loss of volatile flavors during drying is another concern. If exposed to moving air, desirable flavor compounds will evaporate along with the water. Thus, the longer the drying and the higher the temperature, the greater the loss. This is why air-dried vegetables and fruits just do not taste as good as fresh or frozen products.

**METHODS
OF DRYING**

Sun Drying

Sun drying, where fruits or vegetables are laid out on racks in the sun, can take three to four days. This is because the supply of solar energy is limited and, of course, at night the supply is nonexistent. Air flow is also very slow compared to a commercial mechanical dryer. Sun drying is still used today because it is cheap. For example, grapes are sun dried to make raisins. Prunes are also sun dried. The process is so inefficient that over one acre of drying area is needed for every 20 acres of raw crop. Microbial growth is a drawback in this drying process because the air temperature does not get very high, thus the time required for drying makes it possible for molds, yeast, or bacteria to grow on the surfaces of these foods. In addition, rodents, insects, and birds can attack and contaminate the foods in the drying field. One foreign country with a large fish-drying industry has had major contamination problems in one plant. Some 10% of the weight of the finished dry product was fly larvae deposited on the fish during the drying process. This certainly would be unacceptable in the United States on the basis of HACCP principles.

Chemical and enzymatic reactions occurring during sun drying are important in the production of flavor and the dark color for grapes and prunes but are undesirable during drying and storage of most other dried foods. Sun drying causes the largest loss of vitamins of any drying process, due to the length of time necessary to dry the food. For example, peaches can lose 50% of their vitamin C during sun drying. Many people have tried to use sun drying at home to produce products such as beef jerky. This should be discouraged because of the possible microbiological hazards and the high losses of nutrients. However, sun drying can be used for spices and condiments and some acid fruits with fewer problems. Sun drying is best when you have direct sunlight and the air does not exceed 20% RH. These conditions are found in only a few places in the United States such as in California.

Grain and animal feed, such as hay, constitute the greatest volume of sun-dried products. Farmers use the sun because it is cheap. They need to dry the grain fast enough to reduce the percent ERH below 60% to stop microbial growth. If rainy weather occurs at harvest time, they have to use gas-heated dryers, which increases food prices. Sun drying is a process at the mercy of the weather.

Commercial Tray and Tunnel Drying

About 60 years ago, food technologists looked for ways to dry food without using the sun, especially because of large losses of fruit crops due to rain during harvest time. Thus tray drying and tunnel drying were developed. The sun is replaced with hot, dry air blown at high velocity in various directions around and over the food. The air supplies the heat to evaporate the water and the air carries the water away. In tray drying, racks with trays containing food are placed in the air chamber. In tunnel drying, the food is placed on a belt or on trays that move through a tunnel through which the air blows. In a closed system such as this, bird, insect, and rodent contamination is prevented.

The humidity of the air in the dryers must be low for dehydration to take place rapidly. The air velocity must also be controlled so that the food is not blown off the tray or belt. A typical process is shown in Figure 19.2. Because it is hard to control piece size exactly, the food is often removed after six to eight hours and transferred to a bin through which air at low humidity and slow velocity is passed. This further reduces the moisture to the desired level.

Tray drying and tunnel drying can accomplish in six to eight hours what takes several days for sun drying. However, the drying cost is about two to three cents per pound of water removed, about four to five times more costly than sun drying. Even though the temperature is higher than in sun drying, the shorter drying time does not cause as many adverse chemical reactions or destroy as many nutrients as sun drying does. A better quality food results.

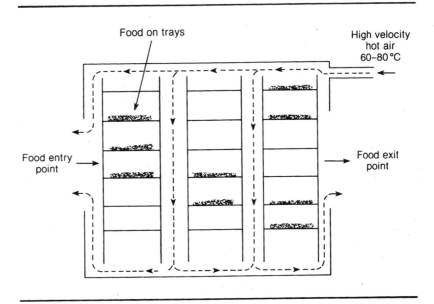

FIGURE 19.2 Tunnel/tray dryer for foods

This is similar to the high temperature–short time canning concept. Less than 10% of the vitamin C in fruits is lost with this process. Less than 20% of the vitamin A in carrots is destroyed. The big problem with tray-dried foods is that they shrink and are hard to rehydrate. This is because the capillaries in the food collapse as the water is lost. Commercially, tunnel and tray drying are used to produce dried vegetables, some fruits, spices such as garlic and onion powder, and pasta. Many of the dried products are not sold as such but are used by food processors as ingredients in food mixes such as dried soups. Pasta is probably the largest selling air-dried food that consumers purchase directly.

Home Dehydrators

Purchased home food dehydrators and portable convection ovens fitted with drying trays provide better control over climatic conditions and food quality than sun drying. Drying foods in a conventional oven gives much less satisfactory results. Home dehydrators and convection ovens are equipped with a heating element and a fan that blows hot, dry air at moderate speeds around the food.

Both countertop dehydrators and portable convection ovens can be used on a 110/120 volt general purpose circuit (15 AMP). The food dehydrators draw 525–800 watts; the convection ovens draw about 1,500 watts and should not be used on the same general household circuit with other heating appliances such as a coffee maker or toaster. This may be an important consideration in view of the fact that convection ovens used for drying may be running for many hours.

Food dehydrators and convection ovens differ in their range of temperature settings and available square feet of drying space. The temperature settings for home dehydrators range from a low of 85°F to 110°F up to a high of 140°F to 145°F. Convection ovens run from about 140°F up to 500°F. The home dryers usually have more racks than a convection oven giving greater capacity, but few can dry more than eight to ten pounds wet weight at a time. Thus, you end up usually with no more than one-half to two pounds of dried food based on its initial moisture content. Convection ovens are limited to two to three pounds wet weight. Drying times vary but range from 16 to 48 hours. A study at the University of Minnesota also found that home drying was more energy costly than home canning (I. Wolf *et al.*, *Drying Foods at Home*, Extension Folder 554–1980, University of Minnesota Agricultural Extension Service 1980). However, it should be safer than home canning. Home drying should be discouraged for any food that fits in the Hazard I category such as eggs, some dairy products, fish, and probably meats. The big problem is how to store home-dried foods, especially if they are susceptible to oxidation and need to be vacuum packaged.

Spray Drying

Spray drying is a process using a large cylindrical chamber, in some cases 60 to 100 feet tall and 20 feet in diameter. Liquid foods, such as milk and coffee, are sprayed into the chamber along with very hot air at high velocity, as seen in Figure 19.3. Drying can be accomplished in seconds because of the high temperature and the very small droplets (if you decrease the size by one-half you reduce drying time by four times). In spray drying, the water is removed in less than two to ten seconds. This results in almost no nutrient loss compared to tray, tunnel, and sun drying. But the process can be used only for liquids. Less than 5% of the vitamin C, which is the most susceptible vitamin, is destroyed in a liquid food such as a citrus drink. Dry milk, instant tea, and most instant coffee are made this way, as is desiccated liver and yeast. The process is expensive,

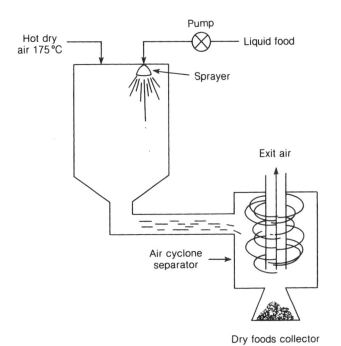

FIGURE 19.3 Typical spray drying process

however, costing three to five cents per pound of water removed. Since skim milk is almost 94% water, it could cost up to 78 cents for every pound of dry milk produced. To reduce the cost, the milk is first passed through a multiple-effect evaporator. This evaporator device is a vacuum chamber that can boil off the water from the milk at low temperature without chemical damage or nutritional losses. It was originally developed by Gail Borden in the mid-1800s. Commercially, milk, tea, and coffee are concentrated to 30–40% solids at a cost of about 0.1 cents per pound of water removed. For milk, evaporation would then cost only 7.4 cents. Since, only three additional pounds of water per pound of solids would need to be removed in the spray dryer at a cost of 10–15 cents, the total cost would be less than 20 cents. In 1983 over five billion pounds of spray-dried dairy products and more than three billion pounds of spray-dried instant coffee were produced. Figure 19.4 outlines the steps in the production of dried nonfat milk showing the MCCPs and QCCPs. Of interest is the step where steam is added to instantize the product. In the first drying step, the lactose in milk solidifies in a form (called amorphous form) that is highly hygroscopic, that is, it readily takes up moisture. In addition, the particles are very small and do not wet easily when added to water. The steaming causes the lactose to recrystallize and form bridges. The particles become larger and dissolve more rapidly when water is added. In addition, they are much less hygroscopic and caking will not occur in storage, so a lined box can be used for storage. This is not done with instant tea or coffee because in the recrystallization much of the flavor would be lost. Tea and coffee are usually distributed in glass jars.

In the milk-drying process fat is first removed. This is because dry whole milk is very susceptible to oxidation and requires very expensive vacuum packaging to keep it for even a short time. In looking at all the steps involved, it should also be obvious to us that one cannot spray dry at home.

Drum Drying

The drying of very viscous food pastes and slurries such as mashed potatoes or tomato paste is achieved by drum drying. Drum drying is used because these pastes are too difficult to spray. One method of drum drying uses two rotating cylinders with a very small space between them, as seen in Figure 19.5. Steam at high temperature (120 to 140°C) is passed inside the cylinders and the slurry is dripped between the cylinders onto the outer surface of the cylinders. The slurry sticks to the cylinder surface, forms a thin layer, dries out, and is scraped off by a blade as the cylinder rotates. Drying is accomplished in two to three minutes because the layer is usually less than

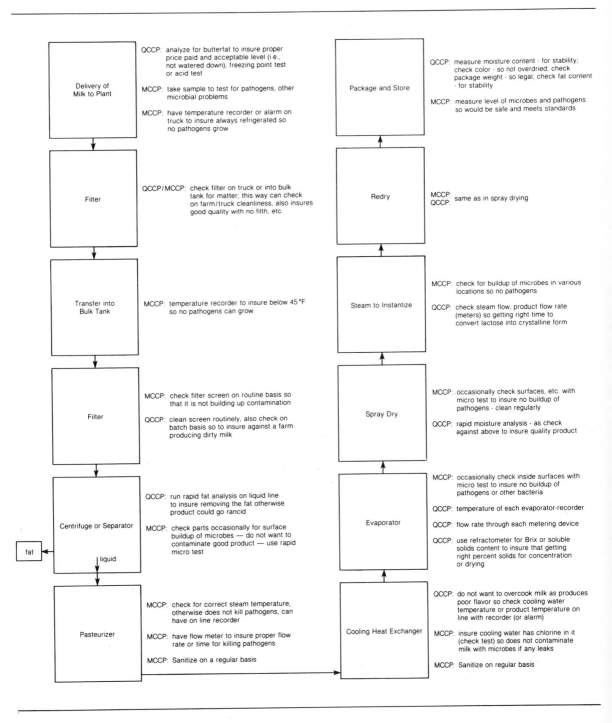

FIGURE 19.4 Instantized dry milk process

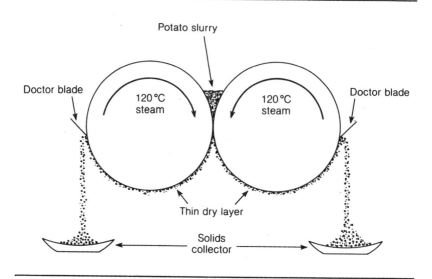

FIGURE 19.5 Typical drum drying process

0.1 inch thick. Nutrient losses are greater than in spray drying but less than in tray drying and sun drying. This is because of the combination of higher temperatures and a short drying time. Drum drying costs about one to two cents per pound of water removed, so it is cheaper than spray drying.

Freeze Drying

Freeze drying is the best dehydration process available at the present time for preventing chemical changes and minimizing nutrient losses during the process. In the production of freeze-dried coffee, for example, coffee is poured to about one-fourth of an inch deep into stainless steel trays. The trays are placed in blast freezers at −40°C (−40°F) and, when frozen, are transferred into a chamber connected to a vacuum pump. Heat is applied to the frozen layers in this chamber after the vacuum is pulled. The heat supplies the energy to sublime (evaporate) the ice directly into a vapor. A vacuum of less than 1.5 mm Hg is needed to prevent the ice from melting. This is based on the same principle as dry ice which at normal pressure sublimes directly into a gas. The ice cannot melt at the pressure created by the vacuum in the chamber, just as dry ice does not melt at atmospheric pressure. The evaporated water travels into a second chamber where it is refrozen on a condenser surface. The vacuum not only prevents the ice from melting but also pulls out residual air so that the water vapor can move rapidly to the condenser surface. The vacuum does not suck out the water, as is commonly thought. The advantage of freeze drying is that the food is kept frozen solid so that it does not shrink as in tray or tunnel drying. This makes rehydration much easier and gives a higher quality product. The process design is shown in Figure 19.6.

Because the food is frozen and is at a low temperature during freeze drying, about six to eight hours are needed to dry food of only one-fourth-inch thickness. In spite of the long time necessary, however, the low temperature results in little nutrient destruction. For example, less than 1% of the vitamin C in fruits is destroyed and less than 5% of the thiamin in dried pork is destroyed. The process is not used extensively, however, because it is prohibitively expensive. It costs much more to operate the four stages of a freeze dryer (freezing, heating, running a condenser, and pulling a vacuum) than it does to tray, tunnel, drum, or spray dry. Freeze drying costs about 30 to 50 cents per pound of water removed. Thus, it is used only when it can provide a distinct advantage such as for coffee, camper foods, and pharmaceuticals. There are no home freeze dryers, although small ones are available but cost anywhere from $8,000 to $10,000 compared to the $30–$150 for a home air dryer.

Other Drying Methods

Many other procedures are used to dry foods. Juice slurries can be dried at low temperatures on belts in a tunnel under vacuum to prevent a cooked flavor. Another juice-drying process uses air blown up from the bottom through a liquid foam (foam mat drying).

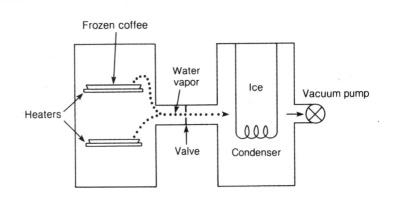

FIGURE 19.6 Typical freeze drying process

These methods are used relatively infrequently because demands for the products are small.

Microwave energy can also be used in drying. When a food is heated during drying, heat must pass from the surface through the dry layer to the water where it can cause evaporation. This is a rather difficult process since the dry layer transmits heat almost 10 times more slowly than the wet food does. This is one reason why drying slows down as the food dries out.

Microwaves operate on a different principle of heat transfer. Water molecules have a charge separation that can be considered like the opposite poles of a magnet. With a magnet, opposite poles attract and like poles repel. A microwave cooker generates a field that changes polarity at a rapid rate. The field can penetrate throughout the food. The water molecules try to move in opposition to the charge of the field. As the water molecules move rapidly, energy is generated and is released as heat. Because the microwaves can penetrate rapidly through the food, whether dry or not, the food heats up quickly. If the food is in a dry air steam, the heated water can evaporate and the food dries out. This process has been tried for many different foods but is fairly expensive.

Deep-fat frying is another drying process. The hot oil replaces the hot air as a drying medium. As water boils out of the food being fried, the oil enters the pores. This can create a new food such as potato chips.

In osmotic dehydration, fruit pieces are tumbled in a bed of solid sugar crystals. The sugar can bind water and thus pulls it out of the pieces. This process is becoming more prevalent for production of fruit leathers.

Extrusion drying is used for many cereal and snack products. In this process, a slurry or cereal dough is passed through a tube that is heated on the outside by steam. The tube is hollow and contains a screw that passes down the center. This screw fits up tightly next to the inside heated wall and turns slowly to carry the dough through so that it is cooked by the high heat of the hot walls. The end of the tube is blocked except for a hole of the desired size. As the very hot mixture comes out, it expands from the high pressure and water flashes off. This gives the fluffy texture found in snacks such as corn curls. The same process is also used to prepare dry dog foods as well as intermediate-moisture dog foods. In the latter case, lower pressures are used so expansion does not occur. The cooking produces the desirable soft texture and also pasteurizes the product.

Lastly, baking can be considered a drying process. Water is driven out of the food during the process, which lowers the ERH to the desired level. The longer the bake, the drier the product and the longer the shelf life. Crackers, for example, are baked to an ERH of 20–30%.

DRY FOOD STORAGE

After dehydration, foods must be carefully packaged to prevent any further quality and nutritional losses. The package must act as a barrier to both oxygen and water. The types of chemical deterioration taking place during storage will be discussed in more detail in Chapter 22, but some principles should be listed here:

1. As little air space as possible should be present. Vacuum packaging is best.

2. The package should be opaque to light. Cans or foil-covered jars would be best but are heavier and more expensive than plastics.

3. The package, can, or jar, should not allow moisture gain.

4. The food should be dried to an ERH of at least 30%. This gives the longest shelf life. Unfortunately, it is almost impossible to estimate when the food reaches this level in a home dryer.

5. Packaged food should be kept in cool, dry places.

One problem with many dry foods is that as they pick up moisture, physical changes can occur. For example, crackers and potato chips will lose their crispness when they reach an ERH of 40–50%. Salt and sugar will cake and not flow when the ERH is over 75–80%. It is very important to seal opened packages carefully to maintain quality and prevent these changes. If proper precautions are taken, the shelf life of many dried foods may be anywhere from 6 to 18 months, which is still much shorter than the three years for canned foods. Many manufacturers of home dryers claim an indefinite or infinite shelf life! This is not true.

SUMMARY

Many foods such as instant coffee and instant milk are prepared by dehydration. The principle of drying is to use heated air to supply energy that removes the water from the food. By this process, the ERH of the food is decreased to a low enough value to prevent microbial growth and chemical reactions.

Sun drying is the oldest method of food dehydration. It is still used extensively today for prunes and raisins. It is the slowest process and causes the most nutrient losses. Because of this, most dehydrated vegetables and meats are prepared by mechanical means in hot-air tunnels. Liquids such as coffee are dried by a spray process that uses very hot air but causes little nutrient destruction. Food slurries such as mashed potatoes are dried on hot drums; this causes greater nutrient loss. The least damaging process is freeze drying. However, it is very expensive and is used for very few foods. Dehydrated foods have a long shelf life if they are protected from moisture and oxygen during storage. The initial quality of most dried vegetables and other products is fairly poor compared to other processes, but consumers use the products for convenience.

Multiple Choice Study Questions

1. Water activity is a measure of
   A. the amount of water in a food
   B. the viscosity or texture of a food
   C. the availability of water in a food
   D. the rate of loss of water from a food

2. Dehydrated foods have a water availability (water activity) of
   A. 1.0
   B. 0.8 to 1.0
   C. 0.7
   D. less than 0.6

3. Which food component is least affected by dehydration?
   A. vitamin C
   B. vitamin A
   C. vitamin B_1
   D. protein

4. In drying foods to make them safe from all microbiological decay you need to dry them to below what % ERH?
   A. 60%
   B. 75%
   C. 80%
   D. 85%
   E. 90%

5. In packaging a dry food that is high in unsaturated fats, the primary concern of the package should be to
   A. prevent oxygen from coming into the pouch
   B. prevent water from coming into the pouch
   C. prevent loss of CO_2 from the food so that senescence is decreased
   D. hold in ethylene gas to insure ripening

6. Which of the following causes the greatest deterioration of dehydrated foods?

    A. rancidity
    B. microbial growth
    C. loss of water
    D. enzyme decay

The following is a list of drying processes. Use it to answer questions 7 through 16.

    A. drum drying
    B. freeze drying
    C. air drying
    D. spray drying
    E. sun drying

7. Which one is the most expensive?

8. Which takes the longest time?

9. Which is used to produce potato flakes?

10. Which is used to make the normal type of instant coffee found in vending machines?

11. Which causes the greatest amount of nutrient loss?

12. Which one results in the least amount of nutrient loss?

13. Which one is performed in a tunnel process to make diced vegetables?

14. Which is used to produce many spices?

15. Which one requires the use of a vacuum?

16. Which is used to make instant milk powder?

17. A good place to store dehydrated foods at home is
    A. under the sink
    B. in the cabinet over the stove
    C. in a cabinet near the sink
    D. in a separate pantry

18. In terms of availability of water for microbial growth which process would be considered most like dehydration?
    A. flash 18
    B. freezing
    C. vacuum packaging
    D. filtration

*Essay Study
Questions*

1. What is the major principle of drying?

2. What are the advantages and disadvantages of sun drying foods?

3. How are liquid foods dried?

4. Contrast home drying to commercial tunnel drying.

5. What are the problems with dry-food storage?

6. Describe the freeze-drying process.

*Things
to Do*

1. Make some thin slices of peaches, plums, or apples. Place them on a screened tray and cover with cheesecloth. Dry them outside in the sun. How long does it take? What is their quality?

2. Determine which foods in your home were prepared by drying and by what methods.

3. Slice some very lean beef into thin slices. Place in an oven at the lowest setting and keep the door ajar. A fan blowing into the space will help. How long does it take to dry? What is the quality? If you have access to a home dryer, try it in there instead.

4. Dry some apple slices as in # 3. Before drying, dip them in a solution of vitamin C (about 10 tablets of 100 mg each dissolved in a quart of water). Remove some slices every hour and put them in a sealed plastic bag or jar. Hold them at room temperature. Which ones have developed mold after one to two months? It might help to inoculate them with some spores. You can guess the water activity of the slices by putting them in the four fish tanks previously prepared for the microbiology experiments. Put two slices of the same drying time (and cut to exactly the same weight) into each tank. Weigh before and after being in the tank for 24 hours. Plot the weight change versus the water activity (% ERH) on graph paper like this.

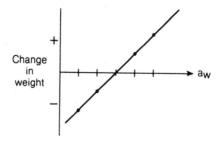

Connect the values. The intersection point at zero weight change is the % ERH of the food. This method can also be used for other foods such as breads, figs, fig newtons, etc.

Chapter 19. Answers to Multiple-Choice Study Questions: **1,** C; **2,** D; **3,** D; **4,** A; **5,** A; **6,** A; **7,** B; **8,** E; **9,** A; **10,** D; **11,** E; **12,** B; **13,** C; **14,** E; **15,** B; **16,** D; **17,** D; **18,** B.

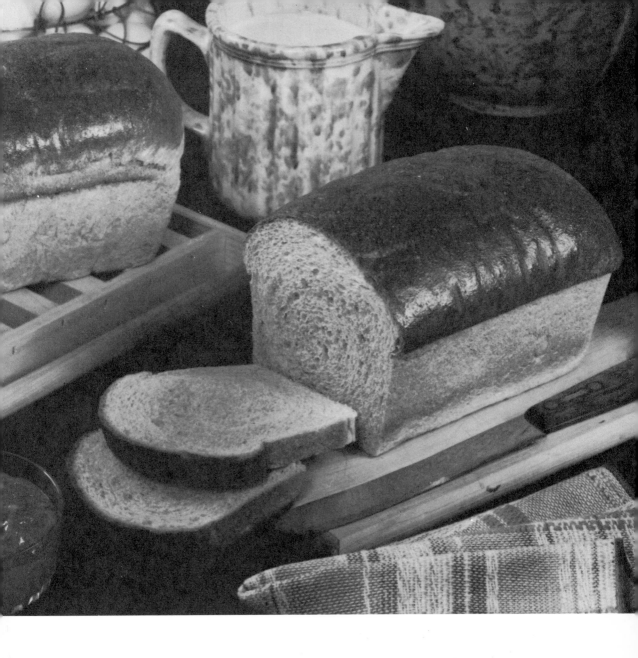

FOOD FERMENTATIONS:
THE USEFUL GERMS

20

As with many other processes, there is little information about how fermentation was discovered. At some point a villager may have put berries in a jar, and the right microorganism may have caused it to turn into an interesting bubbling juice. The same may have been true for milk fermentations, carried out in the stomach skin of an animal and left out in the sun. It was not until the 1860s when Louis Pasteur was trying to solve spoilage problems in the French wine and beer industry that the understanding of fermentation came about.

PRINCIPLES OF FERMENTATION

The basic principle of fermentation is the conversion of unstable food components into a more stable form by the use of microorganisms. To avoid totally using up the food, fermentation is carried out under conditions that produce amino acids, acids, alcohols, other small organic compounds, and various gases. This is much like the incomplete breakdown of glucose in muscles when oxygen is limited.

If done properly, the process also eliminates the chances of the growth of pathogens in many foods. This is because most food poisoning organisms cannot grow in very acid conditions or in alcohol. For example, *Clostridium botulinum* is prevented from growing at a pH of less than 4.6, *Salmonellae* species at a pH less than 4.8, and *Staphylococcus aureus* at around pH 4.2. Using desirable microorganisms to produce enough acid in milk converts it to cheese, which then becomes a safe product. Since most spoilage organisms cannot grow in alcoholic or acidic conditions, the shelf life of the product is extended. A second basis of fermentation is the production of an aesthetically acceptable new food product from the raw material. Wine from grapes or Camembert cheese from goat's or cow's milk are two good examples, as is sauerkraut from cabbage and bread from wheat.

TYPES OF FERMENTATIONS

There are many different kinds of fermented products that use natural fermentation, which means that the useful organisms are already in the starting material; conditions only need to be set up to get the process going. Natural or "wild" fermentations include sauerkraut, pickles, and olives. Many soy products, poi, coffee, tea, and cocoa all have a natural fermentation step. Wine can also be made by wild fermentation, but it is hard to get an acceptable product every time. In some natural fermentations salt is added as the first step. Since salt acts to bind water, it lowers the a_w and prevents the undesirable organisms from growing while allowing the "wild" type organisms to take over.

The other type of fermentation is a "controlled" type in which a large inoculum of the desired organism is introduced into the food material. This inoculum is called a starter culture. Most people who practice home fermentation use commercially prepared starters. A large number of organisms is used so that they don't have to compete with the other natural organisms present. Most fermentations of cheese, yogurt, bread, wine, beer, vinegar and sausage are carried out this way. For beer, wine, or bread, a yeast of the *Saccharomyces* genus is used, whereas most dairy fermentations use lactic acid producing bacteria such as the *Streptococcus* and *Lactobacillus* species. Typical starter cultures are either frozen or dried. One area of interest in genetic engineering is to create starter organisms that are hardier under adverse environmental conditions, metabolize and produce the desired end products faster, and are resistant to any potential inhibitors that may be present.

To get the desired end product in either type of fermentation, the environmental conditions of the food must be controlled. These include temperature, amount of inoculum, concentration of initial food material (for example, the sugar level in grapes), pH, water activity (by adding salt or sugar), and the oxygen level. For example, sauerkraut needs to be covered during fermentation. This not only prevents mold growth but also sets up an anaerobic (low oxygen) condition for the organisms that will then produce the desirable fermentation acids. Salt is also added to lower a_w and start the process.

TYPICAL FOOD FERMENTATIONS

To understand fermentation better, we will discuss two typical processes.

Bread

The manufacture of bread from flour is a controlled fermentation that uses a starter culture. There are numerous ways in which it can be carried out. The basic process used in the home is the straight dough procedure. Flour is mixed with water and various dry ingredients such as sugar (sucrose), milk solids, salt, and fat. Then yeast is added to this mixture. To make the yeast more active, especially if the dry form is used, it is dissolved initially in water. The yeast solution is kept at room temperature for 3 to 60 minutes to allow the yeast to recover from the previous injurious effects of drying and is then added to the flour/ingredient dough and mixed thoroughly. The mixture is held at 25 to 35°C at high humidity to prevent drying out. The yeast begins to break down the sugar, producing carbon dioxide, alcohol, and some acid. The yeast also excretes some enzymes (amylases) that digest the starch into sugars that they then can also ferment. At the same time, the flour protein is being oxidized (reacted upon by various constituents) so that it can form a continuous network to hold in the gas. The added salt binds water and prevents other organisms from growing during the fermentation so the yeast does not have to compete against them. The dough is punched down several times and held until the protein has been developed. At home this may require six to eight hours. It can then be rolled, panned, and baked. The baking kills the yeast so that fermentation is stopped. As the bread is heated, the gases and water vapors expand inside the loaf and give it the desired texture and the heat causes chemical reactions to give the desired flavor and color.

Cheese

Milk initially has a pH of around 6.6 to 6.8 so most organisms, including food poisoning types, can grow rapidly in it. The milk is first pasteurized to reduce the natural bacterial load and kill pathogens. It is then added to a large vat. A starter culture that produces lactic acid from lactose (*Streptococcus lactis*) is introduced into the milk. The mixture is held at about 30°C in the vat. Rennin, an enzyme that can coagulate the milk protein under acid conditions, is also added. The acid and rennin work together to form the curd, which is the coagulated protein casein. One can also coagulate milk without using a starter culture just by adding some acid along with the rennin. As the curd forms it is cut so that the liquid (whey) drains out. As this is going on the acid level is continuously checked to make sure the culture is working. Once the desired pH level is reached the liquid whey is drained out of the vat. The curd is cut up, squeezed, and held at about 37 to 38°C for further fermentation. It is cut and squeezed again and more whey is removed. Not only is fermentation going on but the curd is being dehydrated. The more water that is removed, the drier and harder is the cheese.

At this point the curd is essentially cottage cheese. It has a pH of around 5.0. Salt is added and the cottage cheese is put into a hoop where more water is squeezed out. It is held for at least 60 days at refrigerated temperature to cure it. After this aging, it can be sold as cheddar cheese.

Another type of microorganism may also be added before hooping the cheese. This method is used to produce the desired flavors and textures of the many special cheeses we know. For example, a mold is added for bleu cheese and roquefort cheese. The chopped curd with the added microbe is put in a hoop and water is squeezed out as in the cheddaring process. The hoops are held at the temperature and humidity necessary for the second organism to carry out its fermentation. Eventually the cheese is packaged to prevent further drying out.

A NEW FERMENTATION IDEA FOR THE FUTURE

Protein supplies are low in some parts of the world, and the lack of protein can lead to malnutrition. Scientists have been studying the use of fermentation processes to produce protein more rapidly than by using agriculture or animal husbandry. A typical process would be the fermentation of undesirable waste material by a yeast. The substrates (the material to be fermented) being studied are sewage, raw petroleum, grass and leaves, waste from paper mills, waste from food processing plants, as well as many other fermentable substrates. The idea is to produce more organisms, not to make the substrate into an edible form. To produce these organisms, the mixture must usually be violently agitated and possibly aerated so that maximum growth and division takes place.

Since the organism is the desired end product, one must be chosen that can be eaten by humans or animals. Yeasts are usually used since they have a high protein content that is of good quality. Examples are the *Candida* or *Torulopsis* strains. After fermentation, the yeasts are separated out by centrifugation, then dried by spray drying to form a powder called SCP (single-cell protein), which can be added to various foods. One problem is that the cell wall may have to be broken to increase the digestibility of the protein. In addition, the nuclear material, RNA and DNA, may have to be removed because consumption of large amounts can lead to deposition of uric acid crystals in the joints or kidneys of a human body.

Russia has successfully carried out this process and uses the product for feeding pigs and cattle. The Amoco Food Company in the United States produces dried yeast that can be used in human foods. They grow the yeast on alcohol derived from cereal grain. Because of FDA restrictions on the presence of toxins, raw sewage or crude petroleum cannot be used as the substrate. In the future, however, this may be changed if the world food situation gets worse. One obvious advantage of the process is that it is not at the mercy of the elements because the whole production of food is within a building. The disadvantage is that people don't eat microorganisms as such. Somehow the product will have to be made into a food we would be willing to consume.

SUMMARY

Fermentation is the process by which foods are acted upon by microorganisms. Some of the food constituents are converted into acids, alcohol, and flavor components. If enough acid or alcohol is formed, decay by other microbes and growth of pathogens is prevented. In addition, the process creates a new, aesthetically pleasing food. The fermentation can be brought about either by natural organisms present on the food or by addition of a starter culture. Environmental conditions must be controlled to allow for the correct fermentation. This is done in making bread and cheese. In the future, waste materials may be fermented to produce yeast protein that can be used for animal or human consumption.

Multiple Choice Study Questions

1. Which food is not a fermented food?

A. vinegar
B. olives
C. marinated mushrooms
D. bread

2. The primary basis of food fermentation is to

A. use up the nutritional value of the food to produce bacteria
B. to produce amino acids that kill bacteria
C. to produce acids or alcohol that inhibit pathogens
D. dehydrate the food
E. none of the above

3. Sauerkraut is the result of

A. a natural fermentation of two yeasts
B. a natural fermentation of a mold
C. a natural fermentation of three bacteria
D. the fermentation of an added bacteria
E. none of the above

4. What best describes why yeast do not grow in bread after baking?

A. the acid produced in fermentation inhibits them
B. the calcium propionate inhibits them
C. the % ERH becomes too low for them to grow
D. the salt present binds water so they can't grow
E. the baking kills them

5. In the making of cheese

A. the culture produces alcohol that prevents mold growth
B. the acid is added to prevent yeast
C. salt is added to prevent the bacteria from producing acid
D. the acid causes the calcium to be removed
E. rennin and acid cause the curd to form

6. In cheese making which describes the solid mass?

A. curd
B. whey
C. SPC

D. rennin

E. bacteria

7. New protein sources for future consumption will probably include

A. SCP

B. FDA

C. EDA

D. USDA

E. none of the above

Essay Study Questions

1. What is the basic principle of processing foods by fermentation?

2. What types of fermentations are there? Give examples of each.

3. Describe the process of bread fermentation.

4. How are cheeses made?

5. What is single-cell protein? How is it made?

Things to Do

1. Obtain bulletins from your local county experiment station office for preparation of yogurt, sauerkraut, cheese, or other fermented foods. Prepare one of these foods. The *Science Experiments You Can Eat* book has a yogurt experiment.

2. Using a cookbook make bread from scratch. You can vary the process by first freezing and also drying the yeast and determining the effects on the usefulness of the yeast.

3. Try to list the types of fermented foods found in your home. Are they natural or controlled fermentations?

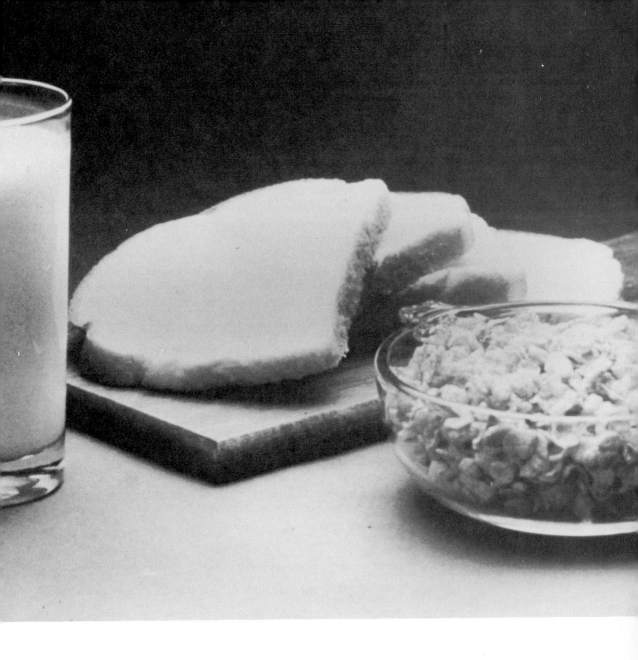

THE USE OF CHEMICALS FOR PRESERVATION AND OTHER PURPOSES

21

As with other food preservation techniques, the use of chemicals to preserve food has a long history. Perhaps one of the oldest processes is the practice of smoking and drying foods. Of course, at that time no one knew the basis of smoking as a chemical preservation process. Today it is recognized that the surface drying and the chemicals in the smoke deposited on the surface of the food help prevent the growth of deteriorative organisms. Fermentation is another ancient practice that was not well understood by its users. This process also is a chemical preservation technique; a desirable organism grows and produces substances such as acids or alcohol that inhibit the growth of undesirable microbes.

Salts and spices were also used to preserve meats. On expeditions, many early explorers carried a salted, partially dried meat that had the consistency of jerky. The combination of salt, some spices that had antimicrobial properties, and fermentation helped preserve these foods in early times.

Chemical preservation can be divided into two categories according to function: (1) the use of chemicals to control or prevent growth of undesirable microbes and (2) the use of chemicals to control nonmicrobial deteriorative reactions such as rancidity. By the nature of some of these chemicals, the foods also become flavored. Other additives are used to improve the aesthetic properties of a food such as color, flavor, and odor. Those that improve texture are called functional additives. Finally, nutrients can also be added to foods to improve nutritional value.

Chemical additives cannot be added solely at the will of the producer. Controls are necessary. As we will see in Chapter 25, specific tests must be performed to prove their safety. Chemicals can be added only if:

1. They serve a useful purpose.

2. They are effective for the job for which they are intended.

3. They do not conceal disease or decay or any other faults.

4. They are safe for humans as determined by appropriate tests.

5. They are noted on the food label, unless regulations do not require it.

All food additives come under the regulatory authority of the Food and Drug Administration. They will be discussed in Chapter 25. It should be noted now, however, that not all chemicals added to foods are food additives in a legal sense.

CHEMICAL PRESERVATION BY FERMENTATION

Fermentation is the best known method of natural chemical food preservation. As discussed in Chapter 20, during fermentation conditions are set up for the partial metabolism of the components of a food. When sugar is metabolized incompletely, instead of only carbon dioxide and water being produced, many intermediates are formed that can act to preserve the food. Acetic acid is the principle acid formed in vinegar, and lactic acid is the principle acid formed in dairy products. In grape or barley malt fermentation, ethanol is formed. These acids and alcohol prevent the growth of undesirable organisms and thus make the food more stable. It is interesting to note that, because metabolism is incomplete, the energy value of the food is not reduced to any great extent by fermentation.

CHEMICAL MICROBIAL INHIBITORS

Many foods cannot be preserved by the fermentation method. Microbial inhibitors may be added to these foods to impart stability if they are not processed by canning, drying, refrigeration, or freezing. The most commonly used microbial inhibitors for foods are table salt (sodium chloride) and sugar (sucrose). Sugar and salt inhibit microbial growth by binding the water, thus making it less available for biochemical reaction. This is the method used in making jams, jellies, and cured hams. Other chemicals that do the same job are glycerine and propylene glycol, which are added to the soft, moist, burger-type pet foods and to toaster tarts.

Various types of acids are good microbial inhibitors, especially against pathogens. Typical acids added to processed foods include citric acid, acetic acid, and phosphoric acid. They are used to lower the pH to a value where pathogenic organisms cannot grow. Thus, mayonnaise has vinegar (acetic acid) added to it so that it does not have to be sterilized by heating at high temperatures. In fact, if properly made, mayonnaise needs no heat treatment. Phosphoric or citric acids are typically added to carbonated beverages as microbial inhibitors. These acids probably prevent certain enzyme reactions from occurring that are important for growth of the microbe.

Some inhibitors directly affect the metabolic processes of microbes, thus preventing their growth. An example is benzoic acid, which is found naturally in high concentration (about 4–5%) in cranberries. It is used in many carbonated beverages. Other examples are calcium propionate, which is added to bread, and sorbic acid, which is added to beverages and to semi-moist pet foods; both prevent mold growth. Some spices, such as garlic and pepper, are felt to have a similar antimicrobial effect.

Synthetic metabolic inhibitors, such as the paraben compounds, are incorporated in fresh food wrappers to prevent surface growth of molds. Antibiotics, another form of growth inhibitor, have been used in some food processes to prevent spoilage; an example is a dip for fresh fish. The regulation allowing the use of antibiotics for this purpose was finally revoked by the FDA because many processors were relying on the dip rather than on good sanitation. Antibiotics are still used in animal feeds. There they prevent pathogenic organisms from causing disease in animals that are kept in close quarters. The law requires that there be no residue of the antibiotic in the meat or milk when it is consumed. Keeping antibiotics out of raw milk is also important to the cheese industry. If milk contains the antibiotic penicillin, it will inhibit the growth of the starter culture, thus spoiling the batch.

One of the most controversial additives is sodium nitrite. It is used in meat curing to create the pink color we associate with hams, hot dogs, and bacon. Nitrite also helps prevent, the out-growth of *Clostridium botulinum* spores during processing and storage. It has been shown that nitrite can react with certain amino acids of the cooked food to produce a chemical (nitrosamine) that can cause cancer. Thus a certain risk is involved. The issue of which risk is greater, death from food poisoning or cancer, will be covered in Chapter 26.

Many other chemicals are used as sanitizing agents, that is, they are used to sterilize food contact surfaces, the inside of bottles, and process equipment. A common sanitizing agent is the iodophor compounds that have unfortunately contributed to an excess of iodine in the diet. Another compound, chlorine, is used in water to sterilize it for both processing as well as drinking water. In fact, in processes where water contacts food directly, such as in a blancher, measurement and control of the free chlorine level is a HACCP procedure. Anyone who has been in a pool has noted the use of chlorine to prevent spreading of diseases.

ADDITIVES THAT PREVENT CHEMICAL DETERIORATION

In the next chapter we will discuss some of the chemical reactions other than microbial decay that destroy food quality. One particular common reaction is rancidity. Many synthetic chemicals can be used to slow down the process, including propyl gallate (PG), butylated hydroxytoluene (BHT), butylated hydroxyanisole (BHA), and tertiary butyl hydroquinone (TBHQ). In addition, processors may use ethylenediamine-tetracetic acid (EDTA) and vitamin E for a similar effect. Although the names may sound unusual and possibly dangerous, these chemicals, which are legal food additives, help prevent food losses. They can be used only at certain levels established by the Food and Drug Administration. You will find these chemicals listed on the labels of foods such as cereals, snacks, and dehydrated products.

Sulfite, in various forms such as sulfur dioxide or sodium bisulfite, is used to prevent browning in sun-dried fruits and in frozen fruits and vegetables. Sulfite is also used in wine production as an antimicrobial agent. Introduced into the crushed wine juice to inhibit bacterial growth, it does not affect growth of the yeast starter culture.

FUNCTIONAL ADDITIVES FOR TEXTURE

Many different types of additives and chemicals are used to impart physical stability to foods during processing and storage.

Emulsifiers

Emulsifiers and surfactants are chemicals with surface-active properties that help both to create an emulsion and to preserve the structure of the food material. For example, in the manufacture of salad dressing, a surfactant is added to help separate the oil into small droplets in the water phase. Monoglycerides and diglycerides are common surfactants added to foods for this purpose. Other types used are Tweens and the Spans, which are synthetic chemicals that have the same function. They are nontoxic to the body because they are not digested. They are used quite often since they are cheaper than natural emulsifying agents. A natural type of surfactant is lecithin. It is extracted from egg yolks and soybeans. It has a charge and adsorbs on the oil drop surface slowing coalescence. Mustard powder helps in a similar way and is added to stabilize mayonnaise. Surfactants such as the mono-and diglycerides and sodium stearyl-lactylate are also used in the manufacture of bread to prevent staling during storage. They keep the bread soft. In addition, surfactants can be used in juices to prevent settling and in coffee creamers to prevent separation.

Anticaking Agents

Anticaking agents are chemicals that, when added to dry foods, such as salt or powdered sugar, absorb water preferentially so that the product does not stick together. This allows the material to be free-flowing. Silicates are added to salts to prevent caking and to yield an easy-pouring material. Cornstarch is usually added to powdered sugar for the same reason. This is a problem in the food industry where huge storage bins are used. Without the starch, the sugar would not flow. Dextrose may be added to salt for this same purpose.

Oxidizing Agents

Oxidizing agents are chemicals added to flours to create a more elastic protein. This results in a bread that will retain its structure after rising and baking. Bromate, iodates, and vitamin C are some of the chemicals that are used for this purpose.

Water Binders and Thickeners

Binding and thickening agents are made from proteins, gums, and starches. When added to food they help bind water as well as impart a thick gravy or heavy syrupy texture. For example, the manufacture of cream-style corn requires the addition of a starch to produce the creamy texture. Many natural starches and gums lose their ability to hold water during heat processing or freezing, thus some starches and gums have been chemically modified to give heat or freezer stability that improves functionality. Some of the major carbohydrate thickeners include corn starches, wheat starches, micro-crystalline cellulose derived from wood pulp, and carboxy methylcellulose (CMC). A recently approved one (in 1981) is polydextrose, a long chain compound made from glucose but with chemical bonds that are not digestible by human enzymes. It is completely soluble. Polydextrose can serve as a thickener, as a viscosity agent, and as a non-nutritive filler (for use in reduced-calorie foods). It can be added to salad dressing to increase viscosity (fluid thickness) without increasing calories. Increasing the viscosity also decreases the rate at which the oil phase separates out.

Major protein functional ingredients are whey solids, casein, and soy protein. They can be used to bind water, to impart a desired gel-like texture, or to replace some of the animal protein used in a formulation.

Gums come from a variety of sources. The seaweed gums include carrageenan and agar. The major gum from fruits is pectin. Plant gums include agar, locust bean, and tragicanth. A common gum that is being used more often by the food industry is xantham. It is produced by a bacteria in a fermentation process. All these gums have a basic carbohydrate structure similar to starch, but the sugars in the structure may be different (e.g., galacturonic acid in pectin) and the sugars may have substitute compounds attached to the -OH groups. Most are nondigestible by humans so they also function as dietary fiber as we discussed in Chapter 4.

Phosphates and polyphosphates are added to some foods, especially processed meats, to help retain water. Meat, when cooked, loses water and becomes tougher. The polyphosphates prevent water loss by interacting with proteins and calcium. Calcium, magnesium, and aluminum salts added to vegetables that are to be processed help maintain crispness after canning or freezing.

Enzymes

Certain enzymes can also be used to impart a change in texture. For example, pineapple contains a very heat-stable enzyme called bromelin, which tenderizes meat such as chicken during cooking. Other useful enzymes that have similar properties are papain from papaya fruit, zingabain in ginger, and ficin from figs. Meat tenderizers used in the home contain these enzymes. One meat company has devised a process to inject the animal with tenderizing enzymes just before slaughter to produce a very tender meat. Other enzymes are used to clarify apple juice (amylases).

**FUNCTIONAL
ADDITIVES
FOR AESTHETIC
PURPOSES**

Flavoring Agents

Sugar and Salt. Many food additives are used for purposes other than preventing the growth of organisms or obtaining physical effects. Salt and various sugars are frequently used to enhance flavor because of their obvious salty and sweet flavors. Sucrose consumption (disappearance) in the United States amounts to about 90 pounds per person per year. Other sugars, such as glucose, corn syrups, and the newer high fructose corn syrups, account for another 40 pounds per person per year. Salt disappearance amounts to 10 to 15 pounds per year. All other chemicals and food additives, including spices and proteins, account for less than another 10 pounds per person per year with about 3,000 of these making up only two pounds.

Artificial Sweeteners. Artificial sweeteners have had an interesting and sobering history. Dulcin, which was used in the early 1900s, and cyclamate, which was used up to 1969, were removed from the market because later research showed they might produce cancer. The major artificial sweeteners allowed today are saccharin and aspartame. Aspartame was approved only in late 1981. Although aspartame is somewhat unstable in solution, it can be used in soft drinks as well as in dry food mixes or as a powdered table sweetener. The history of saccharin will be discussed in the last chapter because of its unique legal and safety aspects. Aspartame has also had a difficult history. It is essentially a molecule made from two amino acids—aspartic acid and phenylalanine. Some animal studies seemed to suggest that if fed in high enough levels aspartame could produce brain damage. After 10 years of controversy, many animal studies, and public hearings, the FDA finally approved the compound but required a warning label on any food it is used in to indicate that people with a rare genetic disorder called phenylketonuria (PKU) should avoid the product. These people do not have the right enzymes to metabolize phenylalanine totally so that toxic byproducts may build up in the brain.

Other sweeteners derived from foods are being worked on, for example, several proteins from artichokes and miracle fruit. Grapefruits, despite their bitterness, also contain dehydrochalcone, a compound that induces sweetness. Although the foods themselves can be eaten, extraction and sale of specific compounds derived from them is illegal since they are unapproved food additives under the law.

Artificial sweeteners are important for diabetics and others on sugar-restricted diets, but the necessity for the average person to consume large amounts of artificial sweeteners is nutritionally dubious. Advertising and snacking habits have greatly increased the consumption of foods with artificial sweeteners. Of course, if people cannot control their appetites, it may be better to drink carbonated diet beverages rather than many cans of sugar-sweetened ones a day that add excess calories to the diet.

Organic Flavors. There are many companies that produce flavor compounds for foods. These flavors can be produced either by extracting the natural flavor from a food, by fermentation, or by synthesizing it from other organic molecules. In the latter method, trained chemists can identify many of the components of a natural food flavor simply by tasting or smelling a flavor and by using high-powered chemical analysis equipment. Instruments called gas or liquid chromatographs are used. These separate the odor and flavor of a food into its various organic components, which are then analyzed on more complicated instruments such as a mass spectrometer. These instruments can be used to identify many of the components in a flavor. For example, an analysis of coffee flavor shows that it is made up of over 400 different components, tea has more than 200, and cocoa has over 300. The instruments can be used in production as well. Since the flavor of roasted coffee beans can vary from batch to batch as well as from variety to variety, a gas chromatograph is used to determine the combination of raw beans necessary to maintain a uniform flavor in the final coffee product.

This way you can always be sure that you are getting the same coffee flavor in your favorite brand.

Because of their ability to identify the flavor characteristics of the various constituents of a food, chemists can make up a given flavor from a few individual chemical compounds. It is very difficult to get the exact flavor because flavors can be made up of hundreds of different compounds and occur in quantities as minute as several parts per million or less. Some of these compounds would be toxic if consumed in large amounts but are harmless when present in traces. For example, acetone occurs in the natural extract of coffee flavor at less than one part per million and is necessary for the flavor. By itself acetone is the principal ingredient in nail polish remover and would cause severe liver damage if consumed in large quantities.

After the chemist isolates and identifies the various chemicals from the natural flavor, the compounds are mixed together to simulate the natural flavor. Making artificial flavors is necessary because natural flavors are very expensive to produce in large quantities. For example, it takes five tons of bananas to produce one pint of banana oil, which gives banana flavor. It is easier and cheaper to mix together synthetic organic ingredients to get the same flavor.

One of the principle flavoring agents used in foods is MSG (monosodium glutamate). It enhances the flavor of meat and adds meaty flavor and "mouth feel" to soups. We consume about one and one-half pounds of it per person per year. MSG is the sodium salt of the natural amino acid, glutamic acid, but is usually produced by a microbial fermentation rather than by extraction from food. Vanillin is the synthetic compound used to simulate natural vanilla flavor. In the United States we consume so many products that are vanilla flavored that if it were all to come from natural vanilla beans, we would use up the world supply in one day.

Spices. Spices are used to enhance the flavor of foods. The quest for spices, especially salt, was the major reason for much early exploration. Many spices have metabolic effects that aid in the preservation of foods by preventing microbial growth and rancidity. Spices are added in the home as well as in industry to aid in food acceptance.

Coloring Agents
There are two different types of food coloring agents: natural coloring agents, which are extracted from foods, and synthetic

coloring agents, which are usually synthesized from various organic petroleum products. Carotene extracted from carrots is an example of a natural coloring agent. Violet # 1 is an example of a coloring agent made synthetically. It was used for stamping the grades of meat on animal carcasses until some tests showed it to be carcinogenic to rats. It was then removed from use in foods. Many other color derivatives have been proven to be unsafe according to the best available data. It should be noted that today there are very few approved synthetic food coloring agents used compared to the 695 used in 1900. Most of these were made from coal tars and were known as coal tar dyes. Synthetic coloring agents are present in less than 10% of the food we consume and amount to a very low intake level since they need only be used in small quantities. Every synthetic (artificial) color must go through the safety testing procedures before it can be approved by the government (FDA) for use in food. In addition, every time the manufacturer makes a batch of the chemical, samples must be sent to the FDA so that the purity can be checked. Once checked and found to meet the standards the chemical can be used in the food supply. This second test is called certification.

Each certified color has its own special letter/number code. For example, FD & C # 5 is yellow # 5 or the chemical tartrazine. The FD & C means it can be used in foods, drugs, and cosmetics. If you read the labels on such cosmetics as hair shampoo, you might see some certified colors listed such as D & C Green # 5. This is an approved, certified color that can be used only in drugs and cosmetics. The natural pigments used as food colors, such as carotene, saffron, paprika, and caramel, are exempt from certification but still must be proven to be safe as a food-color additive. Certification is testing only for purity, not for safety.

One example of the use of synthetic food-coloring agents is with Florida oranges. When these oranges are picked at the proper state of ripeness, they are a mottled green color. If the oranges were held until they turned orange they would spoil because of senescence. Thus, the oranges are sprayed with a synthetic color to create an orange color that the consumer feels is desirable and uses as an index of ripeness. People might be confused by ripe green Florida oranges since California oranges are naturally orange in color when optimally ripe. If people did not mind eating oranges with green skins, the added color would not have to be used. Many people feel this practice is deceptive. It should be realized, however, that the nutritional value of a food not eaten is zero. Thus the green orange, if not eaten, would have no true value. In addition, all the energy and labor used to produce it would be wasted. Floridians would grow the other variety of orange if it could withstand the Florida climate, but this is not yet possible. It is to be hoped that there is enough information available to assure that each cosmetic additive used is safe and that in the future the Florida orange can be genetically manipulated to have the desired color.

Some compounds are used to stabilize or maintain a color in food. One of the most important is sodium nitrite. When added to meat, especially pork, it combines with the meat pigment to produce the familiar pink color found in frankfurters, bacon, ham, and other cured sausage. Nitrite also adds some flavor and has some antimicrobial action. It has been found that nitrite both reduces the heat resistance of *Clostridium botulinum* spores and inhibits their outgrowth, so less heat processing is needed. Thus it helps preserve the texture and nutritional value of the food, produces the desirable flavor and color, and insures safety.

Other compounds used to stabilize food color are the various forms of sulfite. Sulfite compounds are applied to fruits and vegetables to inhibit the browning reaction. Vitamin C has a similar effect. Benzoyl peroxide is used to whiten flour by bleaching the natural plant pigments.

NUTRITIONAL ADDITIVES: VITAMINS, MINERALS, PROTEINS, AND AMINO ACIDS

Many ingredients are used specifically to increase the nutritional value of the product. The addition of nutrients to foods is based on policies set by the National Academy of Sciences and the Food and Drug Administration. Some general concepts for the addition of nutrients are:

1. *Restoration.* This is the addition to a food of nutrients that were lost during processing, thus restoring the food's original value. An example would be adding vitamin C to canned tomato juice or to dehydrated mashed potatoes. The FDA suggests that when a food is restored all vitamins that are lost should be added, not just one.

2. *Enrichment.* Enrichment is the addition of nutrients to a food for which specific legal standards have been set. For example, enriched flour and enriched bread have a standard of identity that requires the addition of thiamin, riboflavin, niacin, and iron in order to be sold as such. These standards were established as a health measure to help decrease deficiencies in the diets of Americans in the early 1940s. There is no national law that requires enrichment, only standards of nutrient addition if you want to call a cereal or bread an enriched product. About 20 states, however, require enrichment with the above four nutrients for all cereal grain products sold in their state.

3. *Fortification.* Fortification is the addition of one or more nutrients to a food for a special dietary purpose such as for a health reason. An example would be the fortification of margarine or skim milk with vitamins A and D to help prevent nutritional disease. In certain states where this is required by law, it could be considered enrichment. Many cereals today are fortified to supply 25% of the RDA for many nutrients. Since the terms enrichment and fortification can be confused, the Food and Drug Administration makes no legal distinction between them.

4. *Nutrification.* Some foods are sold as total meal replacers or as substitutes for common foods. If a claim is made that they "are as good as food X," nutrients must be added to be equal or better than X as required by regulation. This is usually done on the basis of the ratio of nutrients to calorie level. Technically there is no difference between this and fortification. Another use of nutrification is to get around the requirement of labeling a product as an imitation food. The FDA regulations require the imitation label only if the product resembles and is a substitute for the real food but is nutritionally inferior. By adding nutrients to reach the same level as in the "real" food, the word imitation is not required.

It should be mentioned that the nutrient addition policies of the FDA were set to prevent over addition of nutrients so that no dietary imbalance or harm will occur. However, the FDA has very little control of over-the-counter vitamin/mineral preparations advertised for nutritional purposes. A question still remains today as to whether snack foods should be fortified to supply vitamins, minerals, and protein in relationship to calories. Many people feel that this is unnecessary because even snack eaters get enough of the other nutrients from their regular foods. The FDA discourages the practice, but fortified snacks are not technically illegal.

AN EXAMPLE OF A FOOD WITH ADDITIVES: WHITE BREAD

A discussion of the additives found in commercial white bread can be used to summarize the kinds and functions of additives used in foods. When flour is milled it is yellow in color, makes an unstable, inelastic dough, and produces bread of low loaf volume. This flour must be oxidized in order to develop the protein necessary to a good texture bread. This can be done by storing the flour in air for several months or by the use of additives to develop the protein. For example, the addition of ascorbic acid (vitamin C) modifies the protein in the flour to help in dough development. Potassium bromate and iodate can also be added to develop the protein. To bleach the flour pigments, hydrogen peroxide, benzoyl peroxide, or lipoxidase are added. This gives bread a white color.

Milk solids can be added to increase the nutritional quality of the protein since wheat gluten is low in lysine and the milk protein provides sufficient lysine. The milk solids also help increase the elasticity of the dough. The sugar found in milk solids, lactose, is important for forming the crust flavor and color. During baking and toasting of bread, the lactose reacts with the protein to produce the desired darkening and flavor.

Besides being added for its flavoring capabilities, salt is added to help control bacterial growth so that only the yeast can grow during fermentation. The salt also helps toughen the dough so it is easier to work with. Sugar is added not only for flavor but also as food for the yeast during the fermentation process. Lysine could also be added to bread to increase the protein nutritional value, since the protein present in bread is a poor quality protein.

Functional additives used in bread include emulsifiers such as the diglycerides that help to prevent staling. Antioxidants can be added to lengthen the shelf life during storage. Calcium propionate is added to bread to prevent moldiness and ropiness, the latter caused by growth of undesirable bacteria. Certain B vitamins and iron must also be added if the bread is to be labeled "enriched." Many chemicals can be added to commercial white bread to increase its shelf life and improve its quality.

SUMMARY

Chemical preservation of foods is done both to control or prevent the growth of undesirable microorganisms and to control or prevent chemical deteriorative reactions. Chemicals used in foods are controlled by the FDA and can be used only if they are proven food ingredients with a long history of use or they have been tested for safety and efficacy. The fermentation process is a natural chemical preservation technique in which acid or alcohol as well as flavors are produced by microbes. Many synthetic acids as well as other chemical inhibitors such as benzoic acid, sorbate, and propionate prevent growth of undesirable microbes. Antioxidants are used in foods to prevent rancidity, and sulfite is used to inhibit browning.

Other types of chemical additives are used to impart desirable physical or appearance characteristics. For example, emulsifiers prevent oil separation in a salad dressing. Other chemicals include anticaking agents, oxidizers, thickeners, and water binding agents. Sugars and salt are the major flavoring agents and account for almost 95% of the total weight of compounds added to foods in the United States. Most artificial flavoring agents are chemicals that are the same as those found in food flavors naturally; the only difference is that they are made synthetically. Other synthetic and natural agents are used to color foods. These cannot be used to deceive the consumer, for example, to conceal damage or decay. They improve the aesthetic value of a food and thus make it more appealing.

The last major category of food additives are nutrients. Certain standards control the addition of nutrients to food. These include restoration of nutrients lost in processing, enrichment as required by law, fortification for special dietary purposes, and nutrification of substitute foods.

Additives are used only when physiological safety has been proved at the levels consumed. All chemicals or foods can cause harm if overconsumed. Proper use should not be a problem. The Food and Drug Administration also requires that additives cannot be used to disguise spoiled or poorly processed foods and that they should be effective in their intended purpose. As a last note it should be remembered that the nutritional value of a food not eaten is zero. Thus aesthetic coloring and flavoring agents do have their place in our food system.

Multiple Choice Study Questions

1. The per capita consumption of chemical compounds added to food (other than sugars and salt) amounts to

  A. more than 100 pounds per year
  B. less than 10 pounds per year
  C. one pound per year
  D. 50 pounds per year
  E. none of the above

2. Which food ingredient is used in the greatest quantity?

  A. salt
  B. sugar
  C. nitrite
  D. propionate
  E. citric acid

3. The use of nitrites in vacuum-packaged bacon does not result in

  A. inhibition of chemical deterioration
  B. inhibition of botulism
  C. possible formation of secondary amines that are carcinogenic
  D. more rapid breakdown of the cured meat pigment
  E. none of the above

4. Sulfite can be used in processing

  A. to destroy thiamin
  B. to prevent rancidity
  C. to prevent fat oxidation
  D. to retard browning
  E. it cannot be used

5. Which food additive is not used to prevent rancidity?

    A. BHA

    B. BHT

    C. EDTA

    D. citric acid

    E. Tween 20

6. Which one of the following additives does not help to prevent microbial growth?

    A. salt

    B. propionate

    C. lecithin

    D. nitrite

    E. sugar

7. Tween, Span, and lecithin are

    A. used to fulfill GRAS list standards

    B. unregulated additives

    C. surfactants

    D. antimicrobial agents

    E. bleaching agents

The following are the regulatory categories for nutritional addition to a food. Use this list to answer questions 8 through 12.

    A. restoration

    B. fortification

    C. enrichment

    D. nutrification

8. The present addition of four nutrients to bread comes under which category?

9. If you wanted to add vitamins to breakfast cereals which regulation category would be applicable?

10. Which category applies to enhancing the nutrient content of a food to make it more competitive against other foods (e.g., adding vitamin C to Tang ® to make it better than orange juice)?

11. In the manufacture of orange juice, which principle is used to bring the level of vitamin C back to the level in fresh juice?

12. A breakfast meal replacer advertised to be as good as eggs, bacon, toast, and juice would come under which category?

13. Which additive helps develop color rapidly when bread is toasted?
   A. non-fat dry milk
   B. sucrose
   C. iron
   D. calcium propionate

The following is a list of additives that can be used in bread. Choose the best one for questions 14 through 18.
   A. sodium propionate
   B. benzoyl peroxide
   C. sodium chloride
   D. iron
   E. sodium iodate

14. Enrichment standard of identity.

15. Bleaches flour pigments.

16. Acts to bind water to prevent bacteria growth during fermentation but to enhance yeast growth.

17. Inhibits mold growth.

Essay Study Questions

1. Into what categories can chemical preservation be divided? Give some examples.

2. List some examples of microbial inhibitors and give an example of where they are used.

3. For what purposes are functional food additives that control texture used? Give some examples.

4. List some other functional food additives and give reasons for their use.

5. What kinds of natural and artificial flavoring agents are used in foods? How great is their use?

6. How are artificial flavors made?

7. Discuss the use of chemicals that are used to color foods.

8. What are the various standards for adding nutrients to foods? Give specific examples.

9. Using white bread ingredients as an example, discuss the function of each additive.

1. Copy down ingredient lists of various foods found in your home. Indicate the individual food additives and ingredients and try to determine their function in the food.

2. Do the experiments in sections 3, 5, and 6 in *Science Experiments You Can Eat.*

3. Make some fresh white bread with and without 0.2% propionate (obtain from pharmacy) or use a commercial white bread. Put slices in plastic bags and observe when mold growth occurs.

Chapter 21. Answers to Multiple-Choice Study Questions: 1, B; 2, B; 3, D; 4, D; 5, E; 6, C; 7, C; 8, C; 9, B; 10, D; 11, A; 12, D; 13, A; 14, D; 15, B; 16, C; 17, A; 18, E.

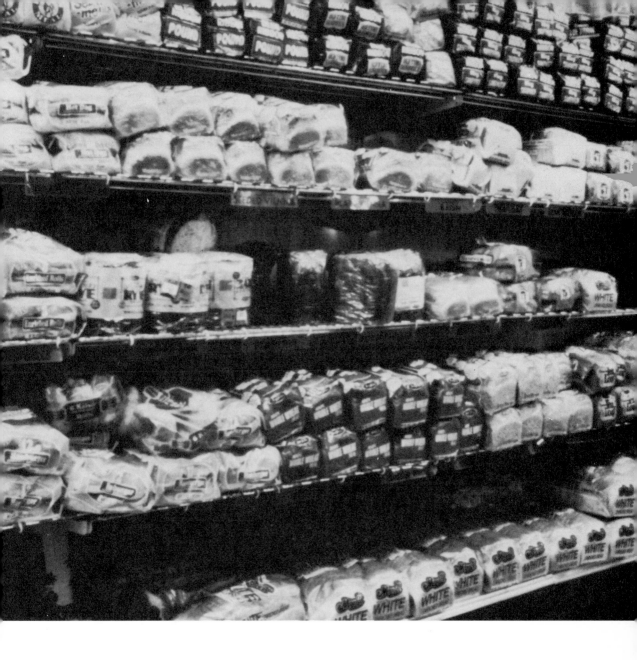

NUTRITIONAL LOSSES DURING STORAGE OF PROCESSED FOODS

GENERAL CONSIDER-ATIONS ON NUTRIENT LOSS

Some nutrients are subject to certain chemical reactions that can result in their chemical loss or loss of bioavailability during processing and storage. Fats, for example, can oxidize in the presence of air, resulting in the loss of linoleic acid, which is an essential fatty acid. However since only a little oxidation is needed to make the food rancid in flavor, the amount of linoleic acid lost is negligible; the problem is that since the food smells bad the value of the food as a whole is lost if it is not eaten. This represents an economic loss to the person who purchased the food. Proteins can react with carbohydrates through nonemzymatic browning at moderate temperatures thereby reducing biological availability. These two reactions, oxidation and browning, will be discussed later in this chapter. Minerals are generally stable to processing and thus not subject to loss unless they are leached out of the food. However some recent work suggests that various constituents of some foods (such as the phytate and some fiber constituents in whole-grain cereals) can interact with some essential minerals such as iron and zinc during manufacture of an engineered food. The mineral then becomes of lower bioavailability, that is the body cannot absorb or utilize it. There is considerable concern since people are using more whole grains and adding fiber to their diet. The USDA is funding major research projects on bioavailability of nutrients in food.

Because of its chemical structure, vitamin C is the most labile (unstable) vitamin. It can be readily oxidized in the presence of water and air and thus will be lost. High temperatures can speed this loss (at a rate of two to three times faster for every 10°C higher temperature). In the dry state vitamin C is much less reactive and much less sensitive to higher temperatures. Vitamin A and its carotenoid precursors, as well as vitamin E, are also subject to oxidation but are more stable than vitamin C. Thiamin is another reactive vitamin but is generally more stable than either vitamin A, C, or E. In enriched cereals, for example, it may take two years for a 25% loss of vitamin B to occur at 25°C and 50% RH, but a 50% loss of vitamin C could occur in several months under the same conditions. Riboflavin is generally stable to heat and moisture. No loss of riboflavin was found in cereals or pasta held at over 120°F and over 50% RH for up to three months as long as it was held in the dark. However, when exposed to light, especially fluorescent lighting, even at room temperature, a 50% loss occurred in one day, especially at the surface of the cereal. Storage of cereals in the dark is advisable.

According to the available literature, the other vitamins are much more stable to processing and storage conditions. A recent book (T.P. Labuza, *Open Shelf-Life Dating of Foods*, Food and Nutrition Press, 1982) gives more details on nutrient losses during processing and storage. The next few sections will look at some of this data. In foods, the reaction leading to nutrient loss is usually due to the fact that when a food is processed the tissues are damaged. This causes the interaction of the nutrient with some other factor and results in an undesirable chemical reaction. Since we have no choice but to process if we want to make foods available year round, we have to accept some nutrient loss. It is this comparison between the risks of some nutrient loss and the benefits of food availability that processing results in the direction of a benefit by insuring year-round availability of all the needed nutrients.

FRESH FOODS   Freshly harvested fruits and vegetables and fresh tissue foods such as meat and fish deteriorate by several different mechanisms—microbial growth, senescence, and physical change. Fresh foods have the highest nutritional value but are subject to some losses as a result of storage and natural aging. The shelf life for most of these fresh products is less than 7 to 14 days so nutrient loss is usually not of great concern. Some other mechanism will usually cause the food to become unacceptable before the nutrient loss would be important in terms of the total diet. For example, when celery loses only 3–5% of its water due to evaporation, it becomes unacceptably soft, that is, it is no longer crisp and will be rejected. Although this water loss damages the tissues and results in a 10–30% loss in vitamin C, that amount of nutrient loss would be of no concern since the product wouldn't be eaten anyway. Some other product would generally be substituted for the celery. Of greater concern is improper refrigeration. At higher temperatures the food metabolizes faster causing reactions leading to nutrient loss. Many green vegetables can lose 50–80% of vitamin C if held at 77°F (25°C) for two to three days. Under these conditions the product may still be edible but the nutrient loss would not be visible. With meats, fish, or milk, on the other hand, holding for that long (24–72 hours) at 77°F would result in such off-flavors that the product would be inedible and any loss of nutrients would not be of consequence to one's well-being because the spoiled product would be replaced with another food. This nutrient loss would be of consequence, of course, when other foods are not available and the whole value of the food is lost, or when one is poor and cannot afford to buy a substitute food.

Table 22.1 shows some data for shelf life of fresh produce. Very little data is available for nutrient loss, and much of it is from old studies that were not very well controlled. Table 22.2 gives some data for beans and spinach. The results indicate that temperature control is very important if loss of vitamin C is to be minimized. It should be noted that spinach, which has almost two weeks' shelf life, could probably lose most of its vitamin C even under refrigeration.

TABLE 22.1 Shelf life of fresh produce

Commodity	Recommended temperature °F	Approximate shelf life
Vegetables		
Asparagus	34	2–3 weeks
Beans (green)	40	7–10 days
Broccoli	32	10–14 days
Cabbage	32	3–4 months
Carrots	32	4–5 months
Cauliflower	32	2–4 weeks
Corn (sweet)	32	4–8 days
Cucumbers	45	10–14 days
Lettuce	32	2–3 weeks
Mushrooms	40	3–4 weeks
Peppers (sweet)	45	2–3 weeks
Spinach	32	10–14 days
Tomatoes	45	4–7 days
Fruits		
Apples	30	3–8 months
Bananas	56	1–2 weeks
Grapefruit	50	4–6 weeks
Grapes	31	2–8 weeks
Lemons	32	1–6 months
Oranges	38	3–8 weeks
Peaches	32	2–4 weeks
Pears	29	2–7 months
Strawberries	32	5–7 days

TABLE 22.2 Loss of vitamin C in fresh vegetables

Commodity	Temperature °F	% Loss in 24 hours	% Loss in 48 hours
Greenbeans	40°F	22	34
	54°F	26	40
	68°F	36	50
Spinach	40°F	27	33
	54°F	41	51
	68°F	56	79

CANNED FOODS

Canned foods have the longest shelf life of all the processed foods, up to several years in some instances. However, the nutritional value, particularly the vitamin content of canned foods, is initially lower than fresh foods because of the high temperature needed in processing to make them safe. In vegetables, for example, 30–50% of vitamin C can be destroyed by the heating process. Canned foods cannot offer the textural quality of fresh foods either, because the heating process changes the texture unless some of the newer HTST methods are used.

Once a food is canned and stored, however, very few changes in nutritional quality or texture take place because of the protection afforded by the can. Holding at high temperature (80–100°F) will defeat this protection as the reaction rates speed up. Figure 22.1 shows how long it takes for a 10% loss in vitamin C to occur in various canned juices and in canned green beans and apricots. It is plotted on a special scale (semi-log scale) to make the data fit a straight line. This plot is called the shelf-life graph. At room temperature (68 to 75°F), a 10% loss of vitamin C in green beans occurs in eight or nine months. This is very long compared to the 50% loss in several days for fresh beans at the same temperature. If the canned foods are held at temperatures near 100°F (37°C) the nutrient losses occur much more quickly. For example, tomato juice loses 10% of its vitamin C in one and one-half months at 100°F.

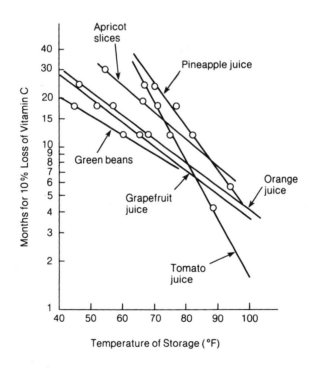

FIGURE 22.1 Time required for a 10% vitamin C loss in canned foods held at different temperatures

Many food scientists use the Q_{10} factor to determine how susceptible a nutrient is to a temperature rise. The Q_{10} is based on how much faster a chemical reaction goes if the food is put at a 10°C (18°F) higher temperature. It is a property of the interaction of the nutrient with the food and is based on how steep the line of log shelf life vs. temperature is. Thus in Figure 22.1 the tomato juice is seen to have a much higher susceptibility to temperature change than orange juice. The Q_{10} for tomato juice is about 5 (shelf life at 60°F, which is about 50 months divided by shelf life of 10 months at 78°F), while for orange juice the Q_{10} is about 1.5. An 18°F increase in storage temperature causes vitamin C to be lost 5 times faster for tomatoes but only 1.5 times faster for orange juice. This does not mean however that vitamin C is more stable in orange juice than in tomato juice. In fact if one examines Figure 22.1 it can be seen that below about 80°F vitamin C is more stable in canned tomato juice than in canned orange juice and vice versa above 80°F. This is called a crossover effect of reaction rates, and is due to the fact that temperature is not the only factor related to nutrient stability. Other important factors are the pH of the food, the trace minerals that may act as catalysts, other chemicals such as sugar, and the moisture content. One cannot take data from one food and use it to project the extent of nutrient loss in other foods. This crossover effect is also important in canning. Since microbial spores are more susceptible to temperature change (they have a Q_{10} of 10 to 40), one can process at high temperature in a short time, kill the botulinum spores, and end up with a high nutrient content. This is the basis of the HTST/UHT processes discussed in Chapter 17.

Canning generally causes no loss in protein quality. In fact, canning may increase the bioavailability of the protein. During canning there is no loss in carbohydrate and no loss in lipids. Lipid oxidation ceases during storage since no oxygen is present in the can. Some loss in vitamins A and thiamin may occur because of the heat treatment but the loss is less than for vitamin C. Heating will not cause a loss of trace minerals, although some will be leached out in washing, cutting, trimming, and blanching.

Because of the difference in reaction rates, quality changes such as color, texture, and loss of flavor generally occur before significant nutrient losses appear during storage of canned foods. With proper storage in a cool dry place, canned foods, are a good nutrition buy, although they start out at a lower nutrient level than fresh foods. With the newer forms of thermal processing, they will certainly have a distinct nutritional advantage. Table 22.3 lists the time for nutrient loss in some canned foods. If canned foods are kept below 70°F, less than 10–20% of the important nutrients are lost in one year, which is the normal holding time for these products.

TABLE 22.3. Vitamin stability in canned fruits and vegetables

Canned commodity	Storage temperature °F	Nutrient loss time for x% loss		
Apricots	70°F	vitamin C	20% loss	14 mos.
	88°F		20% loss	4.5 mos.
	70°F	thiamine	20% loss	3.8 mos.
	88°F			2.1 mos.
	70°F	vitamin A	10% loss	12 mos.
Asparagus	50°F	vitamin C	10% loss	33 mos.
	70°F	vitamin C	10% loss	14 mos.
	90°F	vitamin C	10% loss	6 mos.
	70°F	vitamin A	10% loss	13 mos.
Beans (green)	40°F	vitamin C	10% loss	20 mos.
	70°F	vitamin C	10% loss	9 mos.
	40°F	riboflavin	10% loss	33 mos.
	70°F	riboflavin	10% loss	5.5 mos.
Corn (sweet)	45°F	vitamin C	10% loss	28 mos.
	70°F	vitamin C	10% loss	12.5 mos.
	50°F	thiamin	10% loss	28 mos.
	55°F	vitamin A	10% loss	27 mos.
	70°F	vitamin A	10% loss	15 mos.
Peaches	40°F	vitamin C	10% loss	24 mos.
	70°F	vitamin C	10% loss	10 mos.
Peas	45°F	vitamin C	10% loss	32 mos.
	70°F	vitamin C	10% loss	15 mos.
	45°F	vitamin A	10% loss	26 mos.
	70°F	vitamin A	10% loss	13 mos.
Tomatoes	45°F	vitamin C	10% loss	28 mos.
	70°F	vitamin C	10% loss	13 mos.

FROZEN FOODS

Frozen foods generally have the highest overall nutritional quality if consumed within their shelf-life period, when they are kept at 0°F or below. The lower the temperature during storage, the longer the acceptable shelf life and the greater the retention of nutritional quality.

In general, loss of protein nutritional quality, carbohydrates, minerals, and most vitamins except for vitamins C, E, and A is negligible. Loss of linoleic acid can occur due to oxidation. This makes the food inedible due to rancidity before the loss is significant. Of greatest nutritional concern is vitamin C loss.

Figure 22.2 shows data for the shelf life of some frozen vegetables along with the time for a 10% loss of vitamin C during frozen storage of green beans.

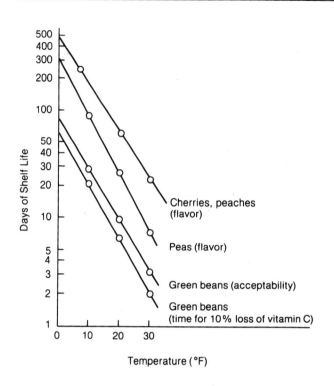

FIGURE 22.2 Shelf life (days) of frozen foods held at different temperatures

Even though the temperature is much lower for frozen green beans than for storage of the canned green beans (see Figure 22.1), loss of vitamin C occurs much more rapidly. For example, a 10% loss occurs in two months at 0°F while for the canned beans a 10% loss occurred in one year at 60°F and about four months at 100°F. The reason for the more rapid loss in the frozen foods is because the oxygen that can act to destroy vitamin C is not removed during freezing while it is removed in canning. With respect to vitamin C the canned food is more stable than the frozen food. The other line for green beans in Figure 22.2 indicates the time at which the beans become unacceptable to an expert sensory panel evaluating color changes. It takes longer for the beans to become unacceptable than it does for a 10% loss of C to occur. Studies show that it would take the consumer two to three times as long as the expert panel to find the beans unacceptable in color. Thus at 0°F (−18°C), which is around the temperature of a normal deep freeze, the beans have about six to nine months' shelf life. During that period a 30-45% loss in vitamin C would occur. This is different than in fresh foods or canned foods where organoleptic quality is generally lost first. One must then balance loss of vitamin C with the usually high quality of the frozen food. Times for loss of quality of some other frozen foods are shown in Figure 22.2. This information is based on various studies of flavor, odor, and color changes that are due to the chemical reactions occurring during storage. The book mentioned earlier has a lot more data for frozen foods. Table 22.4 lists times for shelf life and loss of vitamin C in some frozen foods.

DRY FOODS

Dehydrated foods are subject to similar losses of nutrients because of various chemical reactions. The loss that occurs is a function of both the water content of the food and the storage temperature. The rates of loss increase with increasing moisture contents but reach a maximum in the intermediate water activity range (a_w 0.65 to 0.85). The loss rate then falls again because of dilution effects. Of interest in dry foods is the nonenzymatic browning reaction between essential amino acids, especially lysine, and sugars; this reaction results in loss of protein quality. This will be discussed in more detail later and some information given as to protein quality losses. Lipid oxidation is also enhanced in the dry state, with the minimum occurring at lower a_w (0.2 to 0.3).

Minimizing water pick-up by using impermeable packaging is essential to maintain nutritional quality and avoid nutrient losses in dehydrated foods. For every 3–4% increase in moisture content the rate of nutrient loss can generally increase by two to three times or even much more in some foods. For example, a 5% loss of vitamin C occurs in nine months at 35°C for a powdered orange drink such as Tang® when it is at 1% moisture. At 4% moisture content, however, over 50% of the vitamin C would be lost in less than one week. If

TABLE 22.4 Nutrient loss and shelf-life of some frozen foods at 0°F

Food	Nutrients	Percentage Loss	Shelf-life time for loss	Quality life
Beans (green)	vitamin C	10%	14 mos.	15 mos.
	vitamin C	25%	8 mos.	
Broccoli	vitamin C	10%	28 mos.	10 mos.
		25%	36 mos.	
Peas	vitamin C	10%	16 mos.	10 mos.
		25%	44 mos.	
Spinach	vitamin C	10%	6 mos.	8 mos.
		25%	12 mos.	
Strawberries	vitamin C	30%	64 mos.	24 mos.

the dry juice is not protected and picks up moisture, the loss accelerates. Thus proper packaging—in this case a jar—is needed to protect dry foods.

Temperature is also an important factor in the destruction of vitamins during storage of dry foods. The higher temperature of storage, the faster is the loss of nutritional quality. For example, the pork in a dried soup mix would lose 50% of its thiamin in 70 days if held at 80°F, whereas the same loss occurs in less than one month at 100°F. This is a Q_{10} of about 3 times. If the dry soup mix were inadvertently held in the trunk of a car in the summer where it reached 120°F, the same loss would occur in just over one week. Low-temperature storage as well as good packaging is needed for dry foods. Most people at home store dry foods near the sink or stove, which are probably the worst places because of the warmth and moisture present. A cool dry space is best but, unfortunately, cannot usually be found in the home. The graph in Figure 22.3 shows data for some vitamin losses in a few dry foods. In dry mashed potato over 25% loss of vitamin C can occur in one month at 80°F. This is why dry potatoes are fortified with extra vitamin C and are dried to very low moisture contents to slow the reaction. Table 22.5 lists data for vitamin loss in other dried foods.

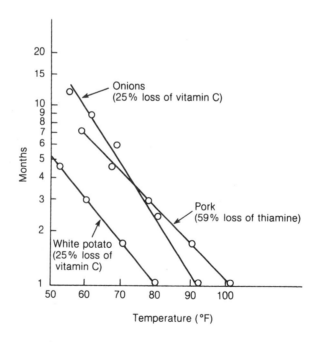

FIGURE 22.3 Time in months for a certain percentage loss of vitamins in dehydrated foods held at different temperatures in moisture-proof packages

TABLE 22.5 Times for nutrient losses in dry foods

Dried Food	Temperature	Nutrient	% Loss	Time for Nutrient Loss
Pasta	77°F	thiamin	50%	8.6 years
	95°F	thiamin	50%	2 years
Peas	70°F	vitamin A	50%	6 mos.
		vitamin B$_1$	10%	7 mos.
Peppers (green)	60°F	vitamin C	10%	1 mo.
Pork	70°F	thiamin	50%	9 mos.
Potato (flakes)	70°F	vitamin C	10%	2 weeks
			25%	1 mo.
Tomato powder	70°F	vitamin C	30%	32 weeks.

CHEMICAL REACTIONS CAUSING QUALITY LOSSES IN FOODS

Many different chemical reactions result in the deterioration of processed foods. Canned foods can have flavor, color, and textural changes during storage. The same is true for frozen or dry foods. The mechanisms of a few of these reactions have been researched in detail, the most important of which are rancidity and browning. They are of critical importance since they either make the food totally inedible or result in significant nutrient loss.

Rancidity

Rancidity caused by oxidation of the unsaturated fats contained in foods is a major problem in frozen and dried foods and in cooked meats. The unsaturated fats in the food react with oxygen very rapidly. Trace metals present in the food such as myoglobin act as catalysts to make the reaction go faster. In this process free radicals and peroxides are produced that can destroy many vitamins such as A, C, and E. The nutritional value of protein is also lowered by reaction with the peroxides. Peroxides destroy natural pigments, bleach the food, produce toxins or carcinogens, and cause the typical off-odors and off-flavors of rancid foods. However, some degree of rancidity is accepted in certain dry sausages and potato chips because we have become used to the flavor that develops.

Rancidity reactions in foods can be prevented by several means. Because light catalyzes the reaction, an opaque package should be used. Removing oxygen by vacuum packaging is an important factor in the preservation of dried foods, although it is hard to do if you dry foods at home. Removal of oxygen prevents lipid oxidation in canned foods. Keeping temperatures low and controlling water content are also important. If the food is overdried, it will become rancid more rapidly than at an a_w of 0.2 to 0.3. If it is not dried enough it will also become rancid. An optimum moisture content must be found for best stability. For most dry foods this is around an ERH of 25–35%. Since there are no cheap devices to measure this, the proper ERH is hard to obtain during home drying. The addition of antioxidants, which react with the free radicals and peroxides, slows down the development of rancidity in both frozen and dried foods. Vitamin E (tocopherol) is a natural antioxidant but is not used often in foods because of its high cost and the fact that it is not a very effective antioxidant. BHA, BHT, and TBHQ are synthetic antioxidants that accomplish the same purpose. They need to be added only at 100 to 200 ppm, since they are extremely effective. Ascorbic acid (vitamin C), EDTA, and citric acid also prevent rancidity by tying up the trace metals so they cannot activate the rancidity reaction. They are called chelating agents and must be on the label of food packages when they are used. These food additives are useful because they slow down the reaction and increase shelf life. Temperature control is also important as it is with all other chemical reactions. The Q_{10} for rancidity is low—in the range of 1.5 to 2.5 times. Thus, although cool storage is important, use of the above methods contributes more to extension of the shelf life.

Nonenzymatic Browning

Nonenzymatic browning (NEB) is a reaction that occurs during storage of dried foods and to a much smaller extent in frozen foods. This browning is the result of a reaction between some types of sugars and proteins or amino acids. This is different from the browning that develops in freshly cut apples or frozen peaches. The latter reactions are enzymatic browning reactions that require oxygen and occur much more rapidly. The undesirable browning reaction that occurs between sugars and protein produces toughening of the food during storage and can result in the loss of the essential amino acid lysine. This makes the protein undigestible, tougher when chewed, or less soluble when dissolved in water. The nutritional value of the protein is decreased. Browning can also result in an undesirable bitter flavor.

The sugars that can react in the browning reaction are called reducing sugars because they can also exist in an open-chain structure with a free aldehyde or ketose group (like the ketone bodies during starvation). These include glucose, lactose, maltose, and fructose (the most reactive). Sucrose is not a reducing sugar and thus does not react. Recently however many food manufacturers began replacing sucrose with high fructose corn syrup (HFCS) because it is sweeter and costs less on a dry weight basis to achieve the same sweetness. This replacement makes the food more susceptible to NEB. Since most natural foods already contain some reducing sugars (e.g., lactose in milk, fructose in fruits) they are all susceptible to browning. Table 22.6 lists the times for loss of protein quality due to nonenzymatic browning in a few dried foods. The essential amino acid lysine is primarily lost in this reaction.

Prevention of nonenzymatic browning can be accomplished by the removal of the reducing sugars such as glucose from dry foods. Unfortunately, this is usually not possible. The reduction of ERH of a food to a value of 25–35% also prevents the nonenzymatic browning reaction. Good packaging to prevent moisture gain increases shelf-life significantly since, as with the other chemical reactions, the rate increases as moisture is gained. A maximum in the browning rate occurs in the water activity range of 0.65 to 0.85. Above that a_w the higher moisture content causes dilution and the reaction rate is less. Of course above that range we are dealing with the problems of a fresh or canned food. Cool storage temperatures are also critical.

The only chemicals that can prevent or slow browning reactions are the various forms of sulfite; however, by law, sulfite can be used only in fruits and vegetables because of the off-flavor created and the fact that sulfite can destroy thiamin. Sulfite cannot be used in meats or dairy products because they are significant sources of thiamin.

USES OF PACKAGING TO CONTROL DETERIORATION

Packaging films can reduce rancidity and nonenzymatic browning reactions in dehydrated and frozen foods by control of water gain or oxygen influx. Opaque packaging prevents or slows reactions that are catalyzed by the presence of light such as riboflavin loss or lipid oxidation. It also protects the food from infestation, insects, microbes, and rodents. Packaging is also vital for aroma protection,

TABLE 22.6. Protein quality loss in some dried foods

Food	Temperature	% Loss	Time for Listed % loss of protein quality	
Fish (dried)	70°F	50%	70 mos.	@50% RH
Milk (nonfat—dry)	65°F	50%	28 mos.	@40% RH
			20 mos.	@40% RH
	85°F	50%	13 mos.	@40% RH
			7 mos.	@60% RH
Pasta	77°F	25%	1 year	@40% RH
			32 weeks	@52% RH
	95°F	25%	42 weeks	@40% RH
			27 weeks	@52% RH

either by keeping the good flavor in or the undesirable flavors out. It also serves as a means of shipping, advertising, providing nutritional information for the product, and giving information about the shelf life of a food. We will discuss the information that must be on a package in Chapter 24.

SUMMARY

All foods deteriorate in nutritional quality during storage. Fresh foods have the shortest shelf life due to microbial decay and chemical and physical changes that reduce quality before significant loss of nutrients during storage. Canned foods have a long shelf life, but initial quality and nutritional value is lower than fresh foods because of the heat processing needed to make them safe. As with fresh foods, quality factors cause loss of acceptability before significant nutritional loss occurs. The loss of vitamin C, the most labile of the vitamins, increases when the canned foods are held at temperatures over 70°F. Frozen foods have the highest initial quality of processed foods. However, because of significant physical factors, nutrient loss in frozen foods occurs much more rapidly than in similar foods that are canned. In fact, significant vitamin C can be lost before the food is organoleptically unacceptable.

In dehydrated foods, quality and nutrient losses are directly affected by moisture content or water activity. The higher the moisture, up to a point, the faster the loss. Increased temperature also increases the loss rate. Vitamins C, E, and A can be lost in significant amounts during storage.

Rancidity is one of the most important chemical reactions that causes deterioration of foods. Of importance is the fact that it can make the food unacceptable before significant nutritional value is lost. It is the result of the oxidation of unsaturated fats. Antioxidants, chelating agents, and vacuum packaging slow the reaction. The other major chemical reaction that deteriorates foods is nonenzymatic browning, a reaction between sugars and amines causing loss of protein quality. The essential amino acid lysine can be lost in this reaction. Control of moisture content, lower temperature, and protective packaging slow the reaction.

Multiple Choice Study Questions

1. Which of the processes below gives the longest shelf life?

 A. canning
 B. air drying
 C. freezing
 D. pasteurizing
 E. spray drying

2. Which method would not prevent rancidity in a food?

   A. keep at low temperature
   B. remove sugar
   C. remove oxygen by vacuum packaging
   D. add antioxidants
   E. add EDTA

3. Rancidity does not cause

   A. the bleaching of pigments
   B. formation of green colors
   C. the destruction of vitamin A
   D. the destruction of vitamin E
   E. the loss of lysine

4. In preserving dry foods to prevent rancidity, antioxidants like BHA or BHT

   A. react with the saturated fats preventing off-flavor
   B. combine with oxygen to reduce the reaction
   C. react with peroxides to slow the reaction
   D. are put in the package liner to prevent it from becoming hard
   E. combine with trace metal catalysts, like iron that slow the reaction

5. Antioxidants like BHA work by

   A. reacting with oxygen
   B. slowing down peroxide breakdown
   C. reacting with trace metal catalysts
   D. reacting with UV light
   E. none of the above

6. Antioxidants like EDTA and citric acid work by

   A. reacting with oxygen
   B. slowing down peroxide breakdown
   C. reacting with trace metal catalysts
   D. reacting with UV light
   E. none of the above

7. Unlike non-enzymatic browning the color that forms in bananas after they are bitten into are the results of reactions

   A. between enzymes, oxygen, and polyphenols
   B. between ethylene and peroxides
   C. between vitamin C and sugars
   D. between sugars and protein
   E. that occur because of high temperatures

8. Nonenzymatic browning is a reaction
   A. that turns apples or bananas brown after you bite into them
   B. between unsaturated fats and vitamin E
   C. between lecithin and lactose
   D. between proteins and reducing sugars
   E. that causes ice to form in packages stored in a freezer

9. To prevent nonenzymatic browning during storage of a dry food, the best package to extend shelf life would prevent _____ from entering the pouch.
   A. oxygen
   B. light
   C. water
   D. bacteria

10. Nonenzymatic browning reactions do not lead to
    A. toughening
    B. loss of solubility
    C. loss of protein nutritional value
    D. bitter flavors
    E. bleached pigments

Answer questions 11 through 16 using the following list of reactions.
   A. growth of decay organisms
   B. growth of microbial pathogens
   C. biochemical reactions
   D. rancidity
   E. senescence

11. From the standpoint of food stability and safety which applies to off-odors appearing in potato chips?

12. Which best applies to green mold appearing on bread?

13. Which of the above choices applies to the aging of fruits or vegetables?

14. Which applies to slime formation on meat?

15. Which one is the most important to prevent?

16. Which applies to the conversion of starch to sugar when potatoes are stored in a refrigerator?

The following are some basic mechanisms of food deterioration. Choose the correct response for questions 17 through 21 that best describes the condition.
   A. senescence
   B. biological destruction
   C. microbiological decay

    D. chemical decay

    E. physical decay

17. Which condition pertains to over-ripening of bananas?

18. Which condition pertains to vitamin C loss in canned green beans?

19. Which condition pertains to wilting of celery?

20. Which condition pertains to mold on cheese?

21. Which condition pertains to plant diseases?

Following is a list of the basic principles for many processes. For each of the processes in questions 22 through 30 pick the principle that best describes the process.

    A. thermal destruction of microorganisms

    B. inhibition of growth by low temperature

    C. inhibition of growth by adding or producing chemical agents

    D. binding of water to prevent growth of microbes

    E. removal of water to prevent growth of microbes

22. Pasteurization

23. Spray drying

24. Home freezing

25. Canning

26. Pickling

27. Freeze drying

28. Appertizing

29. Use of calcium propionate

30. Jam- and jelly-making

The following is a list of typical food processes. Choose the process that best fits questions 31 through 43.

    A. thermal processing

    B. freezing

    C. dehydration

    D. chemical preservation (including fermentation)

    E. refrigeration

31. Which process is used in pasteurization of beer?

32. Which process involves the removal of water by heat?

33. Which process causes the greatest loss of nutrients during the processing itself?

34. By what process is Gainesburger ® made?

35. What process uses both the principle of water removal and lowering of temperature?

36. What process uses both the principle of water removal and raising temperature?

37. Which is the best process to use to store bread?

38. Which process gives the longest food shelf life?

39. Which process is used in pasteurization of milk?

40. Which process involves formation of alcohol?

41. Which process gives the highest quality food for three to six months?

42. Which process has the highest quality but for only a short time?

43. Which process gives the shortest shelf life?

Essay Study Questions

1. Compare the quality, shelf life, and nutritive value of fresh, canned, frozen, and dry foods. Use meat, a fruit, and a vegetable as an example.

2. What is rancidity? How does it occur and how can it be prevented?

3. Describe the process of nonenzymatic browning and the methods used to prevent it.

4. Why do frozen foods lose vitamin C faster than canned foods?

5. How should dry foods be stored to maximize quality and nutritional value?

6. Discuss the effect of processing and storage on mineral losses.

Things to Do

1. Make a list of all the foods stored in your home and their location. Indicate the problems involved in their stability, your guess as to their shelf life, and your estimate of their nutrient quality.

2. Store some potato chips in air at 30°C. Smell them daily. How long does it take for them to become rancid? If you have a vacuum jar pull a vacuum and hold at the same temperature. Does this increase shelf life? Similarly keep some in the dark and in continuous light, and determine the effect. Discuss the shelf life in contrast to the loss of nutritional quality.

3. Put some samples of dry milk powder in each of four fish tanks with the salt solutions prepared previously. Hold at room temperature. Examine daily for darkening. Rank the colors on a scale of 1 to 10 (light to dark brown) on a daily basis and plot. Estimate from the table in this chapter when 25% lysine loss would occur.

4. Seal some fresh potato chips in a paper bag, a cellophane bag, a polyethylene bag (baggies), a zip-lock bag, and a seal-a-meal bag. Use the same size bag and same amount of chips in each. Place them in a large fish tank with a saturated sodium chloride solution at the bottom. (Suspend them on a fishing line with clothes-pins.) Weigh them daily. After seven days open the bags and examine them for crispness. Discuss the loss of crispness with respect to rancidity (Things to Do # 3) and loss of nutritional value.

Chapter 22. Answers to Multiple-Choice Study Questions: 1, A; 2, B; 3, B; 4, C; 5, B; 6, C; 7, A; 8, D; 9, C; 10, E; 11, D; 12, A; 13, E; 14, A; 15, B; 16, C; 17, A; 18, D; 19, E; 20, C; 21, B; 22, A; 23, E; 24, B; 25, A; 26, C; 27, E; 28, A; 29, C; 30, D; 31, A; 32, C; 33, C; 34, D; 35, B; 36, C; 37, B; 38, A; 39, A; 40, A; 41, B; 42, E; 43, E.

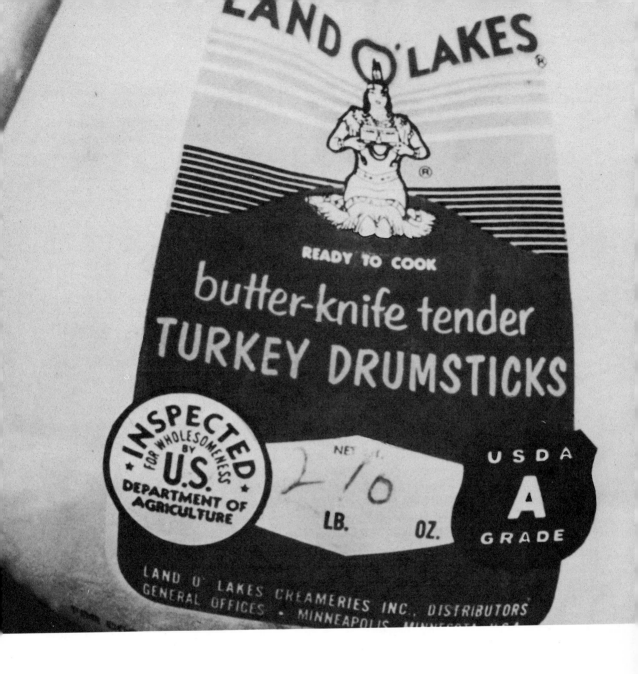

FOOD LEGISLATION AND REGULATION: HOW THE GOVERNMENT PROTECTS OUR FOOD SUPPLY

23

EARLY HISTORY OF FOOD LAWS

There were no federal food laws or regulations in the United States prior to the 1900s except the ones governing meat export and tea import. At that time food companies in interstate commerce could market foods in any way they chose. Many illnesses probably occurred from the addition of untested, harmful chemicals to the food supply, for example, the addition of arsenic or boric acid onto the surface of meat to slow spoilage. Sometimes chalk was added to watered-down milk to make it look white and thus stretch out milk sales. Adding chalk or plaster of paris to bread to extend dirty flour and mixing lard with butter were common practices. Some states, such as Massachusetts, had legislation prohibiting adulteration of foods produced and sold within the state but found it hard to prove wrongdoing.

Harvey Wiley was an M.D. and former chemistry professor at Purdue University. In 1883 he became Chief of the Bureau of Chemistry of the United States Department of Agriculture (USDA). By 1902 Wiley had set up a group to study the problems of adulteration of the food supply. This group, known as Wiley's Poison Squad, was made up of male volunteers who volunteered to taste and eat foods that Wiley suspected of containing poisonous chemicals to see if there was a health hazard. Testing the foods by eating them was not the best or safest method for determining food safety, but at that time no accepted animal test procedures had been established for toxicity testing. Wiley's laboratory also analyzed the foods to try to prove they contained toxic substances. They found many things wrong with some foods and disseminated the information to the public through the media. This caused an uproar as citizens began to suspect they were being poisoned.

At about the same time the Poison Squad was in operation, Upton Sinclair wrote a book, *The Jungle,* which dealt in part with the horrid, unsanitary conditions of the Chicago stockyards and meat-processing plants. After publication of that book, many foreign countries banned the importation of United States beef. In 1906, pressure on the United States Legislature from Wiley and many consumer groups resulted in the passage of two laws on the same day: The *Pure Food and Drug Act* and the *Meat Inspection Act.* Both laws prohibited the manufacture and sale of adulterated or mis-branded foods in interstate commerce. The Meat Inspection Act also provided for continuous inspection of all red meat during slaughter and processing to prevent diseased animals or adulterated meat from entering the food supply. These acts were put under the authority of the USDA. The Pure Food and Drug Act provided for the safety of the food supply in interstate commerce by prohibiting the use of any poisonous or deleterious substance in foods if it rendered the food injurious to health. However, the government had to prove that the substances used were injurious at their level of use in the food.

The USDA, under Wiley, saw fit to publish the results of investigations of food products. Thus there was some impact on consumers when they heard of violations or supposedly harmful substances. However, the act was not very effective, especially since at that time analytical and toxicological methods were primitive. There were few requirements about what had to be on food labels. In the next 30 years, many amendments were added on to patch up the act, especially with respect to food safety and labeling requirements.

THE FOOD, DRUG, AND COSMETIC ACT

In 1931, the Food and Drug Administration (FDA) was created to replace the Bureau of Chemistry and to administer the law. The FDA established precedents as to what was illegal, mainly through court actions, but it had to try each violator to make its point. In 1936, when a drug company improperly formulated a cough medicine with a solvent that killed over 100 people, enough pressure developed to revamp the law, including the food provisions. In 1938, the *Federal Food, Drug, and Cosmetic Act* was passed. The FDA received more powers with respect to regulating the adulteration and misbranding of drugs and foods. In addition, control of cosmetics was added to their authority. The provisions of this law and its amendments will be discussed in the next section. Although it was still the government's responsibility to investigate and prosecute the violators and to prove that a chemical added to food was unsafe or injurious, new drugs first had to be proved safe by the manufacturer before marketing.

The FDA was transferred into the Federal Security Agency during World War II and was relocated in the Department of Health, Education, and Welfare in 1953 which became the Department of Health and Human Services (HHS) in 1980. However, meat inspection remained under the jurisdiction of the USDA and is administered by the Food Safety and Inspection Service. Today several different governmental agencies have authority and regulatory power over the production, handling, and marketing of a single food item. This obviously can create problems as to which agency takes precedence in a particular situation.

OTHER LAWS

In 1954 the *Miller Pesticide Amendment* was added to the 1938 Food, Drug, and Cosmetic Act. This specified the amount of pesticides that could be left on raw agricultural commodities once they entered the marketplace. This amendment was added because of the extensive gypsy moth blight in New York and Connecticut in 1953. The USDA decided to eliminate the gypsy moths by spraying DDT. They contracted local people who owned small planes, shipped them many 100-pound bags of DDT, and told the pilots to spray it over designated infected areas, which included residential areas. Homeowners who had large doses of DDT dropped in their yards opposed the action. Pressure on Congress led to the 1954 pesticides amendment. This law stated that there was to be a zero tolerance level for various pesticides in final food products. A zero tolerance level means that no pesticides could be present at all. Obviously this zero level could change as analytical techniques for pesticides improved and lower levels could be detected, which in fact happened. The agency in power had to set non-zero limits or tolerances similar to the filth guidelines in foods.

Pesticides on raw agricultural foods were first regulated under the USDA and then transferred to the EPA (Environmental Protection Agency) in 1978. With respect to processed foods, the FDA essentially adopted the USDA and then the EPA tolerances on the basis that the tolerance in processed foods would not exceed the limit set for the raw food.

In 1957 the *Poultry Inspection Act* was passed and put under the authority of the USDA. Prior to that time, central locations for the raising of fryer and broiler chickens near big cities were expanding. Before shipping, some poultry raisers were feeding binding agents to chickens that caused them to retain water. This increased their weight at the time of sale. They were also using illegal drugs to increase the weight of the bird. This act specified what was legal to feed a chicken and outlined the practices that were necessary to maintain sanitation in the poultry plant.

Probably the most significant food legislation occurred in 1958 when the *Food Additive Amendment* was added to the original 1938 Food, Drug, and Cosmetic Act. The significance of this act was severalfold. First, it defined what a food additive was. Secondly, the responsibility for proving the safety and efficacy of an additive was assigned to the company that was trying to introduce it rather than to the government. This gave the government the same control that was added for drugs in 1938. Section 409 of the act specified that the company must show that the food additive was safe, by providing overwhelming animal test data as well as estimating the amount that consumers would ingest. They also had to show that the chemical was effective for the purpose (food additive) it was intended to be used for.

Of even greater significance was the addition of the *Delaney Clause* to section 409 that prohibited the addition of carcinogenic additives to food. No chemicals that caused cancer when fed to humans or animals or that were shown by "appropriate tests" to cause cancer could be legally added to foods. Cancer is a disease that is second to heart disease as a cause of death in the United States. In the 1970s there were about 130 deaths per 100,000 population due to cancer compared to 262 per 100,000 for heart disease on an age-adjusted rate basis. Cancer is usually a slow-acting disease that can be very prolonged and painful. People fear it much more than they fear a quick heart attack or stroke. This amendment on carcinogenic additives was easily passed because of this public sentiment, and has played a major role in the design of toxicity tests (see Chapter 25).

In 1960 an amendment concerning color additives was passed. This amendment specified that every batch of an approved synthetic coloring agent had to be tested and certified as being chemically pure within certain limits by the government before the color could be used in foods. It also specified that before being approved for use, all coloring agents had to pass the same pre-clearance safety testing that food additives did. A cancer clause similar to the Delaney Clause was also added. Several coloring additives were taken off the approved list, and others were provisionally allowed until further tests were performed to verify their safety. These tests lasted through 1984, almost 24 years later. Those approved for food use were called certified FD & C food colors.

In 1966 the *Fair Packaging and Labeling Act* was passed, giving the government power to regulate advertising of all packaged items, including foods. The Federal Trade Commission (FTC) has jurisdiction over advertising foods in the media (radio, TV, newspapers, magazines). The FDA has specific control over what can be put on the food package label itself.

The *Freedom of Information Act* (FOI) was passed in 1971. This specified that all actions of government must be public unless they are in the interest of national security. This created much furor since the FDA then had to tell the public that it actually allowed foods to contain such filth as rodent hairs. These guidelines for filth were developed on the basis of what could be expected in foods processed under good sanitary controls.

Several amendments and court cases have held that under the act the FDA has the authority for the whole chain in the food distribution scheme, that is, right down to the consumer level. In only a few cases has the FDA entered a home to seize products (drugs and medical devices). The FDA has generally allowed both state and local public health officials to set standards and control the restaurant and food retail business, but they still have the statutory authority. Imported foods also come under the law, and foreign manufacturers must exercise the same degree of care in manufacturing foods if shipped to the U.S. Some people question whether this is actually true based on the large quantities of adulterated food seized at ports of entry.

RULES AND REGULATIONS

Since 1971 the FDA has promulgated a vast number of rules and regulations to administer the various laws. These regulations are not laws but the courts uphold them as such if they are not arbitrary or capricious. Laws can only be passed by Congress, which is the legislative branch of the government. A rule or regulation is promulgated through an administrative process by the Federal Agency in the Executive Branch, which is given authority to carry out the law. The need for regulation exists because Congress usually only indicates general, not specific, guidelines when passing a law. Proposed rules and regulations must be made public information by publication in the Federal Register, the daily record of the Executive Branch of the government. Usually 60 to 90 days are allowed for anyone to comment on the merits of the proposed regulation. In some cases such as for the approval of an additive or a food standard, a formal hearing in front of the FDA is required. Sometimes the Federal authorities will change the proposed rule because of the public comments. Under due process, if someone really objects, he or she can get the proposed regulation reviewed by the Federal courts, including the Supreme Court of the United States. The FDA operates under Title 21 of the Code of Federal Regulations (CFR Title 21). Some finalized rules and regulations promulgated by the FDA are:

1. *Filth action levels* define the amounts (de minimus) of natural filth allowed in foods marketed in interstate commerce. 21 CFR 110.

2. *Pesticide action levels and tolerances* for foods can result in the FDA seizing the food if the pesticide content goes above the allowed level. 21 CFR 193.

3. *Poisonous and deleterious substance action levels and tolerances* are similar to those for pesticides. Some levels have been set for mercury, PCBs, and aflatoxin. 21 CFR 109.

4. *Standards of Identity Regulations,* which define a standardized food product in terms of either how it can be made and/or what ingredients must be in it. These standards are for the promotion of honesty and fair dealing in the interest of the consumers. The commissioner of the FDA was given authority to set Standards of Identity under the 1938 Act. The regulations are the means to set these standards. Over 300 foods have Standards of Identity. 21 CFR 130 to 169.

5. *Labeling regulations* define the type size and specific information that must be on the food package label to insure that the consumer is not being deceived. 21 CFR 101 to 105.

6. *Regulations to insure safe thermal processing of food* give the specifics in the process. (See Chapter 17.)   21 CFR 113 and 21 CFR 114.

7. *Good Manufacturing Practice Regulations* (GMP) define what methods (HACCP) the processor should use to insure that the food produced is safe and free of harmful or decay microorganisms. (See Chapter 15.)   The general regulation for all industry is in 21 CFR 110; however, specific regulations have been promulgated for certain food industries such as breaded shrimp, confectionaries, and smoked fish.

8. *Nutritional regulations* were put into effect in 1975 after several years of discussion and changes.   These will be discussed in the next chapter.   They define the USRDAs and what can be said on the package about the product's nutritional value.   Recently other regulations dealing with reduced-calorie and low-calorie foods have been added.   21 CFR 101.

9. *Recall procedures* are guidelines that were developed to help a company retrieve foods from the food distribution channel that are in possible violation of the Food, Drug, and Cosmetic Act.   The FDA cannot force the company to remove the food; the action is voluntary.   All the FDA can do is seize the food.   The recall regulations must be followed, however, to insure that the food is properly removed from the marketplace.   FDA forces the recall by announcing a possible violation in the media.   A Class I Recall is a priority procedure in which full press coverage is given because consumption of the food is an imminent health hazard and could cause death.   This category would be used in the case of a batch of canned food contaminated with botulism and was used in the Tylenol tampering incident.   Low levels of mercury or pesticides present in a food as well as filth above an action guideline would constitute a Class II Recall.   There is a danger to health, but it is less serious.   Economic fraud elicits a Class III Recall, although a possible pathogen presence in the food can also be considered a Class III recall if it is not a threat to health.   Wide press coverage is not used for this category.   21 CFR Part 7C.

10. *Common or Usual Name Regulations* provide that the producer must use a product name that accurately describes the product and that pictures of food on the package must not be doctored to look better than what you actually get.   A buttermilk pancake mix must contain the amount of buttermilk solids one would expect, and a juice drink must state the amount of juice present even if it is zero. 21 CFR 102.

Many other rules and regulations have been published by the FDA and will continue to be published. They are all designed to help the government carry out the basic tenets of the 1938 Food, Drug, and Cosmetic Act and other laws pertaining to foods.

Various court cases set precedent for interpretation of the law and of rules and regulation. For example, in 1975 the United States Supreme Court ruled in the *United States vs. Park* case (421 US 658) that a food corporation executive up to and including the president is responsible for the negligence of the employees with respect to sanitation. In this case a company president was given a fine and a jail sentence (suspended) because a warehouse owned by the company, which was used for food storage, was repeatedly found to be rodent-infested, and the president was in a position to insure that it be cleaned although he never visited the warehouse.

ADULTERATION AND MISBRANDING

Basic Principles

The basic principles of the Federal Food Drug, and Cosmetic Act cover foods, drugs, animal drugs, biologics (like blood), cosmetics, and medical devices. The act prohibits the manufacture or selling of an adulterated or misbranded food product in interstate commerce. The act also provides for fines, imprisonment, injunctions, seizure, and public announcement of a violation. Foods are defined as food and drink for both humans and animals (feed for animals and pets) as well as chewing gum. However, alcoholic beverages and chewing tobacco come under the Bureau of Alcohol, Tobacco, and Firearms, which is in the Department of the Treasury, while meat is covered by the USDA.

Food adulteration. Food adulteration is defined as the intentional or unintentional addition of any poisonous or deleterious ingredient or substance to a food. This applies not only to actual chemicals but also to items that are not specifically intentional chemical additives. For instance, if *Clostridium botulinum* or any other pathogen was found growing in canned foods, it would be considered to be a poisonous substance. It would be within the power of the government to ask for a Class I Recall or seize the food, destroy it, and impose penalties. The contamination due to rat feces in food because of mishandling or poor sanitation is also considered food adulteration. Additives over the allowed amount would be in violation as would be levels of pesticides, aflatoxin, or heavy metals such as mercury over allowable tolerance limits or action levels.

If ingredients are in excess of or below the required level or the amount listed on a package, the food product can be seized on the adulteration principle. For example, if the amount of egg in mayonnaise is below that specified in the Standard of Identity for it, the mayonnaise is considered to be adulterated.   Standards of Identity are one of the most controversial areas in food regulation.   By defining how many peanuts should be in peanut butter or how much fruit should be in jam, they prevent companies from using less than those amounts.   However, the addition of lysine to white bread was prohibited, even though the addition would have improved protein quality, because lysine addition was not provided for in the standard for bread.   A new standard had to be set.   A similar problem arose in adding proteins to pasta products to increase protein quality.   To get around the standard, a special allowance was made by the FDA.   This will be more common in the future if the nutritional value of a food can be upgraded by the addition of an ingredient.   FDA now uses common and usual name regulations rather than going through the laborious standard settings that require formal hearings.

Foods that contain levels of filth (insect fragments, dirt, etc.) above the tolerances allowed are considered adulterated.   In 1972 the FDA started publishing filth guidelines stating levels of filth that are acceptable in foods.   For example, in three and one-half ounces of peanut butter, up to 30 insect fragments and one rodent hair are allowed.   Since this filth occurs in the raw nuts themselves, it is hard to prevent all filth unless excessively costly processing procedures are used.   Since commercial processes are designed to reduce the level as much as possible, most products contain filth far below these tolerance levels.   Similarly, vegetables like broccoli can contain up to 60 insect fragments in 100 grams.   The regulations prohibit manufacturers from mixing clean and unclean batches of food to reduce the level below the allowed tolerance level for the unacceptable batch.   Good manufacturing practices should keep the levels well below the tolerances, since sanitary procedures are emphasized.   It should be noted, however, that the courts through the FDA could choose to prosecute the company since the law specifies that no filth can be present even if the process had ground the filth up so fine that it is not detectable by the consumer.   In 1938 in the case of *U.S. vs. 133 Cases of Tomato Paste* (22 F. Supp. 515) the U.S. District Court ruled that the law was set to protect the aesthetic sensibilities of the consumer.   In *U.S. vs. Lazare* (56 F. Supp. 730; 1944) the owner of a very filthy baking operation testified that baking or canning made the food safe.   He even had a physician testify on his behalf that one could eat a canned mouse.   The courts did not accept his argument, but agreed with the FDA that there could be "de minimus" levels present.   In fact the law states, and the courts have upheld under Sec. 402(a)(4) of the FD & C Act, that there is no need to prove that the food is contaminated with filthy, putrid, or decomposed substances.   The mere manufacturing in an unsanitary environment is grounds for a violation, but the FDA will allow for "de minimus" levels.

The use of diseased animals is not allowed in the production of foods. FDA controls any product that contains less than 3% meat (pork, beef, veal, and lamb) or less than 2% poultry and all pet foods, no matter how much meat they contain.

FDA also controls meat sandwiches and cheese/meat snacks with less than 15% meat. All other meat food products intended for human consumption are under the jurisdiction of the USDA through its Food Safety and Inspection Service (FSIS). The Meat Act of 1906 (which was amended in 1967 by the Wholesome Meat Act) is much tougher. Meat processors, whether intra-or interstate, must be under continuous inspection. All processes and procedures must get prior approval. Theoretically no illegal product can leave a meat plant. An inspector who feels a product is being produced under unsanitary or filthy conditions can withdraw inspection, thus preventing the product from leaving the plant. All other food processors are regulated by the FDA, which conducts only random inspections; a plant may be visited only every two or three years. Thus we are at the mercy of the ethical sensibilities of the food industry to insure that a non-meat food product is safe. Past history shows that the food industry in general has respected the law.

The law prohibits the manufacture and shipment of putrid or decomposed foods and ingredients. One of the principles of processing is that food that is unacceptable before processing will not be improved by processing. In some rare cases an unscrupulous manufacturer may use adulterated ingredients and try to hide the adulteration in some way. Eventually the FDA will catch them.

Extraction of a valuable nutrient from a food is considered adulteration. Concealing damage to food by using food additives is also against the adulteration law. This prohibits the adding of color to hide the decay in vegetables that have turned brown. But one can use an additive to prevent the decay from occurring in the first place.

Unsanitary practices in production are also prohibited by the adulteration legislation. Unfortunately the low budget and the small number of food inspectors make yearly inspection of all food plants impossible. The processing regulations set by the FDA are to help food companies do their own policing. We are assured that most food companies will follow this practice since they don't want their name ruined by an unfortunate incident. The FDA still finds unsanitary conditions often enough, but usually in small and sometimes unknowledgeable food companies. The larger food processing companies are more capable of self-policing than smaller companies. They have found the HACCP procedures to be useful in providing safe, high-quality food for the consumer.

Misbranding. The regulations governing label requirements were set up to control false labeling, which is the most obvious violation covered by misbranding. The law implies that a failure to reveal any facts that would be material to the purchase of the food would constitute misbranding. This is in addition to the required specific elements that must be on a food label (see next chapter). The regulations also prevent any health-benefit claims being made for nonessential food ingredients. Substitution is also a violation under misbranding. An example would be the substitution of margarine for butter, which occurred relatively frequently when margarine was first manufactured. Package deception in terms of fill of container is sometimes clarified by statements on packages saying that settling may occur; however, a reasonably sized package must be used or a certain fill is necessary. At present only the net weight (the actual food weight) need be declared on a label. However, some companies also declare the drained weight for canned food products such as peas in brine when the liquid is not consumed. The drained weight would be the weight of the peas. This is common practice for olives because the juice is poured out.

Finally, under misbranding, one cannot offer for sale an inferior product that has a standard for it without declaring that it is below standard or is an imitation. We will see in the next chapter what the word imitation means.

FDA PROCEDURES

The FDA works with both laws and regulatory procedures. In actual practice, the FDA sends inspectors to plants, including foreign manufacturers who offer food for sale in the United States, to determine if foods are being produced under unsanitary conditions. An average food processor will be inspected only once every two to three years unless the company is constantly in violation or the food has a high hazard potential based on HACCP analysis. In 1980 over 17,500 plants were inspected. Various states under contract inspected over 20,000 plants for the FDA. For example, in Minnesota the state inspects all carbonated and nonalcoholic beverage establishments. They share inspection of bakeries, canneries, and warehouses with the FDA. Minnesota also inspects many dairy establishments for the FDA. Other states have similar contracts.

The FDA also does market-basket surveys of food. In 1980 almost 20,000 domestic food samples were analyzed and over 18,000 imported samples were taken. The intake of various additives is based on these samplings. A two-week intake for a 16- to 19-year-old male eating 3.9 kg. of food (8.9 lb.) daily is used as the basis. A normal individual eats 2.2 kg. (4.8 lb.) or less.

If a violation is found and it is minor the FDA will generally send the firm a formal notice of the violation. This is called a regulatory letter and sets a date by which the correction must be made, usually within 10 days. If the situation is not corrected, the FDA can take legal action to institute seizure of the product. Of course, the firm can voluntarily recall the product following FDA guidelines. It will then be either reprocessed, relabeled, or destroyed.

If the firm is processing under filthy conditions, the FDA may also ask the court for an injunction. If granted, the injunction would prevent the firm from dealing further in interstate commerce until it literally cleaned up its act. Finally, if the company does not comply with the requirements after repeated inspections, letters, etc., the FDA can ask the U.S. District Attorney in the Department of Justice to proceed with a criminal prosecution. The penalty for this is up to one year in jail and a $1000 fine for the first offense and three years and $10,000 for further offenses. There is a movement in congress to increase these penalties.

In 1974, the FDA sent 238 regulatory letters, made 272 seizures, had no injunctions, and instituted 92 criminal prosecutions. By 1981 this had changed to 198 regulatory letters, 279 seizures, 13 injunctions, but only 18 criminal prosecutions. The reason for this last change is that the FDA now relies on the industry to recall violative food and for cooperation in using HACCP principles in processing. Prior to 1976 no such recall procedures were formalized. Thus the FDA can spend more time on troublesome companies. Between 70% and 80% of seizure actions are for filth (see Table 23.1).

TABLE 23.1 FDA enforcement history

Types of action*	years					
	1978	1979	1980	1981	1982	1983
Criminal prosecution	21	21	22	18	20	22
Injunction	32	30	21	13	11	28
Seizures	402	541	539	276	212	225
Recalls	1,116	1,290	864	658	709	915
Inspections	28,760	32,787	32,778	36,258	31,359	30,014
Warf exams	51,518	55,794		55,924		
Regulatory letters	422	361	783	198	507	254
Samplings	18,683					
Import samples	5,977					
Import detention	18,487		16,909			
Complaints						
FOI requests			33,179			

* Note that in 1977 there were 1,183 inspectors and this decreased to 903 by 1982.

OTHER REGULATORY AGENCIES

USDA

The USDA is second in power to the FDA in food quality and safety regulation. The USDA is responsible for inspection at the slaughtering and processing level of all meat and poultry products destined for human consumption. The inspectors who check for diseased animals and plant sanitation are part of the Food Safety and Inspection Service (FSIS) of the USDA under the Agricultural Marketing and Inspection Division. Since 1967, state laws for inspection must be equal to the USDA standards. In many cases the USDA has taken over intrastate inspection as well (meats slaughtered and used within the state's boundaries). The USDA also sets guidelines for plant construction, personal hygiene, meat food composition, and labeling.

The grading of beef is a service paid for by food companies and done by the Agricultural Marketing Service of the USDA. Grading puts beef into different categories based on eating quality: prime, choice, good, standard, commercial, utility, cutter, and canner. Grading benefits consumers by telling them what quality meat they are buying. The USDA formulated descriptions of the meat cuts allowed for sale to eliminate the many varied names for the same kinds of meats. The USDA grades vegetables, fruits, nuts, and some dairy products as a service to food companies. The companies must pay for this service since grading is not required. If the product is graded, the quality grade can be used on the food label. This grading generally has nothing to do with sanitation but USDA graders can refuse to grade if the food is being produced under unsanitary conditions.

Other examples of grades are: Poultry—Grades A, B, and C; Butter/cheese—AA, A, B; Fresh fruits and vegetables—Fancy, No. 1, No. 2; Processed fruits and vegetables—A, B, C; Rice—US 1 to US 6; Eggs—quality, AA, A, B, and size, Jumbo, Extra large, Large, Medium, Small, Peewee.

Most consumers do not know that the purpose of the grading is to allow a company to market a product of some known standard quality. Most government food commodity purchases are of graded products. The differences in grading levels for various foods are confusing, but in 1981 the proposal to make all grades of similar lettering (e.g., A, B, C) was dropped.

USPHS

The United States Public Health Service (USPHS) of which FDA is a part used to be responsible for several areas of food regulations, including drinking water standards and control of all foods served on planes, trains, and buses. However, this has been taken over by the FDA and the EPA. The USPHS will, if requested, voluntarily inspect milk for certification as raw milk and certify that shellfish come from non-polluted water. One main function of the USPHS is the investigation of food-borne disease outbreaks. The headquarters for this operation is the Center for Disease Control (CDC) in Atlanta, Georgia.

NMFB

The National Marine and Fisheries Bureau of the United States Department of Commerce sells a grading and inspection service for fish processors much like the USDA grading. However, fish processors are still regulated under the FDA.

OSHA

The Occupational Safety and Health Administration (OSHA) is responsible for setting worker safety regulations in food-processing plants. Problems have been created when safety standards allow unsanitary conditions and when food regulations allow a possibly unsafe condition. For example, a required blade guard over a bandsaw used to cut up a block of meat might allow organisms to grow under it. Another example is that the smooth surfaces of processing equipment may cause noise levels to exceed OSHA standards yet are needed to avoid places where pathogens can grow. OSHA also controls the types of chemical solvents workers can be exposed to in food-processing operations and the degree of exposure to these solvents.

EPA

The Environmental Protection Agency (EPA) regulates pesticide use on raw foods. Pesticide residues left after processing, however, are covered by the FDA under the adulteration regulations. The EPA has also been involved in heavy metal regulation and in determining whether fluorocarbons can be used in food aerosols.

BATF

The U.S. Department of Treasury governs all the regulations concerning the production and sales of wines, beers, liquors, and chewing tobacco through the Bureau of Alcohol, Tobacco, and Firearms (BATF). Alcoholic beverages were originally controlled by the FDA, but they gave up their authority to the BATF. In 1975 the FDA tried to gain back control over the labeling requirements for alcoholic beverages because the BATF did not require alcoholic beverage manufacturers to label the ingredients on their packages. Congress and the courts have seen fit, however, to prevent the FDA from doing this. BATF did write proposed label regulations in 1980–81 but withdrew them when it was felt they would have too inflationary an impact. There is very little control over what ingredients can be added to an alcoholic beverage compared to a food. However, new regulations were proposed again in 1983 but not acted on.

FTC

The Federal Trade Commission (FTC) regulates advertising of foods in all media. In 1975 the FTC promulgated some TRRs (Trade Rules and Regulations) that would cover nutritional advertising and protein advertising. These were withdrawn however as were the proposed TRRs on advertising food to children.

CPSC

The Consumer Products Safety Commission (CPSC) has also dealt with foods. But it deals not with the food itself—it deals with the issue of whether a food container or dispensing device is dangerous to use.

CA

The Codex Alimentarius is an international food regulatory agency to which the United States belongs. This organization is setting up rules to ease export/import of foods throughout the world. The same standards for quality, additives, and safety would apply everywhere. Whether we will accept standards that are lower than those required in the U.S. remains to be seen.

SUMMARY

Early concern about safety and quality of the food supply led to the passage of the Pure Food and Drug Act in 1906. This act was improved upon in 1938 with passage of the *Food, Drug, and Cosmetic Act*. This law, which is in operation today after many amendments, controls the United States' food supply except for meats, which are regulated under the Wholesome Meat Act of 1967. Other laws cover specific ingredients in the food supply such as pesticides, color additives, food additives, and packaging. The most significant amendment added to the act has been the 1958 Food Additives

Amendment that outlines the use of additives in foods and puts the onus of proving safety and effectiveness before the chemical can be used on the food manufacturer.

The Food and Drug Administration has basic jurisdiction in administering food laws. To operate under the law they have promulgated a larger series of rules and regulations (Code of Federal Regulations, CFR Title 21). This code covers various aspects of processing, filth guidelines, nutritional guidelines, and recall procedures.

The basic 1938 law covers food, for both humans and animals, including pet foods, that enters interstate shipment. The law specifies two classes of violations, misbranding and adulteration, and lists subcategories of these violations.

Other federal agencies are involved in food laws and regulations. The United States Department of Agriculture (USDA) covers meat inspection and meat plant sanitation. The USDA also grades meat, fruits, and vegetables as a service. Other involved agencies are the United States Public Health Service, the Environmental Protection Agency, the Bureau of Alcohol, Tobacco, and Firearms, and the Federal Trade Commission, all of which control foods to a certain extent.

Multiple Choice Study Questions

1. A food regulation

    A. is a food law passed by Congress

    B. is the interpretation of the law by processors

    C. is only a guideline

    D. becomes law when initially published in the Federal Register

    E. is none of the above

2. Who was the first U.S. food-law administrator?

    A. Upton Sinclair

    B. James Lind

    C. Nicholas Appert

    D. Harvey Wiley

    E. Alexander Schmidt

3. The first Federal Pure Food and Drug Act of 1906 required processors to

    A. test the safety of their additives

    B. disclose the additives used

    C. not use injurious substances in food

    D. prove the efficacy of the additives used

4. A certified food color means

    A. that the U.S. government passed it for safety

    B. that the U.S. government passed it for use in 1958

    C. that the U.S. government passed it for purity

    D. that it has zero toxicity

    E. none of the above

5. The Delaney Clause specifically prevents the use of food additives that are

    A. carcinogenic

    B. teratogenic

    C. mutagenic

    D. toxic

    E. nutritious

6. The Miller Amendment prohibits

    A. the use of uncertified colors

    B. the use of pesticides on food

    C. the presence of pesticides on food above their tolerance

    D. the use of uncertified additives

    E. the use of noncertified GRAS substances

7. GMP stands for

    A. general marketing procedures

    B. gross malpractice procedures

    C. good manufacturing practices

    D. glucose mono-propionate

    E. general manufacturing purposes

8. A FDA inspector finds rodent droppings and urine on a package of food in a warehouse. The first action would be to

    A. destroy all the product with a similar code

    B. use a Class I recall because of the imminent health hazard

    C. ask the company to make a Class II recall of all products with a similar code and clean up the place

    D. take the warehouse owner to court for criminal action

    E. close down the warehouse

9. The use of polyvinyl chloride containers for alcohol was banned because the monomer vinyl chloride leaked into food. This action was taken under the FDA act covering

    A. adulteration with intentional additives

    B. non-intentional poisonous and deleterious substances

    C. misbranding by not having the monomer content labeled

    D. the Delaney Clause

    E. improper use of colors

The following are violations of the 1938 Food, Drug, and Cosmetic Act. Choose which category of violation items 10 through 12 best fit under.

    A. adulteration
    B. misbranding
    C. neither of the above

10. Mercury in food over the tolerance limit

11. No nutritional label on the product

12. Improper picture on front panel

The following are Federal agencies responsible for food actions. Choose the best one for questions 13 through 17.

    A. OSHA
    B. FDA
    C. USDA
    D. BATF
    E. FTC
    F. CPSC

13. This agency sets standards for allowance of environment contaminants in foods.

14. This agency is responsible for control of media advertising not on a food package.

15. This agency has control over industrial safety problems.

16. This agency has control over alcoholic beverages.

17. This agency has authority over potentially dangerous package shapes.

Essay Study Questions

1. What did the 1906 *Pure Food and Drug Act* accomplish?

2. What are the basic provisions of the 1938 *Food, Drug, and Cosmetic Act?*

3. What is the Delaney Clause?

4. What is the difference between law and the rules and regulations of an administrative body?

5. Describe some of the FDA regulations.

6. List some violations covered under the adulteration and misbranding principles with respect to food.

7. What other federal agencies regulate foods? What are their functions?

8. What authority does the USDA have with respect to food safety?

9. Define adulteration and misbranding of foods and give some examples.

10. What is a product recall?

11. What does certification of a color mean?

Things to Do

1. Write your local and state regulatory agencies for copies of their food regulations. How do they compare to federal laws?

2. Try to find references in the news to FDA violations. Good sources are the *FDA Consumer Magazine,* available from the FDA for $20/year, and *Food Chemical News,* available from a large library. The FDA also has an electronic bulletin board on Compuserve (GO FOI).

3. Visit a local food-processing plant and discuss how they comply with FDA and USDA requirements.

Chapter 23. Answers to Multiple-Choice Study Questions: 1, E; 2, D; 3, C; 4, C; 5, A; 6, C; 7, C; 8, C; 9, C; 10, A; 11, C; 12, B; 13, B; 14, E; 15, A; 16, D; 17, F.

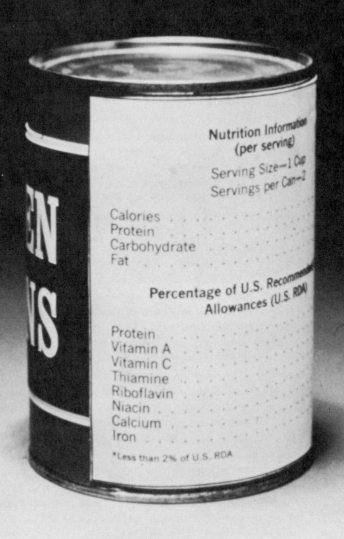

**READ THE LABEL AND
SET A BETTER TABLE**

24

We eat every day. We purchase food, open jars, cans, packages, and boxes, but do we ever take time to read what is printed on the label? The package label provides required information as well as some educational information if we take the time to read and understand it. As one previous U.S. government pamphlet stated, "Read the Label. Set a Better Table."

The labeling of foods, except for meats, is controlled by the Food and Drug Administration under the misbranding section (Section 403) of the Federal Food, Drug, and Cosmetic Act (FFDCA) and under the Fair Packaging and Labeling Act (FPLA). Meats and meat-food products for humans (not pet foods) are covered under the Meat Inspection Act (MIA) and the Wholesome Meat Act (WMA), and are under the control of the Food Safety and Inspection Service of the USDA. The MIA and the FFDCA say about the same thing with respect to misbranding. In general both acts declare illegal those foods whose packages bear false or misleading labels, including labels that fail to reveal facts that are material to the purchase of the product (e.g., how much juice there is in a juice drink). Also covered under the laws are provisions on false names, not using the designation of "imitation" if a product is an imitation, slack fill, required information as to contents, weight, etc., and other information. These provisions will be considered in more detail in this chapter. The labeling must also be done in such a manner that the ordinary individual can read and understand the label under customary circumstances of purchase and use. Type size requirements, cents-off labeling, economy size packages, etc., are covered in the FPLA, which is administered by both the FDA and the USDA in their respective jurisdictions. Requirements also specify where the information must appear on the label. It should be remembered that any information on a label other than that which is required is technically considered advertising and falls within the jurisdiction of the FTC. However, the FDA or the USDA could take action if they felt the information was false or misleading and could affect purchase.

No meat-food product can be made in a processing plant until the label is submitted to the USDA for prior approval, whereas under the FDA the control would come about only by consumer and competitor complaints asking the FDA to investigate an illegally labeled product. The FDA has promulgated general regulations as to what a food should be called under the common and usual name regulations. On the other hand, the USDA, although promulgating some general labeling regulations, relies on an internal labeling review manual that lists specific types of foods with specific recipes (e.g., pork sausage, corned beef hash, meatballs with spaghetti). In areas of labeling not spelled out, such as with nutritional labeling, the USDA mostly follows the FDA rules and regulations. To examine label contents we will go around the package by area to see what we can find.

**THE FRONT
PANEL OF A
FOOD PACKAGE**

The Name of the Food

The front of a box, flexible pouch, can, or bottle (40% of the area) is called the principal display panel (PDP). It is the area most likely to be displayed on a market shelf. The major piece of information required on the PDP is the identity labeling, i.e., the legal name of the product. This legal name or statement of identity can be either (under 21 CFR part 101 for the FDA):

1. a product for which a Standard of Identity (i.e., a government-prescribed formula) has been set,

2. a common or usual name, or

3. a fanciful name commonly used by the public.

If there are optional forms of the product (e.g., slices versus dices) it must also be part of the name.

Standards of Identity

The name of a food based on a Standard of Identity is for foods for which the U.S. government has set a basic formula under 21 CFR Parts 130–169. Not all foods have Standards of Identity and, in fact, in recent years the FDA has spent less time on standards as they take too long to develop and/or change. Standards which exist for food products under both FDA and USDA are listed in Table 24.1. Few people even know that these standards exist or where to find them. An example from the list is peanut butter. Several years ago the standard required 95% peanuts in peanut butter. The industry petitioned to get it changed to 90% peanuts. Because of the legal process that required formal hearings, the final change took almost 10 years of hearings with over 100,000 pages of documents. The FDA feels it has better things to do than waste time on long hearings like this.

The original idea of Standards of Identity was to promote honesty and fair dealing in the interest of the consumers. It all started because of a product seized by the FDA called Bread Spread (*US vs. Ten Cases Bread Spread* 49 F. 2d 87, 1931) in which gelatin was mixed with artificial strawberry flavor and color, and grass seed was used to imitate strawberry seeds. The courts held that the product was legal because it did not purport to be jam, since jam was not in the name. The courts however admonished Congress to add something to the law to prevent this, and Section 401 on Standards of Identity was added to the 1938 Act.

Table 24.2 contains the actual Standard of Identity for mayonnaise and the beginning part for salad dressing with some critical points underlined. Mayonnaise must contain at least 65% oil while salad

TABLE 24.1 Foods that have a standard of identity (FDA classification)

21 CFR Part 131   Milk and milk products

131.110 Milk.
131.115 Concentrated milk.
131.120 Sweetened condensed milk.
131.122 Sweetened condensed skimmed milk.
131.123 Lowfat dry milk.
131.125 Nonfat dry milk.
131.127 Nonfat dry milk fortified with vitamins A and D.
131.130 Evaporated milk.
131.132 Evaporated skimmed milk.
131.135 Lowfat milk.
131.145 Skim milk.
131.147 Dry whole milk.
131.149 Dry cream.
131.150 Heavy cream.
131.155 Light cream.
131.157 Light whipping cream.
131.160 Sour cream.
131.162 Acidified sour cream.
131.180 Half-and-half.
131.185 Sour half-and-half.
131.187 Acidified sour half-and-half.

21 CFR Part 133   Cheese and related cheese products

133.102 Asiago fresh and asiago cheese.
133.103 Asiago medium cheese.
133.104 Asiago old cheese.
133.106 Blue cheese.
133.108 Brick cheese.
133.109 Brick cheese for manufacturing.
133.111 Caciocavallo siciliano cheese.
133.113 Cheddar cheese.
133.114 Cheddar cheese for manufacturing.
133.116 Low-sodium cheddar cheese.
133.118 Colby cheese.
133.119 Colby cheese for manufacturing.
133.121 Low-sodium colby cheese.
133.123 Cold-pack and club cheese.

133.124 Cold-pack cheese food.
133.125 Cold-pack cheese food with fruits, vegetables, or meats.
133.127 Cook cheese, koch kaese.
133.128 Cottage cheese.
133.129 Dry-curd cottage cheese.
133.131 Lowfat cottage cheese.
133.133 Cream cheese.
133.134 Cream cheese with other foods.
133.136 Washed curd and soaked curd cheese.
133.137 Washed curd cheese for manufacturing.
133.138 Edam cheese.
133.140 Gammelost cheese.
133.141 Gorgonzola cheese.
133.142 Gouda cheese.
133.144 Granular and stirred curd cheese.
133.145 Granular cheese for manufacturing.
133.146 Grated cheeses.
133.147 Grated American cheese food.
133.148 Hard grating cheeses.
133.149 Gruyere cheese.
133.150 Hard cheeses.
133.152 Limburger cheese.
133.153 Monterey cheese and Monterey jack cheese.
133.154 High-moisture jack cheese.
133.155 Mozzarella cheese and scamorza cheese.
133.156 Low-moisture mozzarella and scamorza cheese.
133.157 Part-skim mozzarella and scamorza cheese.
133.158 Low-moisture part-skim mozzarella and scamorza cheese.
133.160 Muenster and munster cheese.
133.161 Muenster and munster cheese for manufacturing.
133.162 Neufchatel cheese.
133.164 Nuworld cheese.
133.165 Parmesan and reggiano cheese.

133.167 Pasteurized blended cheese.
133.168 Pasteurized blended cheese with fruits, vegetables, or meats.
133.169 Pasteurized process cheese.
133.170 Pasteurized process cheese with fruits, vegetables, or meats.
133.171 Pasteurized process pimiento cheese.
133.173 Pasteurized process cheese food.
133.174 Pasteurized process cheese food with fruits, vegetables, or meats.
133.175 Pasteurized cheese spread.
133.176 Pasteurized cheese spread with fruits, vegetables, or meats.
133.178 Pasteurized neufchatel cheese spread with other foods.
133.179 Pasteurized process cheese spread.
133.180 Pasteurized process cheese spread with fruits, vegetables, or meats.
133.181 Provolone and pasta filata cheese.
133.182 Soft ripened cheeses.
133.183 Romano cheese.
133.184 Roquefort, sheep's milk blue-mold, and blue-mold cheese from sheep's milk.
133.185 Samsoe cheese.
133.186 Sap sago cheese.
133.187 Semisoft cheeses.
133.188 Semisoft part-skim cheeses.
133.189 Skim milk cheese for manufacturing.
133.190 Spiced cheeses.
133.191 Part-skim spiced cheeses.
133.193 Spiced, flavored standardized cheeses.
133.195 Swiss and emmentaler cheese.

TABLE 24.1 Foods that have a standard of identity (FDA classification) *(Continued)*

133.196	Swiss cheese for manufacturing.

21 CFR Part 135   Frozen desserts

135.110	Ice cream and frozen custard.
135.120	Ice milk.
135.130	Mellorine.
135.140	Sherbet.
135.160	Water ices.

21 CFR Part 136   Bakery products

136.110	Bread, rolls, and buns.
136.115	Enriched bread, rolls, and buns.
136.130	Milk bread, rolls, and buns.
136.160	Raisin bread, rolls, and buns.
136.180	Whole wheat bread, rolls, and buns.

21 CFR Part 137   Cereal flours and related products

137.105	Flour.
137.155	Bromated flour.
137.160	Enriched bromated flour.
137.165	Enriched flour.
137.170	Instantized flours.
137.175	Phosphated flour.
137.180	Self-rising flour.
137.185	Enriched self-rising flour.
137.190	Cracked wheat.
137.195	Crushed wheat.
137.200	Whole-wheat flour.
137.205	Bromated whole-wheat flour.
137.211	White corn flour.
137.215	Yellow corn flour.
137.220	Durum flour.
137.225	Whole durum flour.
137.230	Corn grits.
137.235	Enriched corn grits.
137.240	Quick grits.
137.245	Yellow grits.
137.250	White corn meal.
137.255	Bolted white corn meal.
137.260	Enriched corn meals.
137.265	Degerminated white corn meal.
137.270	Self-rising white corn meal.
137.275	Yellow corn meal.
137.280	Bolted yellow corn meal.
137.285	Degerminated yellow corn meal.

137.290	Self-rising yellow corn meal.
137.300	Farina.
137.305	Enriched farina.
137.320	Semolina.
137.350	Enriched rice.

21 CFR Part 139   Macaroni and noodle products

139.110	Macaroni products.
139.115	Enriched macaroni products.
139.117	Enriched macaroni products with fortified protein.
139.120	Milk macaroni products.
139.121	Nonfat milk macaroni products.
139.122	Enriched nonfat milk macaroni products.
139.125	Vegetable macaroni products.
139.135	Enriched vegetable macaroni products.
139.138	Whole-wheat macaroni products.
139.140	Wheat and soy macaroni products.
139.150	Noodle products.
139.155	Enriched noodle products.
139.160	Vegetable noodle products.
139.165	Enriched vegetable noodle products.
139.180	Wheat and soy noodle products.

21 CFR Part 145   Canned fruits

145.110	Canned applesauce.
145.115	Canned apricots.
145.116	Artificially sweetened canned apricots.
145.118	Canned apricots with rum.
145.120	Canned berries.
145.125	Canned cherries.
145.126	Artificially sweetened canned cherries.
145.128	Canned cherries with rum.
145.130	Canned figs.
145.131	Artificially sweetened canned figs.
145.134	Canned preserved figs.
145.135	Canned fruit cocktail.

145.136	Artificially sweetened canned fruit cocktail.
145.140	Canned seedless grapes.
145.145	Canned grapefruit.
145.170	Canned peaches.
145.171	Artificially sweetened canned peaches.
145.173	Canned peaches with rum.
145.175	Canned pears.
145.176	Artificially sweetened canned pears.
145.178	Canned pears with rum.
145.180	Canned pineapple.
145.181	Artificially sweetened canned pineapple.
145.185	Canned plums.
145.190	Canned prunes.

21 CFR Part 146   Canned fruit juices

146.110	Cranberry juice cocktail.
146.111	Artificially sweetened cranberry juice cocktail.
146.113	Canned fruit nectars.
146.114	Lemon juice.
146.115	Lemonade.
146.120	Frozen concentrate for lemonade.
146.121	Frozen concentrate for artificially sweetened lemonade.
146.125	Colored lemonade.
146.126	Frozen concentrate for colored lemonade.
146.130	Limeade.
146.133	Canned pineapple-grapefruit juice drink.
146.135	Orange juice.
146.137	Frozen orange juice.
146.140	Pasteurized orange juice.
146.141	Canned orange juice.
146.145	Orange juice from concentrate.
146.146	Frozen concentrated orange juice.
146.148	Reduced-acid frozen concentrated orange juice.
146.150	Canned concentrated orange juice.
146.151	Orange juice for manufacturing.
146.152	Orange juice with preservative.

TABLE 24.1 Foods that have a standard of identity (FDA classification) *(Continued)*

146.153	Concentrated orange juice for manufacturing.
146.154	Concentrated orange juice with preservative.
146.185	Canned pineapple juice.
146.187	Canned prune juice.

21 CFR Part 150   Fruit butters, jellies, and preserves

150.110	Fruit butter.
150.140	Fruit jelly.
150.141	Artificially sweetened fruit jelly.
150.160	Fruit preserves and jams.
150.161	Artificially sweetened fruit preserves and jams.

21 CFR Part 155   Canned vegetables

155.120	Canned green beans and canned wax beans.
155.130	Canned corn.
155.131	Canned field corn.
155.170	Canned peas.
155.172	Canned dry peas.
155.190	Canned tomatoes.
155.191	Tomato paste.
155.192	Tomato puree.
155.194	Catsup.
155.200	Certain other canned vegetables.
155.201	Canned mushrooms.

21 CFR Part 156   Canned vegetable juices

156.145	Tomato juice.
156.147	Yellow tomato juice.

21 CFR Part 160   Eggs and egg products

160.100	Eggs.
160.105	Dried eggs.
160.110	Frozen eggs.
160.115	Liquid eggs.
160.140	Egg whites.
160.145	Dried egg whites.
160.150	Frozen egg whites.
160.180	Egg yolks.
160.185	Dried egg yolks.
160.190	Frozen egg yolks.

21 CFR Part 161   Fish and shellfish

161.130	Oysters.
161.131	Extra large oysters.
161.132	Large oysters.
161.133	Medium oysters.
161.134	Small oysters.
161.135	Very small oysters.
161.136	Olympia oysters.
161.137	Large Pacific oysters.
161.138	Medium Pacific oysters.
161.139	Small Pacific oysters.
161.140	Extra-small Pacific oysters.
161.145	Canned oysters.
161.170	Canned Pacific salmon.
161.173	Canned wet-packed shrimp in transparent or nontransparent containers.
161.175	Frozen raw breaded shrimp.
161.176	Frozen raw lightly breaded shrimp.
161.190	Canned tuna.

21 CFR Part 163   Cacao nibs

163.110	Cacao nibs.
163.111	Chocolate liquor.
163.112	Breakfast cocoa.
163.113	Cocoa.
163.114	Low-fat cocoa.
163.117	Cocoa with dioctyl sodium sulfosuccinate for manufacturing.
163.123	Sweet chocolate.
163.130	Milk chocolate.
163.135	Buttermilk chocolate.
163.140	Skim milk chocolate.
163.145	Mixed dairy product chocolates.
163.150	Sweet cocoa and vegetable fat (other than cacao fat) coating
163.153	Sweet chocolate and vegetable fat (other than cacao fat) coating.
163.155	Milk chocolate and vegetable fat (other than cacao fat) coating.

21 CFR Part 164   Tree nut and peanut products

164.110	Mixed nuts.
164.120	Shelled nuts in rigid or semirigid containers.
164.150	Peanut butter.

21 CFR Part 166   Margarine

166.110	Margarine.

21 CFR Part 168   Sweetners and table sirups

168.110	Dextrose anhydrous.
168.111	Dextrose monohydrate.
168.120	Glucose sirup.
168.121	Dried glucose sirup.
168.122	Lactose.
168.130	Cane sirup.
168.140	Maple sirup.
168.160	Sorghum sirup.
168.180	Table sirup.

21 CFR Part 169   Food dressings and flavorings

169.115	French dressing.
169.140	Mayonnaise.
169.150	Salad dressing.
169.175	Vanilla extract.
169.176	Concentrated vanilla extract.
169.177	Vanilla flavoring.
169.178	Concentrated vanilla flavoring.
169.179	Vanilla powder.
169.180	Vanilla-vanillin extract.
169.181	Vanilla-vanillin flavoring.
169.182	Vanilla-vanillin powder.

9 CFR Part 319   Definitions and standards of identity or composition for meat-food products

Subpart A   General

319.1	Labeling and preparation of standardized products.
319.2	Products and nitrates and nitrites.
319.5	Standards for Mechanically Processed (Species) Product.
319.6	Limitations with respect to use of Mechanically Processed (Species) Product.

Subpart B   Raw Meat Products

319.15	Miscellaneous beef products.
319.29	Miscellaneous pork products.

Subpart C   Cooked Meats

319.80	Barbecued meats.
319.81	Roast beef parboiled and steam roasted.

TABLE 24.1 Foods that have a standard of identity (FDA classification) *(Continued)*

Subpart D Cured Meats, Unsmoked and Smoked

319.100 Corned beef.
319.101 Corned beef brisket.
319.102 Corned beef round and other corned beef cuts.
319.103 Cured beef tongue.
319.104 Cured pork products, unsmoked and smoked.
319.105 Chopped ham.
319.106 "Country Ham," "Country Style Ham," "Dry Cured Ham," "Country Pork Shoulder," "Country Style Pork Shoulder," and "Dry Cured Pork Shoulder."

Subpart E Sausage Generally: Fresh Sausage

319.140 Sausage.
319.141 Fresh pork sausage.
319.142 Fresh beef sausage.
319.143 Breakfast sausage.
319.144 Whole hog sausage.
319.145 Italian sausage products.

Subpart F Uncooked, Smoked Sausage

319.160 Smoked pork sausage.

Subpart G Cooked Sausage

319.180 Frankfurters, frank, furter, hotdog, weiner, vienna, bologna, garlic bologna, knockwurst, and similar products.
319.181 Cheesefurters and similar products.
319.182 Liver sausage and braunschweiger.

Subpart K Luncheon Meat, Loaves and Jellied Products

319.260 Luncheon meat.
319.261 Meat loaf.

Subpart L Meat Specialties, Puddings and Nonspecific Loaves

319.280 Scrapple.
319.281 Bockwurst.

Subpart M Canned, Frozen, or Dehydrated Meat-Food Products

319.300 Chili con carne.
319.301 Chili con carne with beans.
319.302 Hash.
319.303 Corned beef hash.
319.304 Meat stews.
319.305 Tamales.
319.306 Spaghetti with meat balls and sauce, spaghetti with meat and sauce, and similar products.
319.307 Spaghetti sauce with meat.
319.308 Tripe with milk.
319.309 Beans with frankfurters in sauce, sauerkraut with wieners and juice, and similar products.
319.310 Lima beans with ham in sauce, beans with ham in sauce, beans with bacon in sauce, and similar products.
319.311 Chow mein vegetables with meat and chop suey vegetables with meat.

319.312 Pork with barbecue sauce and beef with barbecue sauce.
319.313 Beef with gravy and gravy with beef.

Subpart N Meat-Food Entree Products, Pies, and Turnovers

319.500 Meat pies.

Subpart O Meat Snacks, Hors d'Oeuvres, Pizza, and Specialty Items

319.600 Pizza.

Subpart P Fats, Oils, Shortenings

319.700 Oleomargarine or margarine.
319.701 Mixed fat shortening.
319.702 Lard, leaf lard.
319.703 Rendered animal fat or mixture thereof.

Subpart Q Meat Soups, Soup Mixes, Broths, Stocks, Extracts

319.720 Meat extract.
319.721 Fluid extract of meat.

Subpart R Meat Salads and Meat Spreads

319.760 Deviled ham, deviled tongue, and similar products.
319.761 Potted meat food product and deviled meat food product.
319.762 Ham spread, tongue spread, and similar products.

Subpart U—Miscellaneous

319.880 Breaded products.
319.881 Liver meat food products.

dressing needs only 30% oil and thus will generally be lower in calories. Mayonnaise must contain one or more of several optional forms of eggs. The percent is not specified but without the needed amount (usually about 10% egg yolk) the emulsion will not be stable. Salad dressing needs only the equivalent of 4% egg yolk to be stabilized. Both Standards refer to safe and suitable optional ingredients. In the late 1970s as modern food technology advanced the FDA began changing the Standards to allow processors to add ingredients and additives other than what was specified in the

TABLE 24.2 Standard of identity for mayonnaise and salad dressing

21 CFR § 169.140 Mayonnaise.
(a) *Description.* Mayonnaise, mayonnaise dressing, is the emulsified semisolid food prepared from vegetable oil(s), one or both of the acidifying ingredients specified in paragraph (b) of this section, and one or more of the egg yolk-containing ingredients specified in paragraph (c) of this section. One or more of the ingredients specified in paragraph (d) of this section may also be used. The vegetable oil(s) used may contain an optional crystallization inhibitor as specified in paragraph (d)(7) of this section. All the ingredients from which the food is fabricated shall be safe and suitable. Mayonnaise contains not less than 65 percent by weight of vegetable oil. Mayonnaise may be mixed and packed in an atmosphere in which air is replaced in whole or in part by carbon dioxide or nitrogen.
(b) *Acidifying ingredients.* (1) Any vinegar or any vinegar diluted with water to an acidity, calculated as acetic acid, of not less than $2\frac{1}{2}$ percent by weight, or any such vinegar or diluted vinegar mixed with an optional acidifying ingredient as specified in paragraph (d)(6) of this section. For the purpose of this paragraph, any blend of two or more vinegars is considered to be a vinegar.
(2) Lemon juice and/or lime juice in any appropriate form, which may be diluted with water to an acidity, calculated as citric acid, of not less than $2\frac{1}{2}$ percent by weight.

(c) *Egg yolk-containing ingredients.* Liquid egg yolks, frozen egg yolks, dried egg yolks, liquid whole eggs, frozen whole eggs, dried whole eggs, or any one or more of the foregoing ingredients listed in this paragraph with liquid egg white or frozen egg white.
(d) *Other optional ingredients.* The following optional ingredients may also be used:
(1) Salt.
(2) Nutritive carbohydrate sweeteners.
(3) Any spice (except saffron or turmeric) or natural flavoring, provided it does not impart to the mayonnaise a color simulating the color imparted by egg yolk.
(4) Monosodium glutamate.
(5) Sequestrant(s), including but not limited to calcium disodium EDTA (calcium disodium ethylenediaminetetraacetate) and/or disodium EDTA (disodium ethylenediaminetetraacetate), may be used to preserve color and/or flavor.
(6) Citric and/or malic acid in an amount not greater than 25 percent of the weight of the acids of the vinegar or diluted vinegar, calculated as acetic acid.
(7) Crystallization inhibitors, including but not limited to oxystearin, lecithin, or polyglycerol esters of fatty acids.
(e) *Nomenclature.* The name of the food is "Mayonnaise" or "Mayonnaise dressing".
(f) *Label declaration of ingredients.* Each of the ingredients used in the

food shall be declared on the label as required by the applicable sections of Part 101 of this chapter.
§ 169.150 Salad dressing.
(a) *Description.* Salad dressing is the emulsified semisolid food prepared from vegetable oil(s), one or both of the acidifying ingredients specified in paragraph (b) of this section, one or more of the egg yolk-containing ingredients specified in paragraph (c) of this section, and a starchy paste prepared as specified in paragraph (e) of this section. One or more of the ingredients in paragraph (e) of this section may also be used. The vegetable oil(s) used may contain an optional crystallization inhibitor as specified in paragraph (e)(8) of this section. All the ingredients from which the food is fabricated shall be safe and suitable. Salad dressing contains not less than 30 percent by weight of vegetable oil and not less egg yolk-containing ingredient than is equivalent in egg yolk solids content to 4 percent by weight of liquid egg yolks. Salad dressing may be mixed and packed in an atmosphere in which air is replaced in whole or in part by carbon dioxide or nitrogen.
(b) *Acidifying ingredients.* (1) Any vinegar or any vinegar diluted with water, or any such vinegar or diluted vinegar mixed with an optional acidifying ingredient as specified in paragraph (e)(6) of this section. For the purpose of this paragraph, any blend of two or more vinegars is considered to be a vinegar.

standards. However the processors were then required to label all the optional ingredients on the package. Prior to that there was no required ingredient statement, the idea being that consumers knew what was in a Standard, which was really not true. All the Standards under the FDA were rewritten to make all the ingredients optional (e.g., in canned peaches, the peaches are optional since they come in different varieties and could be whole, halves, slices, or diced). In the mayonnaise Standard shown in Table 24.2, it can be seen that the forms of vinegar, egg, and sweeteners are all optional, yet they are required to make the product acceptable. Processors must now list all the ingredients in a standardized food if everything is optional.

As was seen in Table 24.1 there are standards for some meat-food products that the USDA has published in Title 9 of the Code of Federal Regulations (9 CFR 319). Other formulas for meat products are listed in the label review manual of the USDA but have not been published as regulations, although in late 1981–1982 the USDA was being pressured to make them regulations. The only other section pertinent to USDA labeling is 9 CFR 317. Any differences between this section and the FDA sections on labeling will be pointed out in this chapter.

Common and Usual Name

The second major way a name can appear on a food label is as a common and usual name. The FDA decided that food processors could choose their own food name, but that the name must give adequate information as to what the food product actually is. The common and usual name should not be confused with the trade name. For example, Cheerios® and Captain Crunch® are trade names for two cereal products. If you read the front label you will see in smaller type size the words Toasted Oat Cereal for Cheerios® and Crunchy Sweet Cereal for Captain Crunch®. By using the common and usual name the FDA got around having to have long drawn-out hearings to set a Standard of Identity for each product. But even here the FDA ran into trouble. For example, calling a canned juice product in which the juice was diluted, a juice drink fails to reveal facts (i.e., juice content) that would be important in purchase. Thus for some classifications of food the FDA wrote regulations (which did not require a formal hearing) that would insure the consumer received adequate information. Those foods for which there are specific common and usual names are listed in Table 24.3. The USDA has no similar section.

TABLE 24.3 Common or usual names for nonstandardized foods

Subpart A	General Provisions	102.30	Noncarbonated beverage products containing no fruit or vegetable juice.	102.45	Fish sticks or portions made from minced fish.
102.5	General principles.			102.46	Pacific whiting.
102.19	Petitions.	102.32	Diluted orange juice beverages.	102.47	Bonito.
Subpart B	Requirements for Specific Nonstandarized Foods	102.37	Mixtures of edible fat or oil and olive oil.	102.49	Fried clams made from minced clams.
102.23	Peanut spreads.			102.50	Crabmeat.
102.26	Frozen "heat and serve" dinners.	102.39	Onion rings made from diced onion.	102.54	Seafood cocktails.
				102.55	Nonstandardized breaded composite shrimp units.
102.28	Foods packaged for use in the preparation of "main dishes" or "dinners."	102.41	Potato chips made from dried potatoes.	102.57	Greenland turbot (Reinhardtius hippoglossoides).

The general principle for setting common and usual names as stated in Section 21 CFR 102.5 is that the name "shall" accurately identify or describe, in as simple and direct terms as possible, the basic nature of the food or its characterizing properties or ingredients. The name "shall" include the percentage(s) of any characterizing ingredient(s) when the percentage has a material bearing on price or consumer acceptance. These principles apply whether or not there has been a specific regulation for a particular class. For example, Figure 24.1 shows a simulated label for a juice drink. "Reggie's Juice Drink" is the trade name. The legal name is in smaller-size letters and says "Imitation flavored orange and apple juice drink. Contains 10% apple and 0% orange juice." Thus one can figure out that the product was made by diluting apple juice at a 1 to 9 parts water ratio, adding imitation orange flavor and perhaps some sugars to sweeten it. One would have to look at the ingredient statement to see if this were done. Knowing this information, a consumer could decide whether to buy whole apple juice or orange juice or this imitation product by comparing prices and ingredient contents. The imitation is probably cheaper; if not, it would not be a good buy unless it were nutritionally better. Another example is

REGGIE'S JUICE DRINK

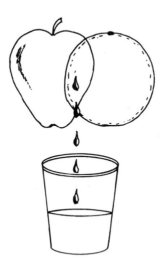

Imitation flavored orange and apple juice drink. Contains 10% apple and 0% orange juice.

Net weight 12 oz.

FIGURE 24.1 Typical front label for a juice drink product

the shrimp seafood cocktail regulation (21 CFR 102.54) that requires that the percentage of shrimp in the cocktail be declared.

Fanciful Name
The last type of legal name that can be used is a fanciful name, one that has been commonly used and accepted by the public. Coca Cola® is such a name. If it were to come under the common and usual name regulation it might have to have the words "carbonated beverage flavored with ...." Another fanciful name is Pork and Beans. In fact, if one examines the ingredient list you will find that beans and water and some tomato paste are the major ingredients with pork near the bottom of the list. It is required by law that the ingredients be in order of predominance. In fact the label will not carry the USDA inspection seal as shown in Figure 24.2 because although pork is the first ingredient in the name it is actually at a level less than 3%. The USDA has jurisdiction over meat-food products containing more than 3% meat. Under 9 CFR 317 it is required that the package have an inspection label showing that the product was inspected and passed for wholesomeness. The number on the seal is the plant registration number. A possible common and usual name might be "small white beans in a water/tomato sauce with less than 3% pork." How many of us would buy the product if we read that and never had consumed it before?

Picture of Food
A picture on the package representing the food is viewed as a part of the name label. It must truthfully depict the contents. For exam-

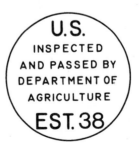

FIGURE 24.2 USDA inspection seal

ple, a slice of frozen cherry pie should contain at least the number of cherries shown in the slice on the front label. Since some consumers are confused about the contents, the processors sometimes put a statement near the picture clarifying it. This is usually as simple as "serving suggestion." Some people might actually think that a box of cereal contains the milk or fruit or that a "Hamburger Helper" type product contains meat if the picture shows these other items.

Imitation and Calorie-Modified Foods

Several other important factors affect the legal choice of the name and can have a bearing on purchase. If the product is an imitation of another food, that is, it resembles another food, is a substitute for it, but is nutritionally inferior, the legal name must include the word "imitation" (21 CFR 101.3(e)). Nutritional inferiority is based on having a reduction of more than 2% of any of the required nutrients used in a nutrition label. The USDA follows the same principles for imitation meat-food products.

Reduction of calories by reducing the fat or sugar content does not make a food an imitation (21 CFR 105.66). A reduced-calorie food is one in which there has been a reduction of more than one-third of the calories compared to the regular calorie food without a reduction in any of the other nutrients. The term "a reduced-calorie food" would become part of the common or usual name on the principal display panel. Thus one could take a mayonnaise and by omitting more than one-third of the oil make it a reduced-calorie mayonnaise. In fact, salad dressing could be a reduced-calorie mayonnaise if all the other ingredients were added to keep all the nutrients at the same level as mayonnaise. In 1981 the FDA suggested that there is some legal confusion about reduced-calorie versus standardized products. It is permissible to make an imitation of a standard that is reduced in calories by removing fat or sugar and that is also reduced in nutrients. There are many imitation jellies on the market that contain little fruit, are artificially flavored, and may have less sugar. These are imitations but even though they are reduced in calories they cannot use the term "a reduced-calorie food" because the other required nutrients have not been added.

A food can be labeled a "low-calorie food" as part of its common and usual name. Legally this is a food for which one serving gives 40 or fewer Calories and which has less than 0.4 Cal/gram. It does not have to be nutritionally equivalent to the food it resembles or replaces. Natural foods can bear this label if properly used. Celery can be labeled "a low-calorie food," but it would be illegal to call it "low-calorie celery" since all celery is low calorie according to the legal standard.

Dietetic Foods

Both low-calorie and reduced-calorie foods can be legally labeled either a diet food, a dietetic food, or an artificially sweetened food if such a sweetener is used. The label diet food or dietetic food does not apply to foods for which salt has been reduced. The term sugar-free can be used legally if sugar is omitted in a reduced- or low-calorie food, although it is also legal to use such a term if the food is neither and the common and usual name says so, e.g., "sugar free . . . not a reduced-calorie food." However, to confuse us further, one can legally use the words "no added sweeteners" as long as sweeteners are not added. Labeling of foods for diabetics requires a special statement so they don't get confused with the "low calorie," "reduced calorie," and "no sugar added" statements. The statement says: "Diabetics: This product may be useful in your diet on the advice of a physician." Food labels can appear to be quite confusing, but getting to know the specific requirements should help immensely in choosing foods, especially for those who are trying to diet.

Artificial Flavors and Colors

A last requirement in the common or usual name is an indication of whether artificial flavors or artificial colors have been added. A blueberry cake mix would use as the common and usual name "artificially flavored and artificially colored blueberry cake mix" if no natural blueberries were used. The designation would also be required in the ingredient list. Many companies use the negative approach on the front label indicating that their products contain "no artificial color" or "no artificial flavor."

Sodium Labeling

Hypertension is a disease that may afflict over 60 million Americans. For some of these individuals, reducing salt intake, or more specifically sodium intake, can help alleviate the condition. Presently the only regulation for sodium labeling is 21 CFR 105.69, which comes under the FDA and applies only if a sodium statement is made. It requires that the processor indicate on the label the amount of sodium both in mg. per serving and per 100 grams of the food (about 3.5 oz.) if they choose to say anything about sodium. Many processors don't want to label both in mg. per serving and per 100 grams. In early 1982 the FDA proposed deleting the requirement from 21 CFR 105.69 for labeling both ways allowing only mg. per serving. Another problem that may confuse some consumers is that the sodium designation is expressed in mg. of the atom sodium and not as table salt, which is sodium chloride. Lastly there is no provision concerning what can be included in the name of the food so that the consumer can identify the product as a low-sodium product.

In 1981 a bill was introduced in Congress to help in naming sodium-containing foods, but it was not acted upon. The FDA has taken the stance that the food industry should not need mandatory regulations but should voluntarily label for sodium using the following suggested critera (21 CFR 105.69 as proposed):

1. Low-sodium food $\leq$ 35 mg./100 g. It may be designated as such in the name.

2. Reduced-sodium food $\geq$ 75% reduction from normal products.

3. No salt added: sodium chloride is not used in processing but the product may contain sodium. This could be misleading, especially for foods naturally high in sodium.

4. Sodium (or salt-) free: product contains no detectable sodium ions. A survey by the FDA in 1983 indicated that over 40% of major brands used sodium labeling.

The USDA had used a different criteria for reduced-sodium foods that specified a 25% reduction, but this has been deleted. They now use the FDA standard. The USDA has no written criteria for no-salt-added or sodium-free products, but does allow labeling of sodium on a mg. serving basis only. One problem with most cured meat products is that because of the way they must be processed they are high in sodium, since salt is a needed preservative to prevent pathogenic organisms from growing. As of 1983, there were no viable substitutes for sodium chloride except for partial replacement with potassium chloride.

Contents Statement

The last requirement for the front of the package is a statement of the quantity of contents. This can be either by weight (ounces or pounds), by measure (fluid ounces, quarts), or by count (e.g., five sticks of gum). The amount must appear in the bottom 30% of the principal display panel in lines parallel to the base of the package unless there are exemptions. For example, it can appear on the cap of a pop bottle.

If the declaration is by weight, the term net weight followed by the weight must be used. Metric measures are allowed but only in addition to the English system. If content is by volume the word "net" is not needed, just the volume must be listed. The regulations also prohibit the use of modifiers such as "jumbo" gallon or "full" quart since legally all gallons are gallons and all quarts are quarts.

For some foods such as olives and pickles the liquid that fills the can or jar is not consumed but is required in processing for heat transfer. So that consumers will know how much solid food they are really getting, the label must bear the term drained weight instead of net weight. This is the amount of actual solid food left after the liquid has been drained off. Some processors are voluntarily adding this information on labels for other canned fruits and vegetables that contain fluids such as peas in brine.

Many consumers wonder about slack fill, especially for dry goods such as cereals and crackers. Manufacturers usually put a statement on the side of the box indicating that "the contents may settle during shipment." In the cases in which the FDA has taken a company to court over slack fill (e.g., *U.S. vs. 174 Cases of Delson Thin Mints*, 287 F. 2d 246) the courts have held that consumers know that it is possible for products to settle and that as long as the net quantity of contents is placed on the package, there is no consumer deception.

THE RIGHT SIDE PANEL

Information Panel Use

The panel of the package that is to the immediate right of the principal display panel is called the information panel (IP). It is on this panel that other required information is usually put, although it may legally be placed on the front panel. Most manufacturers don't place it on the front because it would clutter the display of the information they like to see there. Besides the name of the food, the net quantity of contents, and the placing of the words artificial, imitation, etc., in a name, the only other FDA required information for all foods is the ingredient list, the name and place of business of the manufacturer, packer, or distributor, and the fact that preservatives may have been used in the formula. Nutritional labeling is not mandatory unless certain claims are made.

Ingredient List

For all foods including standardized foods in which optional ingredients are used a list of ingredients in decreasing order of predominance must be placed on the food label in either the PDP or IP area. The order of predominance is based on the weight of the ingredient with the greatest percentage ingredient being listed first. However, the percentage need not be put on the label. A survey in 1981 by the FDA found that many consumers did not realize that the list was by weight, and the FDA has tentatively proposed either to require a statement saying that ingredients are listed by weight or to require the actual percentage.

The name of each ingredient has to follow its common and usual name except that spices, flavors, and colors can be declared as such.

Exceptions exist however. If any artificial flavor is used, not only does it have to be in the label name but the words "artificial . . . flavor" must appear on the ingredient list. Some consumers would like each chemical in the flavor listed, but since the flavor might contain over 200 such items the list would be too long and would not serve a useful purpose. All components added purposefully to color a food are technically artificial colors even if they are a food ingredient such as beet juice or cranberry juice. All intentional coloring agents must be listed collectively as "artificial color," with one exception. The exception is FD & C yellow No. 5 or tartrazine. Because it may cause allergic reactions in some people, it must be labeled by name. All preservatives must be listed, giving their function, for example, BHA (to maintain freshness) or calcium propionate (retards mold). Again, exceptions to labeling of preservatives exist for certain substances. For example, sugar, salt, vinegar, and certain spices actually act as preservatives but have an exemption from being labeled as such. This exception to labeling foods as containing "no preservatives" is misused by some manufacturers who try to get on the natural bandwagon. They may advertise their product as containing "no chemical preservatives," yet the product may have had salt or sugar added to lower the water activity or vinegar added to lower the pH to prevent microbial growth. These functions are true preservative effects.

Sometimes one also sees in the ingredient list the words "vegetable oil (may contain soybean, cottonseed, corn oils)." Since the price and availability of oils vary greatly during the year, food processors like the option of using the least costly one at any time. Thus to avoid the problem of having to make a new label indicating the specific oil/oils added and placing them in the correct order, they are allowed to use a collective term with all the possible oils that might be used. Of course, a consumer who wants to avoid a particular oil would then not purchase the product. For certain ingredients that may contain a mixture of other ingredients, the same procedure is used—parentheses containing the ingredients in their order of predominance—or each specific ingredient can be placed in its own proper place by weight. One can see both ways on labels of products containing enriched flour. An example ingredient list is shown in Table 24.4.

TABLE 24.4 Granola bar ingredient list

Ingredients: Enriched Rolled Oats (thiamin, riboflavin, niacin, iron), Brown Sugar, vegetable oil, may contain Soybean oil or Coconut oil, Almond pieces, Salt, Sesame seeds, Soy lecithin (a natural vegetable ingredient used as an aid in blending), Natural flavor.

Name and Place of Business

The name and place of business must be indicated on the label. This information can be for either the processor, the packer (someone who packs food for another company), or the distributor (someone who hires a co-packer). The address must include the city, state, and zip code. A street address is required if the company is not listed in a telephone or city directory, which is an unlikely occurrence. This information is needed by the FDA in case they find an adulterated or misbranded food and they need to contact the responsible company. Most companies usually use their general office for the address rather than the particular plant where the food was made.

Handling Instructions

The USDA requires a statement on the handling of meat-food products if they require refrigeration (keep refrigerated) or freezing (keep frozen until used). The FDA has no such requirements.

Saccharin Warning Statement

Because of the controversy about the question of whether saccharin causes cancer and because of the potential FDA ban in 1977, Congress passed the *Saccharin Study and Labeling Act*. This act required that further studies be made on the safety of saccharin and that in the interim a warning label be put on all labels of foods that contain saccharin. This warning label states: USE OF THIS PRODUCT MAY BE HAZARDOUS TO YOUR HEALTH. THIS PRODUCT CONTAINS SACCHARIN WHICH HAS BEEN DETERMINED TO CAUSE CANCER IN LABORATORY ANIMALS.

The saccharin statement must be printed as close to the name of the food as possible but can appear on the IP if no other space is available. The law was amended several times including in 1983 to allow continuation of saccharin use for at least two more years. The law also requires retail food stores (not restaurants) to display a notice that they sell foods containing saccharin. The notice must appear at the front door, near the soft drink section, and nearest the area where most of the other saccharin-containing foods are displayed. The notice appears in Figure 24.3. You might notice the next time you go to a grocery store that the original signs are still hanging but are probably both faded and torn.

Nutritional Labeling Requirements

Nutritional information required by the FDA must follow a specific format. However, nutritional labeling is voluntary except in certain

SACCHARIN NOTICE

This store sells food including diet beverages and dietetic foods that contain saccharin. You will find saccharin listed in the ingredient statement on most foods which contain it. All foods which contain saccharin will soon bear the following warning:

USE OF THIS PRODUCT MAY BE HAZARDOUS TO YOUR HEALTH. THIS PRODUCT CONTAINS SACCHARIN WHICH HAS BEEN DETERMINED TO CAUSE CANCER IN LABORATORY ANIMALS.

THIS STORE IS REQUIRED BY LAW TO DISPLAY THIS NOTICE PROMINENTLY.

FIGURE 24.3 Saccharin notice

situations.   The situations that "trigger" nutritional labeling, that is, that make it mandatory, are:

1. any advertising that the food is nutritious, good for you, etc., even if not on the label.

2. making any kind of statement anywhere on the package label that the product is nutritious.

3. adding a nutrient for nutritional purposes.   Any food that is made to substitute for another one, and that doesn't want to carry an "imitation" label, must be fortified to avoid being nutritionally inferior; it therefore will require a nutritional label.   The same applies to reduced-calorie foods.   If the food contains more than 50% of the RDAs of a nutrient it has specific nutritional labeling requirements as a special dietary food (such as 100% fortified cereals whose common and usual names are "multivitamin and iron supplement cereal food products").   See, for example, the labels of Total® or Product 19®.)

Exemptions from the required total nutritional labeling format include:

1. declaration of sodium content alone.

2. infant and junior foods that use special RDAs instead.

3. dietary supplements such as vitamin pills that are not in a food form.

4. iodized salt.

5. a food to which a nutrient is added for technological purposes (e.g., vitamin C used as a preservative).

6. a food with a standardized ingredient in its formula that requires nutrients. The best example is a cake mix with enriched flour. The flour, if enriched, must list the nutrients with it on the ingredient list but this does not trigger a nutritional label.

7. fresh fruits and vegetables.

8. milk that has a percentage-fat declaration as required in some states (e.g., 2% or 1% milk).

9. A statement on the package that says, "For nutrition information send to . . .," that is, a solicitation.

The top line in the required label format, as shown in Table 24.5, indicates that the information is based on a serving size. Immedi-

---

TABLE 24.5 Example of the required nutrition label format for a food

Nutritional information per serving

Serving—5 ounces
Servings per container—2
Calories—406
Protein (grams)—18
Carbohydrate (grams)—52
Fat (grams)—14
*Cholesterol (milligrams)—200
*Calories from fat—30%
*Saturated fat (grams)—4
*Unsaturated fat (grams)—10

* This information is provided for individuals who on the advice of their physician are modifying their dietary intake of cholesterol and fatty acids.
This product contains 250 milligrams sodium per 100 grams. (355 milligrams per serving).

Percent of U.S. Recommended Daily Allowance (USRDA)	
Protein	40
Vitamin A	15
Vitamin C	6
Thiamine	4
Riboflavin	*
Niacin	2
Calcium	8
Iron	10

* Contains less than 2% of the USRDA of this nutrient

ately beneath that is listed the amount of food in a serving and the number of servings per container. Thus one could calculate the amount in the package. In the example, the package has two servings of 5 ounces each so the net weight on the PDP should be 10 ounces.

Calories are listed next and are either based on the Atwater procedure (an oxygen bomb type device) or calculated on the basis of four calories per gram for both carbohydrate and protein and nine for fat. The calorie value may not be exact since the regulations (21 CFR 101.9) require that the label express the values in 2% increments up to 20 calories (i.e., 2, 4, 6, 8 . . . 20), in 5% increments above that up to 50 calories (20, 25, 30 . . . 50), and in 10% increments above 50 (i.e., 50, 60, 70, etc.). Protein labeling must follow to the next nearest gram (note that servings are given in weight or fluid ounces but macronutrients are expressed in grams, which is rather confusing to some). This is followed by the amounts of carbohydrates and fat, also in grams. Variation up to a 20% excess of the label value for protein, fat, or carbohydrate is allowed because of the variability in processing.

Below the fat content one can label, in the same column, the amount of cholesterol in mg. (to nearest 5 mg.) per serving or state in sentence form the amount per 100 grams of food. The amount of unsaturated fat and saturated fat (as triglycerides) in grams per serving (to nearest gram) or per 100 grams may also be included. If the fatty acid content is labeled, the percentage of calories obtained from fat must precede it, as shown in the example. In this case, 14 grams of fat $\times$ 9 calories per gram $\div$ a total of 406 calories $\times$ 100% = 31% of calories from fat (rounded off on the label to 30%). Following this is the required statement that the information is provided for whose who on the advice of their physician are modifying their dietary intake of cholesterol and/or fat. This statement could also be at the bottom of the label. If the food is labeled for sodium, the required sodium statement is usually placed below this, although it can appear anywhere on the PDP or IP. No claims can be made on the label for cholesterol, fats, or sodium with respect to any diseases although they do appear. Why the FDA takes no action against these illegal (but perhaps useful) labels is unclear.

The nutritional label format continues with "Percentage of the USRDA" or "Percentage of the U.S. Recommended Daily Allowance." This is followed by the percent of USRDAs of eight mandatory and several other voluntarily labeled nutrients. The USRDAs are not the same as the NAC/NRC RDAs of Table 2.1. The FDA uses the highest value obtained from any age or sex group for the standard person, exclusive of pregnant women, lactating women, infants, and children under four years of age. For example, the USRDA for iron is 18 mg., which is the requirement for women. The USRDAs were based on

TABLE 24.6 U.S. RDA for nutritional labeling

	Adults and children over 4 yrs	Children under 4	Infants under 13 months	Pregnant or lactating women
Mandatory nutrients				
Protein PER > 2.5	45 grams	20	18	45
PER < 2.5	65 grams	28	25	65
Vitamin A	5000 IU	2500	2500	8000
Vitamin C	60 mg.	40	40	60
Thiamin B_1	1.5 mg.	0.7	0.7	1.7
Ribolflavin B_2	1.7 mg.	0.8	0.8	2.0
Niacin	20 mg.	9.0	9.0	20.0
Calcium	1000 mg.	800	800	1300
Iron	18 mg.	10.0	10.0	18
Optional nutrients				
Vitamin D	400 IU	400	400	400
Vitamin E	30 IU	10	10	30
Vitamin B_6	2 mg.	0.7	0.7	2.5
Folic acid	0.4 mg.	0.2	0.2	0.8
Vitamin B_{12}	6 μg.	3	3	0.8
Phosphorus	1000 mg.	800	800	1300
Iodine	150 μg.	70	70	150
Magnesium	400 mg.	200	200	450
Zinc	15 mg.	8	8	15
Copper	2 mg.	1	1	2
Biotin	0.3 mg.	0.15	0.15	0.3
Pantothenic acid	10 mg.	5	5	10

the NAS/NRC RDA table published in 1968. The USRDA values are listed in Table 24.6 for all age groups. The label that appears on most foods is based on the first column, that is, the values for adults and children over four years of age. The other columns would be used only for foods made specifically for those specific age groups and are called special dietary foods. Parents who serve a product, such as a cereal to their children under four years of age should be familiar with the big differences in the RDA levels.

It can be seen on Table 24.6 that protein is based on the PER (protein efficiency ratio) value that accounts for its quality. A good quality protein source with a PER greater than 2.5 such as meat, milk, fish, or eggs have the USRDA based on 45 grams. In our example from Table 24.5, 18 grams of protein, which supplies 40% of the RDA, would be a high quality protein source because 18 divided by 45 is 40%, which is what appears on the label. If the food has a PER of less than 2.5 the protein USRDA would be 18 divided by 65 or 28%. The label could then show 25 or 30% for protein.

The percentage of the USRDA of the vitamins, minerals, and protein must use the following format:

1. If the level is below 2% it can be labeled with either a zero or an * with a note at the bottom saying "less than 2% of the USRDA."

2. Between 2% and 10% the label can state only 2, 4, 6, 8, or 10%, that is, the amount is given in 2% increments.

3. Between 10% and 50% the information must be expressed in 5% increments (10, 15, 20 . . . , etc.).

4. Above 50% the information must be given in 10% increments (50, 60, 70, etc.)

Nutrients can be listed only at the above values, not at the actual level in the food. Thus the label will tend to underestimate the actual value. Since some nutrients may be lost in storage, the processor will label at some lower value so as not to be in violation of the law. Although the regulation states the levels can be based on the level right after packaging, some nutrients can be lost during storage and it is safer to use the lower value. For example a nutrient calculated at 14% of the USRDA may be shown on the label at only 10%. Because of storage losses, the FDA will not prosecute for a violation unless the level of a natural vitamin in the food falls below 80% of the label declaration. Thus the label number is only an indication of the true nutritional content. For added nutrients, however, the actual level must match or exceed the label value. If the product is generally consumed with another food (e.g., cereal with milk), the manufacturer has the option of adding a second column showing the total nutrient content when consumed with the other food.

The USDA has similar nutritional labeling guidelines for meat-food products that suggests that the label indicate the nutrient content for both the uncooked and cooked product. Cooking instructions may also have to be included if the product is cooked before consumption. Table 24.6 also lists the USRDAs for other nutrients that can appear on the label. These can be put on the label only following the first eight mandatory nutrients.

The nutritional label requirements indicate whether or not certain claims can be made on the package label. A food for which a claim is made, for example, that it is a significant source of a nutrient, must have at least 10% of the USRDA of that nutrient. In addition, a food that claims that it is nutritionally superior to another food in any nutrient must have a USRDA that is greater than 10% or more than the level in the comparison food.

Regulations prohibit claims such as that certain foods can cure or mitigate a disease, that the soil a processed food is grown in may cause nutritional deficiencies, that processing, storage, transportation, and cooking result in deficiencies in the diet, and that natural ingredients are superior to synthetic. The FDA has also promulgated nutritional quality guidelines for frozen heat-and-serve dinners (such as salisbury steak with potatoes and peas). These guidelines (21 CFR 104.47) set the nutrient density (amount) based on 100 calories and also set minimums for certain nutrients such as protein (16 grams). FDA has also published guidelines for fortification/nutrification of foods (45 FR 6131; Jan. 25, 1980). The text in these guidelines traces the history of FDA nutritional labeling regulations and states several important principles the FDA would like processors to follow:

1. It is inappropriate to fortify fresh produce, meat, poultry, fish, sugar, candy, carbonated beverages, and snacks.

2. When restoration of one nutrient due to a loss in processing is done all other nutrients lost should also be restored.

3. When any nutrients are added to a food, they should include all 20 from Table 24.6 as well as potassium and manganese rather than just the eight in the standard nutritional labeling requirement. The addition to the food should be based on the amount adjusted to a 100-calorie intake basis to maximize nutrient density.

4. If nutrients are added for other than restoration or required enrichment, there must be a specific purpose for the addition, for example, to balance the nutrient/calorie ratio or to eliminate the need for imitation labeling.

Pet foods are not included in the above labeling format but are controlled by the FTC and the Association of Animal Feed Control Officials (AAFCO), which comprises the representatives from various states who have set up nutrient requirements for pet foods. Pet foods generally serve as the sole food source in the diet and thus have more strict regulations.

NON-REQUIRED LABEL INFORMATION

The information on the rest of the package, including the end flaps is left to the manufacturer's discretion. It can include ads, games, recipes, etc. However, some information other than advertising can have a bearing on the purchase of the food and will be discussed here.

Sugar and Fiber Information

Since the mid-1970s the public has become more informed about the effects of both fiber and sugar on their health. Because of this some food processors, especially cereal manufacturers, are voluntarily labeling the carbohydrate content of their food in terms of starches, sugars, and carbohydrates. A typical label with carbohydrate information (Most ® high-fiber multivitamin and iron supplement cereal) is shown in Table 24.7. As seen, when the milk is added the lactose from milk is counted with the sugars. There is some controversy about how to determine the fiber content since different analytical methods give different results. If nothing is said except to give the fiber or sugar information, it may not be considered nutrition information and thus would not trigger the required nutritional label statements. The data on carbohydrates cannot be inserted into the nutrition information panel below the grams of carbohydrate but it may appear below the whole format on the information panel.

UPC

The Universal Product Code (UPC) is a series of black and white lines with numbers below (Figure 24.4). The code is a method by which any retail consumer product that is manufactured in the United States can be identified. For grocery products a zero appears to the left of the lines. The next set of lines and the first five numbers below the lines identify the manufacturer of the food. For example, 24000 appears on all Del Monte products and 51000 on all Campbell's products. The next five numbers and and set of lines relate to the size and contents of the package and are in reverse order. The UPC can be passed over an electronic laser beam at a checkout counter of a supermarket that will then identify the product, automatically ring up the price, and send information to check the inventory and keep a record of how much of the product is left. Sometimes the ten numbers can be reduced to six numbers on a small package. On some checkout registers the receipt prints out the name of each food

TABLE 24.7 Carbohydrate information for Most ® cereal

	Carbohydrate information	
	1 ounce	With ½ cup whole milk
Starch and related carbohydrates	12 grams	12 grams
Sucrose and other sugars	6 grams	12 grams
Dietary fiber	4 grams	4 grams
Total carbohydrates	22 grams	28 grams

with the price so you can make sure you got what you paid for. Use of the UPC was originally rejected by many store clerk unions because they felt that this would eliminate stamping the price on each food package, thus eliminating jobs. Although doing away with individual pricing was in fact partly behind the UPC, consumers also objected because they felt that they would not remember the price displayed in the aisle and the store would cheat them when they got to the checkout. Fortunately, none of that came to pass and the UPC is being used more and more by major food chains because it significantly reduces the price errors made by humans.

Code Number

Somewhere on most food packages, usually at the top or bottom, is a set of letters and numbers. They are usually embossed into the package or can so that they cannot wear off. They identify the specific plant and batch where the product was made and include the date of manufacture. This is done by the manufacturer so that in the event of a recall they can easily get products back from the marketplace that were involved in a potential problem. Without the code the manufacturer would have to recall all products of the same type no matter when they were made. Although the FDA would like to make food coding mandatory it is not required except for low-acid canned foods and infant/baby foods.

Open Dating

Demands for various dating policies, for the purpose of marking foods with shelf-life expiration dates, are increasing steadily. At the

FIGURE 24.4 Universal product code

present time, most food packages in interstate commerce have a code stamped or embossed on them indicating the place and the day the food was manufactured. Since there are approximately 10,000 different codes utilized, it is very difficult for a consumer to know when the product was packaged. A consumer group in the state of New York once published a book with all the codes. Many consumer groups have lobbied their legislators to enact laws on the open dating of foods. Table 24.8 lists those states that have enacted open-dating regulations. Most of these are for short shelf-life foods (perishables) such as meat, eggs, or dairy products. Massachusetts tried to enact legislation to require all foods to be open dated but withdrew the pending regulations in 1981 because they were shown to be inadequate. An excellent analysis of open dating appeared in "Open Shelf-life Dating of Foods" available from the U.S. Superintendent of Documents, Washington D.C. 20402, Stock No. 052–003–00694–4 ($4.50). This study shows that from a scientific basis it would be almost impossible to put an exact expiration date on any individual food package so the date must be an educated estimate. This is because it is not known exactly where any one particular

TABLE 24.8 Summary of open-date labeling requirements by states

State/locale	Primary products	Form of open date	Effective since about
Alabama	Dairy	Sell by	1975
California	Dairy	Sell by	1973
Connecticut	Milk	Sell by	1973
District of Columbia	Perishable products	Sell by	1974
Florida	Dairy	Sell by	1976
Georgia	Milk, eggs	Sell by	1973
Maryland	Milk	Sell by	1971
Massachusetts	Perishable products	Sell by or use by	1979
Michigan	Perishable products	Sell by	1969
Minnesota	Perishable products with shelf life <90 days	Sell by or use by	1973
Nebraska	Eggs	Pack	—
Nevada	Dairy	Sell by	1973
New Hampshire	Cream	Use by	1973
New Jersey	Dairy	Sell by	—
New Mexico	Milk	Sell by	1977
Ohio	Perishable products	Sell by	1977
Oklahoma	Meat, eggs	Sell by	—
Oregon	Perishable products	Pack or sell by	1975
Pennsylvania	Milk	Sell by	1975
Virginia	Dairy & infant formula	Sell by	1974
Washington	Dairy & others	Sell by	1974
Wisconsin	Smoked fish	Pack	1971

food package will go and the U.S. environment varies immensely with place and time of year.

The forms that can be used for open dating can vary. The *date of manufacture or pack date* that involves the translation of existing codes into real dates is one form of open dating. This could be done very easily and might benefit the consumer. However, there is no guarantee that a younger product is a better one since the younger one may have been abused by holding at high temperature during distribution. A *freshness or best-if-used-by date* is a date by which the food should be consumed in order to obtain maximum quality from the product. But if the product is mishandled, the date could prove to be meaningless. A *pull or sell-by date* is a date after which the product should not be sold. Many dairy and processed-meat companies are using pull dates at the present time, since they know the shelf life of the food under normal refrigeration conditions for the package system they are using. On the other hand, if the product is abused by holding at high temperature, the date would be meaningless. Finally a *use-by date* indicates the theoretical end of shelf life of a product. In fact it could last longer or shorter than that date.

Open dating of foods should encourage shippers and supermarket personnel to rotate stock. Many times food companies are blamed for producing stale foods when the problem was actually caused by improper handling, that is, restocking shelves from front to back instead of from back to front or stocking refrigerated or frozen foods above the cold line in a supermarket display case.

Consumer rotating of stock to seek the freshest product may not be a problem if consumers can be convinced that stores will rotate stocks correctly to insure the highest quality. A supermarket chain in Ohio that studied open dating on a USDA research project in 1972 found that at first consumers would search for the dates of the freshest foods and pull them out. However, once convinced that the stores were handling the products correctly, they stopped doing this. Consumers generally benefited from higher quality products and higher nutritional value. There was a 50% reduction in returns of foods to the supermarket because fewer foods were spoiled.

The other problem with open dating is related to liability. Where open dating has been used voluntarily today by some manufacturers, there has been a greater return of product both to the supermarket and distributor. The higher return was because people realized product was past the date on the label. This resulted in higher cost to other consumers. Consumers must be educated that the date is not a guarantee and, even more important, that it has nothing to do with food safety from the standpoint of pathogens. When meats are labeled with an open date, the USDA requires that specific holding temperatures be indicated on the label, for example, "keep refrigerated below 45°F." As of 1984 neither Congress nor the FDA has felt that there was enough scientific data available (based on the above-cited U.S. Congress Office of Technology Assessment Report on Open Shelf-life Dating) to insure an accurate dating system. Thus use of a date is voluntary unless a state requires it. Perishable foods are the most logical for the states to regulate since there is more control over them.

Freeze/Thaw Indicator

Frozen food packages may also have a thaw indicator. This indicator could consist of test tapes affixed to the package that would change color if the package was thawed and/or refrozen. Such thaw indicators would encourage shippers, handlers, and retailers of frozen foods to be more careful with their handling practices, thereby benefiting the consumer. In addition, new devices called time-temperature integrators have been developed for frozen foods that integrate the effects of the temperature during storage. They display a number on a line like a thermometer, that indicates the number of days of high quality life left. This is the best type of device because it accounts for any abuse that occurs in distribution. However the device is very costly (over 25¢ each) and much more research is needed to test its applicability for all foods. Generally, these devices are used for drugs.

SUMMARY

The food package label provides the consumer with required and other information about the food. The front panel explains what the product is and how much is in the package, and may give nutritional information when required or volunteered. The name of the food may be a standard of identity, a common or usual name, or a fanciful name. The name may also indicate whether it is a reduced- or low-calorie food and whether the food contains any artificial colors or flavors. If the food is an imitation of another product it must say so in the name. The right side panel must provide both an ingredient list and a manufacturer's address.

The ingredient list must give the contents in descending order of predominance (weight) and must specify what preservatives are present and what their function is. If a nutritional claim is made for the food, specific nutrient information must be given according to the specified format. The nutritional information contains the caloric value and the fat, carbohydrate, and protein values in grams per serving size. Labeling of protein plus seven vitamins and minerals in specific increments of the USRDA is required when nutritional labeling is used. If claims about sodium or sugar addition are made, specific formats must be followed. Other parts of the package may contain information at the discretion of the manufacturer, for example, fiber content, sugar content, and a shelf-life date. Most foods including all pet foods are under the control of the Food and Drug Administration, while meat-food products are controlled by the U.S. Department of Agriculture. The USDA must approve all labels before they leave an establishment, and the labels must bear a USDA seal.

*Multiple
Choice
Study
Questions*

1. The front panel of a food label does not require

    A. the standard of identity name if there is one

    B. a USDA inspection insignia if the food contains more than 3% meat

    C. the net contents

    D. the picture of the food

    E. the common or usual name

2. The UPC is

    A. the Universal Processing Conditions required by the FDA

    B. the Universal Processing Conditions agreed to by the USDA and FDA

    C. the Underwriters Passing Codes that identify companies under FDA inspection

    D. a bunch of black lines on a white background defining product identity

    E. a secret code companies use on their packages that consumers cannot read

3. In the UPC, the zero at the left

    A. lines up the laser beam

    B. identifies the food company

    C. identifies the product as a cosmetic

    D. identifies the product as a grocery item

    E. is not present

Below is a nutritional label for a breakfast bar.   Questions 4 to 13 refer to this label.

Nutritional Information Per Serving

Serving size	5 oz.
Number of servings	4
Calories	300
Protein	15 g.
Carbohydrate	40 g.
*Fat	15 g.
*Cholesterol	50 mg.
Saturated fats	3 g.
Polyunsaturated fats	10 g.
Sodium	45 mg.

*The use of this food will prevent heart disease

Percentage of the U.S. Recommended Daily Allowance (USRDA)

Protein	20%
Vitamin A	20%
Vitamin C	26%
Thiamin	8%
Riboflavin	10%
Niacin	0%
Calcium	10%
Iodine	2%

4. The net weight of the above package is

A. 2 oz.
B. 5 oz.
C. 10 oz.
D. 15 oz.
E. 20 oz.

5. A statement on the label that "The use of this food will prevent heart disease" is

A. legal since the food has a low cholesterol and a good S:P ratio
B. illegal since the S:P ratio should be 1 to 2
C. illegal because it makes a health claim
D. illegal because no foods can be used to prevent heart disease

6. The labeling of sodium is

A. legal and always required
B. legal, optional, but should also include mg. per 100 grams
C. legal, optional, but should be given as a percentage of the USRDA
D. legal, mandatory, but should be given as a percentage of the USRDA

7. The PER of the protein in this food
   A. cannot be determined from the label
   B. must be of good quality based on the percent of the USRDA
   C. must be of poor quality based on the percent of the USRDA
   D. is greater than 2.5%
   E. is greater than 23%

8. The USRDA for iron is based on
   A. men
   B. women
   C. monkeys
   D. the 1974 RDAs
   E. the 1965 RDAs

9. The USRDA for vitamin C
   A. is correctly labeled
   B. should be labeled 25%
   C. should be labeled 20%
   D. should be labeled 35%
   E. is based on the RDA of 45 mg.

10. Assuming that the weights of fat, carbohydrate, and protein are correct, the correct caloric value is
    A. 295
    B. 300
    C. 350
    D. 355
    E. 400

11. The required mineral missing from the list is
    A. iron
    B. zinc
    C. manganese
    D. potassium
    E. phosphorus

12. The saturated to unsaturated fat ratio is
    A. 0.3 to 1
    B. 3.0 to 1
    C. 3.3 to 1
    D. 15 to 13
    E. 10 to 3

13. The reason that the total fat does not equal saturated and unsaturated fat is

   A. total fat includes glyco-proteins
   B. total fat does not include cholesterol
   C. monounsaturated fats are not included
   D. they are equal

14. The ingredient list on a label is required to include

   A. the ingredients in alphabetical order
   B. the ingredients in order of decreasing amount
   C. the ingredients in order of increasing amount
   D. the percentage of each ingredient
   E. the chemical names of each ingredient

15. Which food is not exempt from nutritional labeling?

   A. enriched flour
   B. enriched bread
   C. iodized salt
   D. low-sodium foods
   E. "Product 19" special dietary cereal

16. A freshness date is the date a food product

   A. was packaged
   B. should not be consumed after
   C. should be used by to insure high quality
   D. might result in food poisoning

Essay Study Questions

1. List the specific general requirements of the FDA for labeling of a food product that makes no nutritional claims.

2. Contrast the difference between the FDA and USDA with respect to labeling of foods for humans.

3. Discuss the purpose of a standard of identity.

4. Discuss the common and usual name regulations.

5. Describe a hypothetical nutritional label. Does the label teach nutrition?

6. What kinds of claims can be made for reduced- or low-calorie food.

7. What is the USRDA? What problems may arise in using it?

8. What forms of open dating are used on food packages and what advantages do they have?

9. What is a freeze thaw indicator?

10. What is the UPC used for?

11. What is the purpose of the code that may be placed on a food package?

12. How is the labeling of pet foods controlled?

Things to Do

1. Collect packages of foods and identify for each package which parts of the label are segments of the required labeling.

2. Using the net weights of similar products (e.g., canned peas), make a price comparison by adjusting to a cost per unit weight (e.g., cost per ounce).

3. Examine the nutritional labels of various foods. Do they comply with the regulations? How do the values compare with the values used in your food survey?

4. Make up a hypothetical food from your food composition tables and then construct a food label and nutritional label for it.

5. Check the ingredient listing of various processed foods. Does the order of predominance comply with the actual name of the product (e.g., pork and beans, fruit drinks, beef stew, fruit cocktail)?

6. Obtain a copy of the Standards of Identities of foods from Title 21 of the Code of Federal Regulations. Examine labels of foods that have standards and how they comply with respect to the ingredient list.

7. Make a list of foods that use some form of open dating. Are the values reasonable? What type of labeling is used?

8. Estimate the protein quality of various foods using the nutrition labeling information.

9. Obtain a copy of the booklet "The Sodium Content of Food," which lists the sodium content of 789 foods. This is free from: FDA HFE–88, 5600 Fishers Lane, Rockville, Md 20857. Use it to determine your own sodium intake.

10. The following publications may be obtained from the U.S. Government Consumer Information Center, Department DD, Pueblo, Colorado 81009. They are related to both labeling, home processing, and nutrition.

Computerized Supermarket Checkout. 541J. Free. 4 pp. 1979. How the Universal Product Code checkout system works and affects the shopper.

The Confusing World of Health Foods. 542J. Free. 4 pp. 1979. Discusses the claims for health, organic, and natural foods; compares cost and nutritional value of health versus conventional foods.

Consumer's Guide to Food Labels. 543J. Free. 4 pp. 1978. Discusses ingredient and nutrient listings, open dating, metric units, and symbols used on food labels.

Food Additives. 545J. Free. 7 pp. 1979. Why chemicals are added to foods; how additive use is regulated; steps to take to exert control over what goes into your food; an index of more than 130 additives; and definitions of the major categories.

Food Stamps. 546J. Free. 13 pp. 1979. Food stamp rules: Who is eligible, how to get them, and how you can use them.

How To Buy Economically: A Food Buyer's Guide. 650J. Free. 28 pp. 1981. How to cut costs on meat, poultry, eggs, milk, fruits, and vegetables; months during which you can get the best buys on a variety of fruits and vegetables.

How To Save Money with Large Cuts of Meat. 651J. Free. 6 pp. 1981. Illustrated cutting instructions for vacuum-packed pieces of meat weighing from 8 to 30 pounds; suggestions for cooking; how to wrap meat for freezing; how long it can be kept.

A Primer on Dietary Minerals. 549J. Free. 4 pp. 1979. Describes necessary minerals and best food sources.

Roughage. 547J. Free. 2 pp. 1979. Claims and facts about high fiber diets; effects on health; and good food sources.

Salt. 550J. Free. 6 pp. 1980. How the body uses sodium chloride; ways to reduce salt intake; lists popular foods with high salt content.

The Sodium Content of Your Foods. 202J. $2.00. 43 pp. 1980. Tables showing the sodium content of many common foods and selected nonprescription drugs so you can limit salt or sodium intake.

Some Facts and Myths About Vitamins. 552J. Free. 4 pp. 1979. What vitamins are, how they work, and best food sources; discusses some controversial claims about vitamins.

Sugar. 551J. Free. 4 pp. 1980. How different types of sugar work in your body; caloric and carbohydrate values of various sweeteners; types of sweeteners available such as cane sugar, honey, corn syrup, etc.

Vegetarian Diets. 652J. Free. 2 pp. 1981. Benefits and possible risks; important nutrition considerations for non-meat eaters.

Can Your Kitchen Pass the Food Storage Test? 630J. Free. 6 pp. 1978. Checklist of food storage hazards and how to correct them.

Food Safety for the Family. 653J. Free. 11 pp. 1980. Causes of food poisoning; specific instructions for safe handling of a variety of foods; what to do when the freezer stops.

Food Canning of Fruits and Vegetables. 133J. $1.50. 32 pp. 1979. A comprehensive, illustrated guide to selecting ingredients and equipment, preparation, and processing; specific instructions for 32 fruits and vegetables.

Home Freezing of Fruits and Vegetables. 134J. $2.00. 48 pp. 1978. A comprehensive, illustrated guide for selecting ingredients and equipment, preparation, packaging and freezing; specific instructions for 78 fruits and vegetables.

Ideas for Better Eating. 192J. $2.50. 32 pp. 1981. Menu ideas and recipes to improve your diet; important facts about nutritional needs and popular foods; and menus at different calorie levels.

Storing Vegetables and Fruits. 135J. $1.50. 18 pp. 1978. Making fresh produce last longer by storing in basements, cellars, and outdoors.

Chapter 24. Answers to Multiple-Choice Study Questions: 1, D; 2, D; 3, D; 4, E; 5, C; 6, B; 7, C; 8, B; 9, B; 10, D; 11, A; 12, A; 13, C; 14, B; 15, E; 16, C.

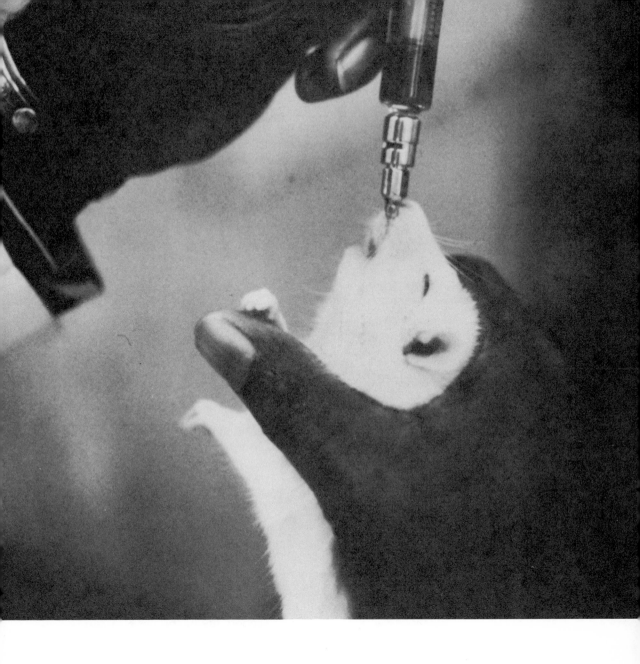

**FOOD SAFETY:
LEGAL BASIS AND
SAFETY TESTING**

25

THE LAWS AND REGULATIONS REGARDING SAFETY OF FOODS

Basic Law

The Food, Drug, and Cosmetic Act declares food adulterated if: 402(a)(1) it bears or contains any poisonous or deleterious substance which may render it injurious to health; but in the case the substance is not an added substance such food shall not be considered adulterated if the quantity of such substances in such foods does not ordinarily render it injurious to health

and

403(a)(2) it bears or contains any added poisonous or added deleterious substance other than one which is:

> (i) a pesticide chemical in or on a raw agricultural commodity
> (ii) a food additive
> (iii) a color additive, or
> (iv) a new animal drug . . . .

These two sections of the act (which are duplicated in the Meat Inspection Act) set the basic principles of food safety regulation. The above sentences mean that a food is unsafe, adulterated, and therefore illegal if it falls in one of the several categories. One such category is food containing substances that came from the environment, either synthetic or natural, that may make it injurious to health when consumed. This refers to certain poisonous substances such as PCBs, DDT, EDB, lead, and mercury that are so prevalent in the environment that it is impossible to have foods without some small amount present. The FDA has used section 406 of the Act to set either action levels, or tolerances for these substances. These action levels and tolerances are limits above which if the chemical is present the FDA will seize the food. Without these limits the Act could be used to condemn almost all foods. An action level can be set for any poisonous or deleterious substance that cannot be avoided in the processing of food but for which there is a chance of new technology that will come about to reduce the level of chemical in food. If the possibility of reduction of the level is remote a formal tolerance can be set instead. Section 406 of the Act also covers the presence of pathogens in foods and any toxins that result from their growth. For example, the FDA has set the action level for aflatoxin at 20 pbb. In many cases the levels are set at or near the level at which chemists can just detect the presence of the compound, that is, the level is not based on how poisonous the chemical is, but rather on its detectability limit.

Although the setting of action levels by the FDA has been challenged in the courts several times (see *U.S. vs. Anderson Sea Food, Inc.* 447 F. Supp. 1151, 1978; *U.S. vs. Boston Farm Center* 590 F.2d 149, 1979), the courts have usually upheld the FDA action levels. The regulations dealing with adulteration from poisonous or deleterious substances (21 CFR 109) disallow the blending of two batches (one with a high level and one with a low level) to achieve a level below the action level. This provision has caused some economic losses, especially to grain farmers, but is enforced to protect the consumer. Furthermore, in 1980 and 1981 under executive order of the President and with the endorsement of the FDA, cereal grain and peanuts with higher levels of aflatoxin than the action level were allowed in feeds for beef cattle, pullets, and pigs because seizure and destruction would have resulted in severe economic loss for farmers in certain regions of the country. This is an example of risk/benefit decision-making, although one may question whether economic benefit should be balanced against toxicological risk. If sections 402(a)(1) and (a)(2) were to be applied worldwide, much food now eaten would be condemned. In fact, the United States has been criticized for setting low action levels, since the low limits prevent less well developed countries from shipping grain to us. This is not an easy issue to resolve when health and safety are concerned.

Natural Toxicants

Section 402(a)(1) is also interpreted to mean that a food can be declared adulterated if natural chemicals produced through metabolism (i.e., not added by the manufacturer), which when consumed may render the food injurious to health. Congress, in its wisdom, realized that almost all foods contain some naturally made toxicants (see next chapter), thus they wrote 402(a)(1) so as to delete from regulation those foods in which the level of natural toxicants is inconsequential if the food as eaten does not ordinarily render it injurious to health. The FDA can use this part of the law to regulate new genetic varieties of grains, fruits, and vegetables for safety. The FDA has informally held that if the natural toxicant level in the new variety of a food is more than 10% higher than that of the normal commodity, they will declare the new food adulterated and therefore illegal. This has, in fact, occurred with a new variety of chipping potato developed jointly by the USDA and Canadian researchers. With the vast increase in genetic engineering research beginning in the 1980s, it is possible that the FDA will have to spend more time in this area. The FDA has also informally declared that new genetic varieties cannot have important nutrients reduced below 80% of the level found in the normal variety.

Added Substances: General Statement

The initial statement of Section 402(a)(1), which was in the 1906 Pure Food and Drug Act, was interpreted to mean that the government had to prove that an added ingredient was injurious. In 1954, 1958, and 1960, respectively, the Miller Pesticide Amendment, the Food Additives Amendment, and the Color Additives Amendment changed that. By adding sections to the act (Sec 402(a)(2) along with Sec 408 covering pesticides, Sec 409 covering food additives, and Sec 706 covering food colors), the law declared all added substances illegal unless they were allowed because of some prior agreement (prior sanctioned), granted an exemption as a substance that was generally recognized as safe (a GRAS list ingredient or chemical substance), or were granted an exemption in a regulation under the appropriate section of the law specifying the function and allowed level of the chemical. The exemption is given only if the chemical is deemed to be safe. The language of the Act provides that the onus of efficacy testing and safety testing is on the food and chemical industry, and not on the government. Later in this chapter, we will cover safety testing in detail.

Pesticides

Several things are of importance in the language of Section 408 of the Food, Drug, and Cosmetic Act. Pesticides are legally pesticides only when they exist on a raw agricultural commodity, i.e., on fresh produce like apples or lettuce. The EPA sets the levels and the FDA can accept the pesticide under Sec 408, once data on its use level, efficacy, and toxicity and an analytical procedure to detect the chemical have been submitted and acted upon. The allowed pesticides are listed in Title 40 CFR Part 180 under the EPA. Once the food is processed, however, a regulated allowed pesticide becomes a food additive and the tolerances are listed under 21 CFR 193, which is controlled by the FDA. A food is declared adulterated if the pesticide level in the finished food product, when ready to eat, is greater than that for the raw food. Drying apples concentrates the pesticides in the food because of moisture loss. If sold to be eaten directly, the apples would be illegal; if sold to be rehydrated for use in pie, the apples might be legal.

Many pesticides such as DDT have been banned from use in the U.S. Unfortunately since some of them are very stable, they have pervaded our environment and they show up at low levels in many foods. This is one way in which the FDA uses Section 406 of the Act to set regulatory guidelines or action levels for the banned pesticides. The case of *U.S. vs. City Smoked Fish Co.* (Civil Action 33989 E. Mich., 1970) upheld the FDA in setting such a tolerance.

Under the EPA, all chemical pesticides must be used by a registered applicator, that is, someone who is trained at the state level in the proper applications procedures so that injury to humans will not occur. One unfortunate part of the law, however, is that manufacture of illegal pesticides is not prohibited in the U.S. if the chemicals are intended and sold for export. Many banned pesticides are used worldwide with the good intention of preventing loss of foods. What happens, however, is that sometimes the use is not controlled well and food we import into the U.S. contains the very chemicals we have banned. Since the FDA cannot check every batch of food at port of entry, we may have a higher risk than we desire (for an excellent review of this problem see J.H. Nicholas, *Food Drug Cosmetic Law Journal* 36, no. 11 pp. 573–595, 1981).

Food Additive Laws

Section 409 of the FFDC Act declares all food additives unsafe unless the additive and its use conform to an exemption or there is a specific regulation for the intended use. The law requires preclearance before use, that is, the industry must petition the FDA for a specific use. As with a pesticide, a company proposing the chemical must submit data as to purity, use levels, effectiveness, an analytical procedure, and results of "safety testing." When evaluating safety, the Secretary of HHS must take into account the potential consumption level, interactions with other substances, and safety factors recognized by experts.

The law does not specify what safety testing is required except that under 21 CFR 110.20 it is stated that the FDA will be guided by current procedures recognized by the National Academy of Science/National Research Council. It specifies that safe means a reasonable certainty that it is not harmful under 21 CFR 170.3(i). New procedures can be added and old ones deleted as toxicologists study what is meant by harmfulness. Some of these tests will be discussed later in this chapter. To insure that the tests are carried out properly and that the data are not fudged or misinterpreted, the FDA requires that all studies relating to food additive petitions follow Good Laboratory Practice (GLPs) under 21 CFR 58. These GLPs specify such things as the animal room environment, calibration of balances, storage of the test diet, and methods of recording data in lab manuals.

The law does have one other specific requirement as to safety and that is the Delaney Clause. The clause, which is Sec 409(c)(3)(A), states that any substance when fed to either man or animals if found to induce cancer (a carcinogen), or as the result of appropriate testing procedures for the evaluation of safety of additives also induces cancer, that substance is to be banned from use in the food supply. This means that there is a zero tolerance level for additives that do not pass these criteria. This law may be difficult to enforce for all additives because of the problems involved in the interpretation of the tests designed for cancer testing. In the 1950s the types of animal tests used showed very few chemicals to be carcinogens. Thus it was easy to conceive of enforcing this clause. However, as more animal tests were added, many chemicals were shown to be carcinogens at some level in the diet. The basic controversy today involves whether a chemical that induces cancer when fed in fairly large doses to animals (such as in the Canadian saccharin study) will really induce cancer in humans at the normally much lower levels of consumption. The law doesn't differentiate between these two levels, and thus in the early 1980s many bills have been proposed to either delete the Delaney Clause or modify it to allow some level of risk (e.g., a potential cancer death rate from the chemical of 1 in 1 million or 1 in 100,000 people for a lifetime). It may be hard to justify any risk when the benefit is purely economic (e.g., with a food color or flavor).

A food additive is legally defined as any substance the intended use of which results directly or may reasonably be expected to result directly or indirectly in its becoming a component of food or otherwise affecting the characteristics of a food. A material used in food packaging materials that could migrate into the food upon contact can be a food additive as well as a substance used in the chemical manufacture of an ingredient for foods. The FDA lists 32 additive categories as shown in Table 25.1. These are further categorized as:

21 CFR 172: Additives for direct addition to a food such as the antioxidant BHA

21 CFR 173: Secondary direct food additives that are substances used in processes that contact foods and can become part of the food. An example is a solvent or an enzyme.

21 CFR 174 to 178: Indirect food additives. For example, those chemicals used in packaging materials that can migrate into food upon contact or chemicals used as sanitizing agents.

21 CFR 179: Food irradiation; a process which is regarded as a food additive.

21 CFR 180: Interim use food additives pending further study. Includes caffeine and saccharine, both under fire because of potential toxicity.

21 CFR 181: Prior sanctioned ingredients are those chemicals that because of use prior to 1958 were granted an exemption from regulatory control. The FDA could legally fight this exemption in court if the substance were shown to be carcinogenic or highly toxic

TABLE 25.1 Food additive categories [21 CFR 170.3(o)]

anticaking	leavening
antimicrobial	lubricants & release agents
antioxidants	non-nutritive sweeteners
color & adjuncts	nutritive sweeteners
curing & pickling	oxidizing and reducing
dough strengtheners	pH control
drying agents	processing aids: clarifying, clouding,
emulsifiers	catalyst, floculants, filter aids,
enzymes	crystallization, inhibitors
firming agents	propellants
flavor enhancers	sequestrants
flavoring agents	solvents & vehicles
flour treating	stabilizers & thickeners
formulation aids: carriers, binders, fillers,	surface active agents
plasticizers	surface finishing agents
fumigants	synergists
humectants	texturizers

at the level of use. Nitrite, used in the curing of meat, is a prior sanctioned ingredient.

21 CFR 189: Prohibited substances such as cyclamate that were once used but are now banned by the FDA. Some of these will be mentioned in the next chapter.

In passing a regulation allowing the use of a food additive, answering the difficult question of risk versus benefit is not required by law. In fact, another part of the law, under 409(c)(3)(A), states that the Commissioner can deny any chemical if the data in the petition fails to establish that under the proposed use the additive will be safe. This is termed the general safety provision and gives wide discretion to the Commissioner irrespective of benefits. In 1981–1982 Congress debated whether to delete this provision as well as the Delaney Clause and make the risk/benefit question part of the regulatory process. How this would be done was not specified however. With drugs there is allowance of more potential risk from side effects if the drug (chemical) can prevent death or cure some dreaded disease. The only additives that might fit into that category are those that prevent the growth of pathogens; the rest provide economic benefits in most respects, for example, they increase food shelf life or help improve eating quality.

GRAS (Generally Recognized as Safe) Chemicals

GRAS chemical additives are a third category of chemicals or substance used in food. They are either food ingredients or chemicals that have a very low toxicity to humans when used in the food supply under normal good manufacturing processes. Technically, they are non-toxic under normal use, but we should remember that anything ingested in high enough levels can cause harm or death, including water. In a cake mix, besides any added artificial flavors or colors, the flour, yeast, shortening, and dry milk powder are considered GRAS substances. All commodities (eggs, fruits, vegetables, cereals, oils) and many of the processed components of these (such as dried milk) foods are implicitly included in the GRAS list since they are safe to use in a normal well-balanced diet and had been used extensively before 1958 when the amendment was added to the Act.

The GRAS list was put together in 1958 by some 300 scientists who, at the request of FDA, submitted the names of food ingredients that could be classified as GRAS. Because some of these substances were subsequently found to have been improperly tested, the FDA rewrote the definitions of the list in 1973 and began examining many of the chemicals on it for reaffirmation of their safety, under an order from then-President Richard Nixon. These categories are spelled out in 21 CFR 170.30.

The GRAS designation under 21 CFR 182.1 technically includes all foods and ingredients of natural biological origin consumed for nutritive purposes and used without detrimental effect prior to 1958. For example, some of the food components (yeast, and flour) of the cake mix previously mentioned would fall in this category. There are so many foods and ingredients that are GRAS that most are not actually listed. Those that are listed include, for example, salt, sugar, vinegar, baking powder, and MSG. Foods chemically modified by conventional processing and used prior to 1958 constitute another category. The chemical modification of starches to impart better gelling ability is an example of this category. Modified gums and gelatin for similar purposes produced by procedures used prior to 1958 would also be included. Table 25.2 lists all those substances for which a GRAS list regulation has been promulgated. In 1981 caffeine was deleted from this list and put on the interim food additive list.

Everything on the GRAS list other than natural food ingredients or components has been under reexamination, scrutiny, and testing for safety and efficacy as required under 21 CFR 170.30(f). This includes foods or chemicals modified by new processes since 1958 and foods or ingredients that have been altered by breeding or genetic selection. An example of the latter is the new variety of tomato that can be mechanically harvested due to its firmer consistency. The FDA is concerned both with possible increased toxicity and with reduction in the nutritional quality of new breeds and varieties of foods. The nutrition concern for the new varieties of fruits and vegetables is because these foods supply 90% of the vitamin C, 50% of the vitamin

TABLE 25.2 GRAS List Substances [21 CFR 182]

PART 182   Substances generally recognized as safe

Subpart A   General provisions

182.1   Substances that are generally recognized as safe.

182.10 Spices and other natural seasonings and flavorings.

182.20 Essential oils, oleoresins (solvent-free), and natural extractives (including distillates).

182.30 Natural substances used in conjunction with spices and other natural seasonings and flavorings.

182.40 Natural extractives (solvent-free) used in conjunction with spices, seasonings, and flavorings.

182.50 Certain other spices, seasonings, essential oils, oleoresins, and natural extracts.

182.60 Synthetic flavoring substances and adjuvants.

182.70 Substances migrating from cotton and cotton fabrics used in dry food packaging.

182.90 Substances migrating to food from paper and paperboard products.

182.99 Adjuvants for pesticide chemicals.

Subpart B   Multiple purpose GRAS food substances

182.1005 Acetic acid.
182.1009 Adipic acid.
182.1033 Citric acid.
182.1045 Glutamic acid.
182.1047 Glutamic acid hydrochloride.
182.1057 Hydrochloric acid.
182.1061 Lactic acid.
182.1073 Phosphoric acid.
182.1077 Potassium acid tartrate.
182.1087 Sodium acid pyrophosphate.
182.1099 Tartaric acid.
182.1125 Aluminum sulfate.
182.1127 Aluminum ammonium sulfate.
182.1129 Aluminum potassium sulfate.
182.1131 Aluminum sodium sulfate.
182.1135 Ammonium bicarbonate.
182.1137 Ammonium carbonate.
182.1139 Ammonium hydroxide.
182.1141 Ammonium phosphate.
182.1155 Bentonite.
182.1165 Butane.
182.1180 Caffeine.
182.1191 Calcium carbonate.
182.1193 Calcium chloride.
182.1195 Calcium citrate.
182.1199 Calcium gluconate.
182.1205 Calcium hydroxide.
182.1207 Calcium lactate.
182.1210 Calcium oxide.
182.1217 Calcium phosphate.
182.1235 Caramel.
182.1240 Carbon dioxide.
182.1320 Glycerin.
182.1324 Glyceryl monostearate.
182.1355 Helium.
182.1366 Hydrogen peroxide.
182.1400 Lecithin.
182.1425 Magnesium carbonate.
182.1428 Magnesium hydroxide.
182.1431 Magnesium oxide.
182.1440 Magnesium stearate.
182.1480 Methylcellulose.
182.1500 Monoammonium glutamate.
182.1516 Monopotassium glutamate.
182.1540 Nitrogen.
182.1545 Nitrous oxide.
182.1585 Papain.
182.1613 Potassium bicarbonate.
182.1619 Potassium carbonate.
182.1625 Potassium citrate.
182.1631 Potassium, hydroxide.
182.1655 Propane.
182.1666 Propylene glycol.
182.1685 Rennet.
182.1711 Silica aerogel.
182.1721 Sodium acetate.
182.1736 Sodium bicarbonate.
182.1742 Sodium carbonate.
182.1745 Sodium carboxymethylcellulose.

182.1748 Sodium caseinate.
182.1751 Sodium citrate.
182.1763 Sodium hydroxide.
182.1775 Sodium pectinate.
182.1778 Sodium phosphate.
182.1781 Sodium aluminum phosphate.
182.1792 Sodium sesquicarbonate.
182.1804 Sodium potassium tartrate.
182.1810 Sodium tripolyphosphate.
182.1901 Triacetin.
182.1911 Triethyl citrate.
182.1978 Carnauba wax.

Subpart C   Anticaking agents

182.2122 Aluminum calcium silicate.
182.2227 Calcium silicate.
182.2437 Magnesium silicate.
182.2727 Sodium aluminosilicate.
182.2729 Sodium calcium aluminosilicate, hydrated.
182.2906 Tricalcium silicate.

Subpart D   Chemical preservatives

182.3013 Ascorbic acid.
182.3041 Erythorbic acid.
182.3081 Propionic acid.
182.3089 Sorbic acid.
182.3109 Thiodipropionic acid.
182.3149 Ascorbyl palmitate.
182.3169 Butylated hydroxyanisole.
182.3173 Butylated hydroxytoluene.
182.3189 Calcium ascorbate.
182.3221 Calcium propionate.
182.3225 Calcium sorbate.
182.3280 Dilauryl thiodipropionate.
182.3616 Potassium bisulfite.
182.3637 Potassium metabisulfite.
182.3640 Potassium sorbate.
182.3731 Sodium ascorbate.
182.3739 Sodium bisulfite.
182.3766 Sodium metabisulfite.
182.3784 Sodium propionate.
182.3795 Sodium sorbate.
182.3798 Sodium sulfite.
182.3845 Stannous chloride.
182.3862 Sulfur dioxide.
182.3890 Tocopherols.

TABLE 25.2 GRAS List Substances [21 CFR 182] (Continued)

PART 182   Substances generally recognized as safe

Subpart E   Emulsifying agents

182.4101   Diacetyl tartaric acid esters of mono- and diglycerides of edible fats or oils, or edible fat-forming fatty acids.

182.4505   Mono- and diglycerides of edible fats or oils, or edible fat-forming acids.

182.4521   Monosodium phosphate derivatives of mono- and diglycerides of edible fats or oils, or edible fat-forming fatty acids.

182.4666   Propylene glycol.

Subpart F   Dietary supplements

182.5013   Ascorbic acid.
182.5065   Linoleic acid.
182.5159   Biotin.
182.5191   Calcium carbonate.
182.5195   Calcium citrate.
182.5201   Calcium glycerophosphate.
182.5210   Calcium oxide.
182.5212   Calcium pantothenate.
182.5217   Calcium phosphate.
182.5223   Calcium pyrophosphate.
182.5245   Carotene.
182.5250   Choline bitartrate.
182.5252   Choline chloride.
182.5260   Copper gluconate.
182.5265   Cuprous iodide.
182.5301   Ferric phosphate.
182.5304   Ferric pyrophosphate.
182.5306   Ferric sodium pyrophosphate.
182.5308   Ferrous gluconate.
182.5311   Ferrous lactate.
182.5315   Ferrous sulfate.
182.5370   Inositol.
182.5375   Iron reduced.
182.5431   Magnesium oxide.
182.5434   Magnesium phosphate.
182.5443   Magnesium sulfate.
182.5446   Manganese chloride.
182.5449   Manganese citrate.
182.5452   Manganese gluconate.
182.5455   Manganese glycerophosphate.

182.5458   Manganese hypophosphite.
182.5461   Manganese sulfate.
182.5464   Manganous oxide.
182.5530   Niacin.
182.5535   Niacinamide.
182.5580   D-Pantothenyl alcohol.
182.5622   Potassium chloride.
182.5628   Potassium glycerophosphate.
182.5676   Pyridoxine hydrochloride.
182.5695   Riboflavin.
182.5697   Riboflavin-5-phosphate.
182.5772   Sodium pantothenate.
182.5778   Sodium phosphate.
182.5875   Thiamine hydrochloride.
182.5878   Thiamine mononitrate.
182.5890   Tocopherols.
182.5892 a-Tocopherol acetate.
182.5930   Vitamin A.
182.5933   Vitamin A acetate.
182.5936   Vitamin A palmitate.
182.5945   Vitamin B_{12}.
182.5950   Vitamin D_2.
182.5953   Vitamin D_3.
182.5985   Zinc chloride.
182.5988   Zinc gluconate.
182.5991   Zinc oxide.
182.5994   Zinc stearate.
182.5997   Zinc sulfate.

Subpart G   Sequestrants

182.6033   Citric acid.
182.6085   Sodium acid phosphate.
182.6099   Tartaric acid.
182.6185   Calcium acetate.
182.6193   Calcium chloride.
182.6195   Calcium citrate.
182.6197   Calcium diacetate.
182.6199   Calcium gluconate.
182.6203   Calcium hexametaphosphate.
182.6215   Monobasic calcium phosphate.
182.6219   Calcium phytate.
182.6285   Dipotassium phosphate.
182.6290   Disodium phosphate.
182.6386   Isopropyl citrate.
182.6511   Monoisopropyl citrate.
182.6625   Potassium citrate.
182.6751   Sodium citrate.
182.6754   Sodium diacetate.

182.6757   Sodium gluconate.
182.6760   Sodium hexametaphosphate.
182.6769   Sodium metaphosphate.
182.6778   Sodium phosphate.
182.6787   Sodium pyrophosphate.
182.6789   Tetra sodium pyrophosphate.
182.6801   Sodium tartrate.
182.6804   Sodium potassium tartrate.
182.6810   Sodium tripolyphosphate.
182.6851   Stearyl citrate.

Subpart H   Stabilizers

182.7133   Ammonium alginate.
182.7187   Calcium alginate.
182.7255   Chondrus extract.
182.7610   Potassium alginate.
182.7724   Sodium alginate.

Subpart I   Nutrients

182.8013   Ascorbic acid.
182.8065   Linoleic acid.
182.8159   Biotin.
182.8191   Calcium carbonate.
182.8195   Calcium citrate.
182.8201   Calcium glycerophosphate.
182.8210   Calcium oxide.
182.8212   Calcium pantothenate.
182.8217   Calcium phosphate.
182.8223   Calcium pyrophosphate.
182.8245   Carotene.
182.8250   Choline bitartrate.
182.8252   Choline chloride.
182.8260   Copper gluconate.
182.8265   Cuprous iodide.
182.8301   Ferric phosphate.
182.8304   Ferric pyrophosphate.
182.8306   Ferric sodium pyrophosphate.
182.8308   Ferrous gluconate.
182.8311   Ferrous lactate.
182.8315   Ferrous sulfate.
182.8370   Inositol.
182.8375   Iron reduced.
182.8431   Magnesium oxide.
182.8434   Magnesium phosphate.
182.8443   Magnesium sulfate.
182.8446   Manganese chloride.
182.8449   Manganese citrate.

TABLE 25.2 GRAS List Substances [21 CFR 182] *(Continued)*

PART 182   Substances generally recognized as safe

182.8452 Manganese gluconate.	182.8628 Potassium	182.8930 Vitamin A.
182.8455 Manganese	glycerophosphate.	182.8933 Vitamin A acetate.
glycerophosphate.	182.8676 Pyridoxine hydrochloride.	182.8936 Vitamin A palmitate.
182.8458 Manganese	182.8695 Riboflavin.	182.8945 Vitamin B_{12}
hypophosphite.	182.8697 Riboflavin-5-phosphate.	182.8950 Vitamin D_2
182.8461 Manganese sulfate.	182.8772 Sodium pantothenate.	182.8953 Vitamin D_3
182.8464 Manganous oxide.	182.8778 Sodium phosphate.	182.8985 Zinc chloride.
182.8530 Niacin.	182.8875 Thiamine hydrochloride.	182.8988 Zinc gluconate.
182.8535 Niacinamide.	182.8878 Thiamine mononitrate.	182.8991 Zinc oxide.
182.8580 D-Pantothenyl alcohol.	182.8890 Tocopherols.	182.8994 Zinc stearate.
182.8622 Potassium chloride.	182.8892 *a*-Tocopherol acetate.	182.8997 Zinc sulfate.

A, 30% of the vitamin B_6, 20% of the thiamin, and significant quantities of essential trace minerals in a normal diet. Some tests indicate that there is a possible 20–30% reduction of vitamin C in the new variety of tomato compared to regular tomatoes. It is not known whether this breeding has caused any toxic chemicals to form. In 1975 a new potato variety bred for better chipping quality was banned from use because it did have a higher content of a dangerous natural alkaloid.

Another class of chemicals or ingredients on the GRAS list being examined is the category including substances that are of biological origin but are not used for nutritive purposes. Coffee, tea, spices, and MSG (monosodium glutamate) are items in this category. Coffee, under certain testing procedures, has been shown to cause chromosome damage (undesirable genetic changes) in rats. It will probably not be revoked from the GRAS list due to its widespread use and its acceptance for hundreds of years. MSG is the sodium salt of an amino acid. It has been shown to damage the brain when injected into the brains of infant mice. But the FDA determined that this was an inappropriate test procedure to determine toxicity of a chemical that is consumed as part of the diet.

The other categories under scientific review for toxicity are distillates, extracts and isolates of GRAS substances, reaction products of GRAS substances, and synthetic (i.e., of non-biological origin) GRAS substances. Once reviewed, these substances can be either banned, put on an interim use list until a food additive petition is submitted, or affirmed as GRAS either as an affirmed direct GRAS substance (see Table 25.3) or as an affirmed, indirect GRAS substance (see Table 25.4).

TABLE 25.3 Affirmed direct GRAS substances [21 CFR Part 184]

Subpart A General Provisions

184.1 Substances added directly to human food affirmed as generally recognized as safe (GRAS).

Subpart B Listing of Specific Substances Affirmed as GRAS

184.1007 Aconitic acid.
184.1021 Benzoic acid.
184.1025 Caprylic acid.
184.1069 Malic acid.
184.1091 Succinic acid.
184.1095 Sulfuric acid.
184.1115 Agar-agar.
184.1143 Ammonium sulfate.
184.1206 Calcium iodate.

184.1230 Calcium sulfate.
184.1257 Clove and its derivatives.
184.1259 Cocoa butter substitute from palm oil.
184.1271 L-Cysteine.
184.1272 L-Cysteine monohydrochloride.
184.1282 Dill and its derivatives.
184.1293 Ethyl alcohol.
184.1295 Ethyl formate.
184.1317 Garlic and its derivatives.
184.1330 Acacia (gum arabic).
184.1333 Gum ghatti.
184.1339 Guar gum.
184.1343 Locust (carob) bean gum.
184.1349 Karaya gum (sterculia gum).

184.1351 Gum tragacanth.
184.1490 Methylparaben.
184.1555 Rapeseed oil.
184.1634 Potassium iodide.
184.1635 Potassium iodate.
184.1643 Potassium sulfate.
184.1660 Propyl gallate.
184.1670 Propylparaben.
184.1698 Rue.
184.1699 Oil of rue.
184.1733 Sodium benzoate.
184.1807 Sodium thiosulfate.
184.1835 Sorbitol.
184.1973 Beeswax (yellow and white).
184.1983 Bakers yeast extract.
184.4560 Ox bile extract.

TABLE 25.4 Affirmed indirect GRAS substances

Subpart A General Provisions

186.1 Substances in food-contact surfaces affirmed as generally recognized as safe (GRAS).

Subpart B Listing of Specific Substances Affirmed as GRAS

186.1025 Caprylic acid.

186.1275 Dextrans.
186.1316 Formic acid.
186.1330 Acacia (gum arabic).
186.1339 Guar gum (technical grade).
186.1343 Locust (carob) bean gum.
186.1551 Hydrogenated fish oil.
186.1673 Pulp.

186.1750 Sodium chlorite.
186.1756 Sodium formate.
186.1797 Sodium sulfate.
186.1807 Sodium thiosulfate.
186.1839 Sorbose.

Food Colors

The last area of chemical additives that can be used in food are the food color additives. According to the Federal Food Drug and Cosmetic Act, Sec 201(t)(1), a color additive is any dye, pigment, or other substance made by a process of synthesis or similar method, or extracted, isolated, or derived from a vegetable, animal, or other source and when applied to a food imparts color unless it is used for reasons other than coloring foods. Sec 706 of the act covers color additives specifically and has a Delaney-type clause (Sec 706(b)(5)(B)). Anything added to color foods is a color additive, must have prior approval, and must have the term ''artificial color'' in the labeling. If it is a synthesized chemical it must also be certified. The regulations on color additives are covered in 21 CFR Part 70 to 82. In Part 70.3(f)(2), the regulations state that food ingredients are not normally color additives but if used deliberately to color foods (such as beet juice to make a food red) the regulations apply. Safety evaluation follows the same procedures as for a food additive. Table

TABLE 25.5 Color additives exempt from certification [21 CFR 73]

73.1 Diluents in color additive mixtures for food use exempt from certification.	73.100 Cochineal extract; carmine.	73.295 Tagetes (Aztec marigold) meal and extract.
73.30 Annatto extract.	73.140 Toasted partially defatted cooked cottonseed flour.	73.300 Carrot oil.
73.40 Dehydrated beets (beet powder).		73.315 Corn endosperm oil.
	73.160 Ferrous gluconate.	73.340 Paprika.
73.50 Ultramarine blue.	73.170 Grape skin extract (enocianina).	73.345 Paprika oleoresin.
73.75 Canthaxanthin.		73.450 Riboflavin.
73.85 Caramel.	73.200 Synthetic iron oxide.	73.500 Saffron.
73.90 β-Apo-8'-carotenal.	73.250 Fruit juice.	73.575 Titanium dioxide.
73.95 β-Carotene.	73.260 Vegetable juice.	73.600 Turmeric.
	73.275 Dried algae meal.	73.615 Turmeric oleoresin.

25.5 lists those natural substances that are color additives but that do not require certification while Table 25.6 lists those color additives that require certification and have an FD & C status. Some are provisionally listed and are under study for their safety.

INTRODUCING A CHEMICAL INTO THE FOOD SUPPLY

To insure that a food or color additive or pesticide is safe and can be introduced into the food supply, four to five years of research may be necessary at a possible cost of between $0.5 million and $10 million dollars. This places a heavy but necessary financial burden on a company. Because of this cost and time, the likelihood that very many new direct food additives will be introduced into the food supply in the future is small. In fact, between 1978 and 1981, only two major direct additives were introduced—aspartame, a new artificial sweetener, and polydextrose, a partially digestible starch.

The first step in the search for an additive is to identify a need to improve the quality, shelf life, or some other factor in a current food product. The primary prerequisite for seeking chemicals to solve the problem is the lack of processing or packaging techniques capable of doing the job. The solution may be sought in several ways. Chemicals already used by the food industry might be one alternative and a search can be made for an already approved additive that would be effective. If it is useful but has not been

TABLE 25.6 FD&C color additives allowed for in food

FD&C color	FD&C color
Yellow # 5 *	Green # 3
Yellow # 6 *	Blue # 1
Red # 3 *	Orange B
Blue # 2	Red # 2
	Red # 40

* Provisionally listed as of 1984.

approved for the specific purpose for which it will be used, a food additive or GRAS petition must be sent to the FDA. These petitions will be discussed later. An example was the petitioning of the FDA in 1974 to allow the use of ethanol (alcohol) to inhibit microbial growth in unrefrigerated pizza crust. Ethanol had previously been approved for use as a carrier of food flavors and was subsequently approved for this new use. A chemical that is available but has not been used in the food industry is another choice. This is more difficult because the biological safety of the chemical may not have been studied by the appropriate tests. A chemical that fits this category is butane-diol. It has been used as a solvent and plasticizer and has potential for use as a food humectant to lower water activity but it has not been approved as a direct additive, although it is effective. A third resource could be the chemistry department of some company. Researchers might be able to synthesize a new substance based on the chemical properties needed to solve the problem. This was done with the new antioxidant TBHQ and with aspartame, a dipeptide approved as a synthetic sweetener in 1981. Again, toxicity would have to be determined. While looking for the right substance it is necessary to convince the management of the company that it is economically feasible to go ahead with the toxicity testing. If the improved market position of the company is not going to bring much more profit, it may not be worth the high cost of testing and the long time necessary to prove safety so that government approval of the additive can be obtained.

ADDITIVE TESTING PROCEDURES

Efficacy Tests

Testing a new chemical is a lengthy process. The first step in the testing is to prove the efficacy of the chemical, that is, to prove that it is suitable for the job intended, such as increasing shelf life of a food or keeping the color during storage. Levels of expected consumption based on the proposed use of the additive in a normal diet would have to be determined. These levels are calculated from the effectiveness level of the additive needed to improve the food and an estimation of the average amount of food containing the additive that an average person would probably consume over the year. Probable consumption of the additive is calculated on the basis of amount consumed per unit of body weight per day (mg./kg./day) so that appropriate animal studies can be designed. A method of analysis for determining the presence of the chemical in foods must also be developed. This analytical procedure must be very specific for the chemical. These specifications are required whether it is a color additive, food additive, GRAS substance, or pesticide.

Toxicity Tests

The most difficult step is to test the chemical for safety. If the chemical is already used in foods, this may not be necessary. Biological testing could require from five years to ten years of research to prove safety. Three specific kinds of toxicity tests are generally used based on NAS/NRC guidelines: acute, subacute, and chronic toxicity testing. Before these begin, the research is usually centered around a few animals. The chemical may be radioactively labeled and fed to them. In this way the scientists can observe the metabolic rate of the chemical and pinpoint the organs in which an adverse effect may possibly occur. One problem is that it may be hard to feed the animal if the chemical makes the diet taste bad. One problem is that a weaning rat gains only five to six grams per day, which is close to 10% of the body weight. If the diet is not balanced nutritionally or consumption level of the diet is low because of a high amount of additive in the food, deficiency diseases could show up and complicate the analysis of toxicity. In comparison, a four- to five-year-old child also gains five grams per day, but because the child weighs about 20 kg., this is less than 0.0025% change in body weight per day. However, we cannot ethically or legally test chemicals in humans.

Acute Toxicity. The acute toxicity test uses two or three species of animals, usually rats and dogs. About 30 to 40 animals of each species are given single doses of the chemical by injection into the bloodstream, by stomach intubation, or by feeding at a single meal. Usually four to five dosages are tested and from the results of statistical calculations the dose level that would potentially kill 50% of the animals within one week after injection or feeding is predicted. This predicted dose is called the LD_{50} (lethal dose for 50% of the animals). The LD_{50} is computed in terms of milligrams of the chemical per kilogram of animal body weight and the value for the most sensitive animal (lowest LD_{50}) is compared with the effectiveness level needed in the food product. If the LD_{50} level was less than the effectiveness level of the chemical, the chemical could not be used in the food supply. For example, if the LD_{50} for compound A (a new antioxidant) in rats is 0.2 mg./kg. and the amount needed in the food would result in a human consumption of 0.3 mg./kg. body weight per day, the proposed antioxidant could not be used. The decision is based on the most sensitive of the animal species tested, and several species are used.

Subacute Tests. The next step is to test at subacute toxicity levels. Animals of two or more species are fed daily for 90 days at levels of the chemical lower than the LD_{50}. There are usually four test groups of animals. One group is fed the chemical in their diet at a level that is somewhat under the LD_{50}. Another group is fed at 10 times the proposed use level in the food. A third group is fed at a level somewhere in between these two extremes and finally there is a control group of animals who get the diet with no chemical added. Rats, guinea pigs, mice, and dogs are the typical animals used; 10 males and 10 females of each animal type are used in each test level. The major evaluation in this study is the observation of the state of health of the animals. Besides monitoring food consumption, the animals are given weekly physical examinations, including weight measurements and chemical analyses of blood and urine. At the end of the study the animals are sacrificed. An autopsy is performed on each animal to determine if changes in any of the tissues and organs have occurred. Tissue slices are taken from over 50 different sites to determine if any adverse effect has occurred. All the tests are aimed at finding the lowest level of the chemical that causes an adverse biochemical or physiological change. Since all chemicals cause some change it is difficult to decide what is an adverse effect. The tests may then be repeated at lower doses until no effect occurs.

The no effect dose (NED)—sometimes also called the maximum tolerated dose (MTD), or the no observed effect level (NOEL)—is that dose that causes no adverse effect to the animal. It is calculated in terms of milligrams per kilogram of body weight. This is the level below the just detectable adverse physiological effect level. This number is then divided by 100 according to 21 CFR 170.82 to set the maximum acceptable level allowed for human consumption. This level is called the ADI or Acceptable Daily Intake for humans and is set in terms of milligrams per kilogram body weight. The most sensitive animal species, that is, the one that gives the lowest MTD in mg./kg. body weight, is used in this regulation setting procedure. The FDA does not, however, set the allowed level at the ADI; it is generally set at the effectiveness level, which should be substantially below the ADI. At the present time there is controversy over the method of determining the safety of a chemical for use in the human diet by using animals. The 100 times safety factor has not been proven to be totally accurate in all cases. One critical area of research in toxicology is establishing a better method of determining a safety factor. In some cases, it may be either larger or smaller than 100. The needed effectiveness level in foods of a chemical additive should be below the ADI, as was true of the LD_{50}. The problem with this type of study is that some changes may go undetected. In addition, effects such as headache or upset stomach could be difficult to determine in an animal. However, past experience indicates that it has been a useful procedure. During the early 1980s a group of industry and academic people formed a Food Safety

Council that developed a set of criteria to try to alleviate these problems but their guidelines have not been accepted by the FDA.

Chronic Toxicity Test. Another major test is the chronic toxicity test procedure that can require up to three years of feeding studies to determine long-term harmful effects. Two or three species of animals (for example, mice, rats, and dogs) are used, usually with a minimum of 25 each of females and males of each species for both the test groups and the control group. The study is carried out long enough so that the effect can be studied over the lifespan of some of the test group animals. The chemical is administered daily in the diet. Physical and clinical examinations of the animals are made at least every three to six months with some animals sacrificed for tissue histopathology. The test levels used are at 10 and 50 times the safety level for humans (ADI) in milligrams per kilogram of body weight but may include higher and lower levels as well. High levels are needed because of the small numbers of animals used.

Examining the health of the animal during the test as well as examining the tissue slices from over 50 sites after sacrificing or death is of great importance. The tissue examinations are geared to look for tumors to comply with the Delaney Clause. Interpretation of the results, however, has led to great controversy. If the studies indicate a higher incidence of cancer in test diets, the additive may not be allowed. But some tests have shown that the controls also have high levels of tumors and that some common foods such as sucrose can produce tumors. It is also difficult to determine the health hazard to humans when the controls have the same number, slightly higher, or slightly lower numbers of tumors than the test group of animals. An even greater problem exists with the low number of animals used because of the statistical interpretation of tests in which "no effect" occurs. For example, if there were no tumors in a group of 100 test rats as well as none in 100 controls, all this means is that at the 95% confidence level, the tumor incident is less than 0.4%; this translates into a potential cancer risk of one million people in the U.S. population if the chemical were allowed. Trying to carry out experiments with a larger number of animals is virtually impossible because of the technical problems involved. Using the currently accepted chronic toxicity test design, over 28,000 tissue slides must be examined by a histopathologist at the end of the study. Most tests are carried out using ridiculously high doses, so that tumors can be induced and some significance can be calculated. Another problem relates to the dose response. If several dosage levels are tested and there is a smaller incidence of cancer as the dose level decreases, can one extrapolate to the theoretical cancer response at the proposed use level of the chemical? Some people suggest a linear relation exists; if even one molecule can cause cancer, any level of use should be banned on the basis of the Delaney Clause. Others accept this theory but suggest we should accept some level of risk (e.g., one cancer in one million people's lifetimes) if there is a proven benefit for the additive. A second theory is that the response decreases exponentially as the dose decreases so that the calculated risk is much less than a linear response indicates. Lastly, some toxicologists suggest that there is a dose cutoff, a level below which the body can handle the chemical with no toxicological effect. The FDA as well as other groups such as the National Toxicology program are testing these theories. It might be possible that everyone is correct in thinking that different chemicals show different responses. The U.S. Department of Health and Human Services is studying this question at the National Center for Toxicological Research (NCTR) in Pine Bluffs, Arkansas. Another problem is that there is the possibility that the present tests will show that almost every chemical can provoke or promote the generation of tumors. Salt, when injected under the skin, has been shown to produce tumors. Sugar when fed to rats increases tumor rates, probably because of increased weight gain.

There are two types of chemical carcinogens, primary type and promoters. Only if the tumor metastasizes (releases cells that cause tumors in other parts of the body) is the chemical causing the tumor considered to be a primary carcinogen since such tumors are malignant. A promoter, on the other hand, does not cause cancer directly but speeds the process if the cancer has already started to form or aids a weak carcinogen in the initiation of cancer. Many oncologists (those who study cancer) believe that even a benign tumor is an unacceptable risk. We need a rapid biological detection test to check chemicals for carcinogenicity that would apply to humans and that would have a high degree of significance. We also need to sift out those chemicals that actually provoke tumor generation from those that only enhance the process when there is a carcinogen in the diet. Some toxicologists believe that the present process is so strict that 50% of the time a compound will be deemed a carcinogen when in fact it is not. This is called a Type I error. This strictness, however, eliminates the other type of error (Type II) in which a tested compound is found to be safe, that is, there are no more tumors than the control, when in fact, the compound is a carcinogen.

Other Tests
Besides testing for cancer, the FDA is also interested in whether the chemicals cause birth defects or mutations. Specific tests are employed to evaluate the safety of a chemical in these areas.

Fertility Test. Fertility testing is carried out in a three-generation mouse study (Figure 25.1). The test is designed as follows: G denotes the generation, with the subscript number indicating which generation: original, first, second, third. The letter A designates the first litter, the letter B the second. The pregnant animals as well as their offspring are fed the chemical daily in the diet. The first litter of each generation, as well as the last litter, is examined, sacrificed, and given complete tissue examinations. The major observations are whether there is a change in litter size, whether there is an effect on the organs of the animals in the litter, and, most important, whether any major birth defect occurs. A chemical that causes a birth defect is called a teratogen. If the chemical adversely affects the host mother, some compromising of the reproductive cycle occurs.

Teratogen Tests. Specific teratogenic tests are usually carried out by giving very high doses of the chemical during the pregnancy of an animal. The pregnant female is usually sacrificed before birth, and the fetuses are examined. Thalidomide, the over-the-counter relaxant drug used in Europe, was a teratogen. It had never been approved for use in the United States because the FDA was not completely satisfied with the animal test results. It is interesting to note that thalidomide caused no birth defects in rats at four grams per kilogram body weight per day, whereas in a pregnant human a single dose of 0.5 milligrams per kilogram body weight at a particular time in gestation produced the horrible birth defect that caused webbed arms and brain damage. This is almost 1/10,000 of the level

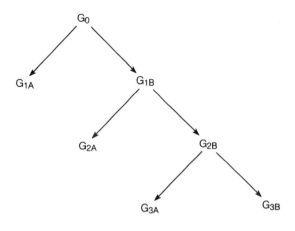

FIGURE 25.1 Fertility test procedure

tested in the animal. Because of this problem, the FDA always insists that several animal species be studied. If three species are used the probability that we can detect a potential teratogen is very high.

Another test for birth defects is the chick embryo assay. A dose of the chemical is injected into the yolk sac of a fertile egg. Afterwards either the hatched chicken or the chick fetus is examined for birth defects. It is interesting to note that aspirin and vitamin A both produce deformities using this test. This shows the problem of extrapolating and interpreting the results with respect to humans. However, this is a very valuable screening procedure.

Mutagenic Tests. Mutagenic chemicals are those that can cause anything from a very minor mutation that may be hard to detect to those that cause cancer or birth defects. If minor, the mutagenic and carcinogenic effects may take as long as 20 to 30 years to become evident in humans. From an evolutionary aspect, animals that mutated were the ones that survived because they were able to adopt to the new environment. One theory is that chemicals may not be harmful because from the adaptive standpoint humans may become resistant to detrimental environments. However, the risks involved prevent us from testing this theory. Many generations or a very large population of animals are necessary to test for a minor mutagenic effect in order for the results to be stastically significant. A teratogenic chemical causes a very obvious mutation since we can readily observe the birth defects when tested in a few animals.

Microorganisms, such as certain bacteria, are most commonly used for testing mutagenic effects. This is because, for several bacteria, the metabolic pathways and genetic makeup of the nuclear material are completely understood and mapped. Since microbes grow rapidly and produce many generations, the mutagenic effect can be observed more easily. The chemical in question is introduced into the growth medium of the organism. The changes, if any, in metabolism and genetic material of the cell are examined. The validity of comparing such tests to humans is questionable because in the human, chemicals are ingested and absorbed through the small intestine, usually passing through the liver first. The liver has many mechanisms for detoxifying chemicals to render them harmless to the body. The metabolites are transported in the bloodstream and eventually excreted in the urine. Bacteria do not have this function. A widely employed procedure developed by Dr. Bruce Ames of Stanford University overcomes this problem to some degree; mammalian liver microsomes are added to the growing medium. These microsomes are similar to the cell systems in the human liver that act upon and convert the toxic chemicals into the form they are carried around in the body. This procedure seems to be a good screening assay for potential carcinogens. About 85% of those compounds that show mutagenic activity in bacteria are carcinogenic in animal studies.

Human tissue cultures can also be used for studying mutagenic effects. Human placental cells grown in special test bottles are observed for mutagenic effects with the introduction of the chemical being used. The effects of detoxification by the liver are not accounted for in these tests as with the microbes.

A more complicated mutagenic test developed during the early 1970s called the *Host Mediated Assay* (HMA) eliminates some of the problems caused by the absence of possible changes in the liver. In this test, bacteria cultures are injected into the cavity between the lungs and the skin of a dog. The bacteria are exposed to the blood and lymph system of the dog and can grow without harming the dog. The chemical being tested is fed to the animal in a large dose. In this manner, the bacteria are exposed to the chemical via the normal digestive functions and liver action of the dog. After ingestion of the chemical, some of the bacteria are removed at several intervals over a certain time period. The bacteria are then grown in cultures to determine if mutations have occurred.

The *Dominant Lethal Test* is a test in which male rats have the chemical in question fed to them or injected into them. Female rats are then bred with these males. Halfway through the pregnancy, the female is sacrificed and the fetuses are examined for genetic changes. Large changes may be the only ones that are evident. However, it is possible to see if any fetuses have died and have been reabsorbed by the mother's system, since a scar will occur on the wall of the uterus. It is presumed that if this reabsorption occurred, a minor mutation took place that caused the fetus to be rejected by the mother.

In the 1970s there was pressure to introduce into law an addition to the Delaney Clause creating a zero tolerance of any chemicals that were shown to be mutagenic or teratogenic. This may have been a good idea, but none of the test procedures discussed here can be reliably applied to humans, and the concept of a zero tolerance is questionable. In the 1980s the issue of whether the Delaney Clause should be retained is still being debated because of the difficulty in assessing the human risk.

APPROVAL OF A CHEMICAL FOR USE IN FOOD

After a proposed new chemical has been put through all the toxicity tests and is found to be safe and effective, the food company may now petition the FDA for a regulation allowing its use. The FDA in turn publishes the information about the new additive in the Federal

Register if it feels that the tests were done adequately enough to insure safety. Over 80% of the petitions submitted to the FDA are initially rejected on the basis of a different interpretation or insufficient data. Once the information is published in the Federal Register, any person in the country can write to the FDA to express an opinion about the published additive. Public response within a 90-day period may delay the allowance of the chemical into the market because further testing is required. Many private consumer health organizations have taken it upon themselves to look for such publications in the Federal Register and to request a public hearing on the evidence since the average citizen usually does not do so. The Center for Science in The Public Interest is one such interest group that follows the Federal Register and requests hearings. Most food company petitions get rejected the first time because the data is usually not adequate to insure safety, thus very few direct food additives have been approved each year.

Some of the issues relating to toxicology that are still not adequately understood are: (1) the human versus animal correlation, i.e., can we use animal data to extrapolate to humans? (2) the fact that some people may be biologically different and may respond more adversely to certain chemicals; (3) the variability of the human diet, that is, some people may ingest more than the ADI; (4) infants and the elderly may be more sensitive to a particular chemical; (5) additives are tested with healthy animals but people with disease may respond differently; (6) the chemical might react with other components in the human diet not present in an animal test diet and form a new chemical that may be more hazardous; (7) the microbial flora in the intestines of a human and a rat are different. These microbes could possibly change the chemical into a more or less toxic form.

The Commissioner of the Food and Drug Administration must weigh all these factors, as well as the toxicological evidence, before giving approval or disapproval. This is where the risk versus benefit decision is finally made. It appears that the right decisions have been made in the past because public health problems related to approved additives have been rare. It must be remembered that the consumer can make the choice not to eat a particular product containing a particular additive. This is an additional personal risk versus benefit decision. However, this decision may be based on illogical evidence or hearsay and not on true facts.

The test procedures, time periods, costs, and legal processes greatly restrict the addition of new additives to the market. If all goes well, the additive can be used. It is hoped that the new and better test procedures will help evaluate the safety of all presently used food additives. In some cases, the regulation for an approved chemical has been revoked because of new evidence and the additive has been removed from the food supply. The next chapter discusses some problem additives and foods that contain naturally occurring toxic substances.

SUMMARY

The safety regulation of chemicals used in the food supply is spelled out in the Food, Drug, and Cosmetic Act, which bans any added, environmental, or natural substance if it is injurious to health. Since Congress recognized that all things can be injurious at some level, sections of the law to approve food additives, food colors, and pesticides were added. In addition, action levels for banned substances present in the food were set. A food additive is anything intentionally added to a food to improve quality, nutrient value, texture, or shelf life. Regulated additives are those chemicals for which a specific tolerance has been set, based on toxicological studies. The use of the additive is based on the benefit of use as compared to the risk to the human population. One risk for which there is a zero tolerance is cancer, as specified by the Delaney Clause. The GRAS list contains those chemicals and food ingredients for which the toxicological risk is very low under normal use.

The basic steps in testing the safety of a chemical proposed for use in the food supply are: (1) determination of the LD_{50} in an acute toxicity test and (2) determination of the maximum tolerated dose (MTD) in a 90-day subacute feeding trial. Based on this latter value divided by 100, the acceptable daily intake (ADI) for humans is established. Further long-term chronic toxicity tests are used to determine whether the chemical causes cancer. Other tests are used to examine effects on reproduction, teratogenicity, and mutagenicity. Only after all this is done can the risk versus benefit be determined for an additive. The benefit would be based on the efficacy of the additive in doing the job it is intended for and its worth to the public. Once this is established, the FDA may approve the use of the chemical as a regulated food additive if the risk from a toxicological standpoint is minor or nonexistent.

Multiple Choice Study Questions

1. The Delaney clause refers to

    A. mutagenic chemicals

    B. teratogenic chemicals

    C. efficacy testing of chemicals

    D. cancer-causing chemicals

    E. the level below the LD_{50} where a chemical is acceptable

2. The risk/benefit concept

    A. is used by the BMR

    B. has been used by the FDA to enforce the Food, Drug, and Cosmetic Act

    C. applies only to food systems

    D. allows the government to set a risk of one case in one million people for cancer

    E. none of the above

3. Efficacy testing of a chemical

    A. establishes the toxic dose

    B. establishes the minimum amount necessary to perform some function in a food

    C. establishes the MTD divided by 100

    D. determines if the chick embryo gets birth defects

    E. relates the additive to the HMA test

4. Efficacy testing of a chemical does not require

    A. the establishment of a method of analysis

    B. the determination of the use level

    C. the determination of a projected consumption level

    D. the establishment of the MTD

    E. any of the above

5. Acute toxicity testing

    A. lasts 7 days

    B. lasts 90 days

    C. determines the cancer threshold

    D. determines the LD_{50}

    E. determines the MTD

6. The LD_{50} is

    A. the dose rate in mg./kg. that kills 50% of a test population

    B. the dose rate in mg. that kills 50% of a test population

    C. the dose rate in mg./kg. that is divided by 50 to get the maximum dose allowed for a food additive

    D. the dose rate in mg./kg. that is divided by 100 to get the maximum dose allowed for a food additive

    E. None of the above

7. Which of the following compounds is the most lethal or toxic?

    A. lead arsenate — $LD_{50} = 100$ mg./kg.

    B. caffeine — $LD_{50} = 200$ mg./kg.

    C. endrin — $LD_{50} = 3$ mg./kg.

    D. warfarin — $LD_{50} = 325$ mg./kg.

8. Subacute toxicity testing

    A. lasts 10 days

    B. lasts up to 3 years

    C. determines the cancer threshold

    D. determines the LD_{50}

    E. determines the MTD

9. Chronic testing is usually done at

    A. 5 $\times$ the MTD

    B. 10 $\times$ the MTD

    C. 5 $\times$ the ADI

    D. 5 and 10 $\times$ the ADI

    E. 10 and 50 $\times$ the ADI

10. Chronic toxicity tests are done

    A. with chronically diseased animals to determine the adverse effect of additives on recovery

    B. for 90 days to get the NED

    C. to satisfy the 1938 food laws

    D. to determine the level that causes cancer

    E. to satisfy the Delaney Clause

11. Which test is not a mutagenic or teratogenic test?

    A. Ames microbe study

    B. dominant lethal test

    C. chick embryo test

    D. acute toxicity test

    E. host mediated assay

12. The Delaney Clause prohibits the use of the suspected chemical

    A. above the level tested in chronic tests

    B. at a level that is above $\frac{1}{100}$ of the minimum physiological response in animals

    C. above the LD_{50}

    D. at any level above zero

    E. if used above the ADI

13. Which of the following would not be considered under the 1958 regulated food additives amendment?

    A. nitrite

    B. water

    C. BHA

    D. sorbic acid

    E. Tween 80

*Essay Study
Questions*

1. What is the difference between a regulated additive and a GRAS list chemical?

2. When is a pesticide a food additive?

3. What is a prior sanctioned ingredient?

4. How are naturally occurring toxins in food handled by the law?

5. What are the various GRAS list categories for food ingredients and chemicals?

6. What does the Delaney Clause specify? Why is it controversial?

7. What is required in efficacy testing of a chemical?

8. What does acute testing establish?

9. How is the ADI (acceptable daily intake) for a chemical established for humans?

10. Describe the steps in chronic toxicity testing.

11. How are reproductive, teratogenic, and mutagenic tests done for chemicals? What do they prove?

12. What are the problems in relating animal toxicity tests to effects on humans?

13. How does an additive get final approval for use in the food supply?

14. Discuss the problems of determining risk/benefit in a legal situation.

15. What are the GLPs?

*Things
to Do*

1. Obtain food ingredient lists. Classify the ingredients according to their specific regulatory status.

2. Interview people about their knowledge of the Delaney Clause.

3. Visit a health food store and look for foods that purport to contain no preservatives but actually have additives.

4. Obtain a copy of *Cancer Rates and Risks* (National Cancer Institute, Bethesda, Maryland, $3.00). Read and discuss the cancer problem.

5. Visit a toxicology testing lab to find out how they handle GLPs.

Chapter 25. Answers to Multiple-Choice Study Questions: 1, D; **2,** B; **3,** B; **4,** D; **5,** D; **6,** A; **7,** C; **8,** E; **9,** E; **10,** E; **11,** D; **12,** D; **13,** B.

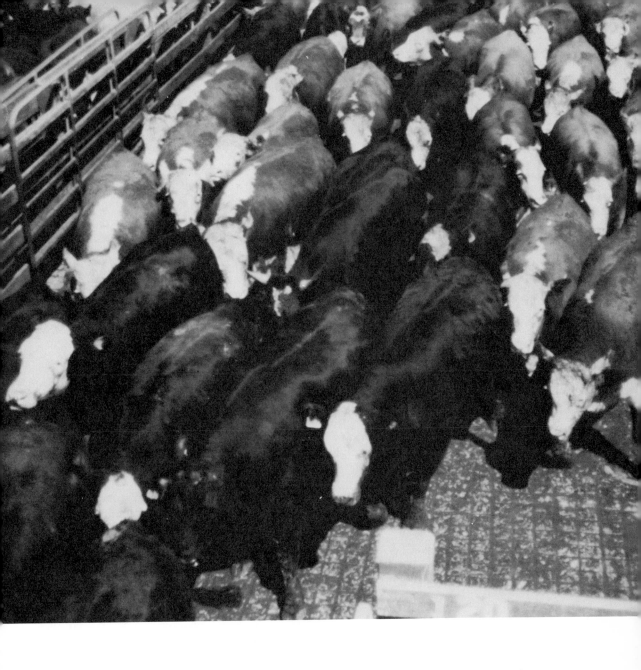

THE FOOD ADDITIVE CONTROVERSY: IS IT OR WAS IT SAFE?

26

Some foods, both natural and processed, as well as food and color additives themselves have been a subject of concern in our daily diet. The concern has been based on scientific evidence, congressional action, as well as public hysteria. We will examine some of these stories in this chapter. But we should first present some principles of toxicology.

1. The toxicity of a substance is related to the dose. At some level toxic factors are undetected or may disappear; it is called a "no effect" dose because the body can handle the chemical, detoxify it, and excrete it. Whether this principle is true for carcinogens is not known at the present time.

2. The toxicities of most substances are not additive, that is, if two food additives are consumed below their individual toxic levels but the sum of the amounts of both exceeds the maximum tolerated dose for either, toxicity generally does not occur. This is because they usually affect different parts of the body or have different metabolic processes. Some toxic agents, in fact, cancel each other out (selenium and mercury, for example). However, a common synergistic type of toxicity is the use of alcohol and certain drugs, such as sleeping pills or tranquilizers. Which chemicals in the food supply are synergistic is not known.

The basic toxicities that do occur can be separated into three areas:

1. The consumption of a toxic chemical, for example, eating seed grain treated with a mercury fungistat to prevent molding during storage or eating the deadly amanita mushroom species.

2. The overconsumption of a chemical by a consumer, for example, eating five to eight pounds of swordfish a day causing some mercury poisoning or overconsuming salt when one has a predisposition to hypertension.

3. The consumption of foods by persons sensitive to a component of that food, for example, a person with lactose intolerance drinking milk or someone with celiac disease eating bread.

In this chapter we will consider both food additives and foods themselves from the standpoint of safety.

CONTROVERSIAL FOOD ADDITIVES

DES

DES (diethystilbesterol) was a synthetic growth hormone (estrogen) that had been originally approved in 1954 for use in the feeds (or as ear implants) of beef cattle for purposes of increasing the feed efficiency of the animal. The animal with DES in the diet can convert a higher percentage of its feed into body protein. DES reduces the cost of feeding cattle and they gain weight more quickly.

In 1962 Congress amended the Food, Drug, and Cosmetic Act to allow the use for animals of feed additives that were carcinogens if the chemical did not adversely affect the animals under the proposed conditions of use and if no residue was found in any edible portion of such animal after slaughter. Thus an exemption to the Delaney Clause was made for animal feed additives and especially for DES since some new animal studies showed that it might be a carcinogen.

In 1971 new evidence showed that there was an unusual number of young women between the ages of 18 and 20 who had developed cervical cancer. It came to light that mothers of these girls had had problems maintaining pregnancy and were therefore given large doses of DES as a fertility drug (approved for testing as such by the FDA) to prevent miscarriage (125 mg. per day). These doses were taken in the 1950s and the cancer showed up in the female children of these women 20 years later, about the length of time that might be expected for chronic cancer development in humans. The doses that were given were extremely high and were presumably not adequately tested for that purpose, but at that time the proposed benefit appeared to outweigh the risk. Subsequent tests showed that DES was not very effective for the prevention of miscarriage, as had originally been thought, and the test application for this use was terminated.

In 1971 the FDA became concerned because DES began showing up at very low levels (2–10 ppb) in samples of beef liver. Cattlemen were made aware of the problem and were instructed to take beef cattle off DES at least seven days before slaughter so it would be metabolized and disappear. Unfortunately, some cattlemen were not convinced that this was necessary, and additional beef liver samples indicated the presence of DES, especially when a new, more exact analytical technique began to be used instead of the one approved in the regulation allowing use of DES. In 1973 the FDA sought a ban on DES, based on the fact that illegal residues were present at the parts per billion level. The cattlemen's organizations and the USDA were upset. They said that a person would have to eat over 50 tons of beef liver per day to reach the levels of consumption that had caused cervical cancer in the daughters of the women who had taken the fertility drugs.

In the case of *Hess and Clark vs. FDA* (495 F.2d 975; 1974) the FDA decision was reversed and the use of DES continued. Cattlemen were allowed to feed or implant DES pellets in the ears of the animals as long as the animals were taken off DES 14 days prior to slaughter. This decision was based on evidence presented by the

Council for Agricultural Science and Technology and by Dr. Thomas Jukes of the University of California. The data suggested that the risk from beef liver was only one cancer per 200 million people per 134 years and thus there was some doubt expressed that the cancers of young women were really due to DES. The FDA did show that at a level of 6.5 ppb in the diet of certain strains of mice, DES did cause a carcinogenic response. Those defending the drug's use calculated that this would require the consumption of almost 19,000 lbs. of beef per day based on its being present at the just detectable level. The court's action was to override the FDA ban.

However, again some cattlemen did not follow the legalized DES feed withdrawal procedure. In 1976 the FDA took steps to revoke the approval of DES for use in animals based on the fact that the original analytical procedure was not specific enough for DES, and there were many more higher levels of illegal residues showing up. Remember that a very specific test procedure must be submitted for approval of a new food additive. Senator Ted Kennedy also introduced a bill in Congress to specifically ban all uses of DES, the first additive for which a bill like this would have been put forward. After a long hearing process in which much testimony was given, the FDA revoked the use of DES on July 6, 1979; after several postponements, the revocation took effect November 1, 1979 (44 FR 42679, 45618, 45764).

In this interim period, one cattleman did implant 273 head of cattle. When they were slaughtered on April 17, 1980, a USDA inspector noticed the ear implants. This resulted in the detention by the USDA of 2,166 boxes of boned beef weighing approximately 154,000 pounds, or close to a million dollars worth of meat. The meat was put into cold storage and a law suit followed (*USDA vs. 2,166 Boxes Boned Beef,* District Court of Kansas Action No. 80–1360, decision made May 7, 1981). Since there is no Delaney-type food additive/feed additive provision in the Meat Inspection Act, the beef was charged in that case as being adulterated because it contained DES as an added poisonous or deleterious substance. In a court of law, the government has the burden of proof to show that the suspect chemical may be injurious to health at the level found in an allegedly adulterated food. The evidence presented by both sides in the DES case makes for interesting reading. One year after the original seizure of the meat, Judge Kelly, after weighing all the arguments, concluded that at the levels of DES present (somewhere between 0.6 to 20 pp trillion) the beef was not injurious to health, an interesting risk/benefit decision. The USDA originally planned to appeal the decision but did not, and the meat was released into commerce in 1982. Where it ended up is not known. This case presents the interesting controversy between science and the law in terms of risk/risk or risk/benefit decisions. As it stands now no beef should contain DES since manufacture of the drug has ceased in this country. But in 1983, veal in the U.S. market was found to contain illegal residues of DES. The cattlemen who were raising these veal calves were getting the DES from Canada and illegally feeding it to calves. It is unfortunate that there are always some unscrupulous people. In fact, these cattlemen are suing the FDA to try to get DES approved again.

Violet No. 1

Violet No. 1 was used until the spring of 1973 for stamping the USDA inspection grades of meat onto beef carcasses. Some Japanese studies published at this time that were widely quoted in the newspapers showed that Violet No. 1 fed at 5% of the diet was carcinogenic. The FDA moved to ban it under the color additives amendment since it was on the interim approval list. The Delaney Clause was not invoked. The FDA merely stated that its safety was not proven. Thus it was removed within one day from the food supply and a different color was used instead.

Subsequent examination of the Japanese data showed that their study was poorly done. Many of the animals contracted pneumonia and were simultaneously given large doses of antibiotics. Most of the animals died. The results showing detrimental effects of Violet No. 1 were based on only a few rats that survived the pneumonia. Violet No. 1 had been used for over 22 years and yet this one obscure, poorly done research study caused its immediate banning. This is a rather interesting way in which the risk/benefit decision is made.

FD & C Red No. 2

FD & C Red No. 2 had been used in the American food supply until January 1975. It was the basic coloring agent used in lipsticks, candy, some foods, and beverages. Sales exceeded three million dollars per year. Red No. 2 was also used to color canned pet foods. This is obviously a purely cosmetic use since dogs are color blind. The red color was there to make the owners feel, at least partially, that they were feeding their dogs raw meat. One reason that Red No. 2 was used to such a great extent was that it was the most heat stable of the synthetic red colors; most natural colors are destroyed by heating.

In 1970 the Russians published a study questioning the safety of Red No. 2. The study showed early deaths and cancer in rats. It must be pointed out that they were not using FD & C Certified Red No. 2 but a more crude form (Amaranth) that contained some impurities. Their study caused much uproar in the press, which pressured the FDA and the manufacturer to do more studies. The color was also on the interim color list established in 1960, thus it was supposed to be reexamined for safety anyway. Prior studies with the color, some for as long as seven years, showed no problems. In fact, it has been stated that Red No. 2 was one of the most studied chemical additives. In any case, a major long-term rat toxicity test was carried out by the FDA at levels of up to 3% in rat diets. Unfortunately, near the end of the study in 1975 the animals from the various test groups were mixed up when the cages were being cleaned and new water bottles put in. Even with the mix-up, the FDA toxicologists felt they were able to separate enough animals to compare the high versus the low doses. They had to base their final decision on about 80 of the original 500 animals. Many non-FDA toxicologists disagreed with this decision. The FDA concluded that there was no difference in the number of tumors found at high and low dose, although feeding at a 3% level showed more of the tumors to be malignant. Based on statistics from this data, the FDA felt that there was at least a 5% chance that Red No. 2 at 3% in the diet was a chemical carcinogen. A level of 3% Red No. 2 in the diet of rats is equivalent to the total amount of coloring in 15,000 12-ounce cans of a cherry carbonated beverage being fed every day to a human. Based on the higher incidence of malignant tumors, the FDA thus delisted the color from the provisional color list as they did with Violet No. 1. If someone wants to go through the expense of long-term testing, Red No. 2 could be brought back since the Delaney Clause was not used. It should also be noted that Canada, given the same evidence, did not ban Red No. 2. In addition, it is interesting to note that if the study were done by a company, and a similar mix-up occurred, the FDA could not legally accept the results and interpretation.

Saccharin and Cyclamates

Saccharin was accidently discovered as a sweetener in 1879 by Dr. C. Fahlberg while he was working at Johns Hopkins University. It was patented for use in 1885 and began to find its way into the food supply with consumption levels of up to 5 g. per day. In 1912 Dr. Harvey Wiley, who was chief of the Bureau of Chemistry at the USDA, tried to get a ban on saccharin based on some studies showing gastrointestinal disturbances. However, then-President Teddy Roosevelt, who was using saccharin, announced at a press conference that, "Anyone who says saccharin is injurious to health is an idiot." Wiley resigned from the government to become Director of the Good Housekeeping Institute. The President then directed a panel of experts to review saccharin's safety. They concluded that levels of 1 g. per day could cause some harm but the normal ingestion of 300 mg. per day was without effect. The USDA, under the Pure Food and Drug Act, issued an order prohibiting its use in foods but after some negotiations the order was postponed. The panel issued a second report again in favor of saccharin and it was approved for use in special foods "intended for invalids."

After 1912 the use of saccharin in "special foods" began to grow, especially during World War I and II when sugar supplies were low. Feeding studies during this period generally showed no problem except for slight toxicity at a 5% level in the diet. In 1955 a NAS report concluded that saccharin was safe for human use. In 1958, therefore, with the passage of the food additives amendment, saccharin along with cyclamate was declared to be a GRAS substance. With this, its use, especially in low-calorie beverages, began to rise and the FDA asked NAS to review its safety again in 1967. The report concluded that it was safe at up to 1 g./day but recommended a maximum ADI of 5 mg./kg. body weight for general consumption. Since cyclamate became available for use in 1950 as an artificial sweetener, the use of saccharin leveled out and was thus of less concern. This was partially due to the fact that cyclamate had a less bitter aftertaste so it was used more.

In 1969, cyclamate was delisted from the GRAS list and therefore technically banned. The study that led to the banning of cyclamate was conducted by the Wisconsin Alumni Research Foundation. One problem of safety testing is that the animals may not eat the food with the levels of test substances researchers want them to be fed because of taste. In this study a cholesterol pellet containing both cyclamate and saccharin in a one to ten ratio (about the same ratio as was used then in diet beverages) was implanted into the bladders of the rats. The idea was that the chemicals would dissolve in the blood at a rate equivalent to the amount that researchers had wanted to feed the rats. This amount was equivalent to the level that someone consuming over 500 12-ounce diet beverages a day would ingest.

Preliminary evidence in 1969 showed more bladder tumors in the test animals than in the controls. Unfortunately, the evidence was released publicly before a scientific evaluation could be made. Such extreme pressure was put on the FDA that they had to do something. They decided to take the cyclamates off the GRAS list, avoiding use of the Delaney Clause. To use cyclamates again, a food additive petition would have had to be made. The FDA later stated that the reason for the ban was not really the test that was publicized, but another one in which it was shown that the bacteria in the gut of one species of rat converted cyclamate into cyclohexylamine, a carcinogen.

Later studies have not proved cyclamates to be carcinogenic. The problem with the WARF study mentioned was that the bladders of the rats were infected with parasites. Any manipulation of the bladder caused tumors to form. The control group actually had a higher than normal incidence of tumors as well.

Much money (estimated over 20 million dollars) and time has been spent on proving cyclamates to be safe since 1969. In a number of hearings the FDA repeatedly rejected the data on the basis that it did not prove the safety of cyclamates. Finally in a court case in 1980 the manufacturer asked for the FDA to rule in favor of the granting of food additive status to cyclamate. The request was rejected and the manufacturer (Abbott Laboratories) decided to stop trying to get cyclamate accepted over 10 years after it lost its GRAS status.

The diet-conscious craze that began in the 1960s and the subsequent delisting of cyclamate gave rise again to an increased intake of saccharin. An FDA-requested NAS report in 1970 concluded that saccharin was safe, based on the available data, but also said that more tests were needed.

In 1972, the FDA removed saccharin from the GRAS list, but gave it immediate interim status as a food additive, something they did not do for cyclamate. The FDA also promulgated a regulation requiring that the label of any product with saccharin state that the product should be used only by persons who must restrict their intake of ordinary sweets. This was implied to mean those who were obese and were on a weight-reduction plan as well as diabetics. The main concern was to reduce saccharin intake by children and teenagers. In another NAS report issued in 1974, and based on new toxicological evidence, there was some concern about the exposure of pregnant women to saccharin, especially because of the possible carcinogenic impurities in saccharin, one of which was orthotoluenesulphonamide (OTS).

Then came the famous Canadian rat study that was reported in 1977. Both OTS and saccharin (at 5%) were fed to rats. The OTS produced no effects but saccharin produced both benign and malignant bladder tumors in second-generation male rats. On March 9, 1977, the FDA issued a statement that saccharin did not meet the standards for food additives, implying that it was unsafe and in violation of the Delaney Clause, the first time the Delaney Clause was invoked for a direct food additive. The Canadian government banned saccharin on that date. Because of the required legal process the ban could not immediately go into effect in the U.S. On April 15 the FDA modified the ban to allow saccharin to be used as a table-top sweetener and to be sold as an over-the-counter-drug if it met the drug standards and carried a warning label. In its risk analysis, the FDA stated that moderate use (one low-cal drink a day) might lead to about 1,200 cases of bladder cancer every year.

Despite this, mail flooded into Congress from industry, physicians, and consumers to try to save saccharin. Finally, as in the feed additive controversy, Congress passed the *Saccharin Study and Labeling Act* (PL 95–203) that President Carter signed on November 23, 1977. It required that further tests be carried out to determine the safety of saccharin and included special warning labels (see Chapter 24). It also stated that this was to be done in two years. The NAS issued another report in November 1978 and concluded that saccharin was a weak animal carcinogen but that the food safety law should be modified to include risk/benefit analysis. In 1981 Congress extended the moratorium on the saccharin ban for two more years and began to seriously look at the food safety issue. The moratorium was again extended in 1983 for two more years. It is anyone's guess what will eventually happen, especially since the new artificial sweetener, aspartame, was approved for use in 1981. If the level of consumption of saccharin stays high (some children were shown to be consuming it near the ADI of one gram per day), it will most likely be banned unless some form of risk/risk or risk/benefit analysis is put into law. Presently its status as an interim use additive is covered under 21 CFR 180.37. When used for weight reduction foods it triggers full nutritional labeling. It also must not exceed 30 mg. per serving in processed foods. Since the FFDCA does not specify an interim use additive category, the status of saccharin is being challenged in the courts by some consumer groups.

Nitrite

Sodium nitrite is a salt that has been used for centuries in curing meat. Its value was probably discovered accidentally. When added to meat at around 150 to 200 parts per million, nitrite causes the natural red color to be fixed during curing to a pink color. This is what occurs in the manufacture of hams, sausage, hot dogs, salami, bologna, etc. Nitrite also helps develop the cured meat flavor.

The nitrite has two other functions as well. It extends the shelf life of meat considerably and prevents the growth of *Clostridium botulinum.* This latter effect is important since many cured meat products are vacuum packaged and the organism can grow under these conditions.

In the late 1960s it became evident from many laboratory studies that nitrite can react with certain types of amine compounds to form nitrosamines. These latter chemicals are extremely potent liver carcinogens. Rats fed five parts per million daily develop liver cancer in several months. Mink fed at two parts per million will die in three weeks.

Nitrite's use in cured meat was then questioned. Samples of cured meat such as ham, bologna, and hot dogs showed no levels of nitrosamines. Bacon fried at high temperatures, however, contained extremely low levels of nitrosamines. It was found that certain of the amino acids in bacon could react with nitrite at the high temperature of frying or under acid conditions, such as in the stomach, to form the carcinogen. Subsequent controlled studies showed that the levels in bacon depended on the degree of doneness: raw or lightly fried bacon had no nitrosamine; microwave cooked had two parts per billion; medium-fried bacon had 15 parts per billion; and well done had 18 to 20 parts per billion.

Other studies then pointed out that 60-65% of the nitrite in the intestinal tract or stomach may have been produced by the bacteria in our mouths or intestines from nitrates whereas only 20-30% came from cured meats. The nitrates participating in this reaction are found naturally in vegetables. To eliminate nitrites entirely, we might have to totally ban both cured meat and vegetable consumption. Deaths have occurred from nitrite itself due to accidental ingestion of large doses at home where it was being used to prepare cured meats. It looks like salt and some people foolishly put it in a shaker for easier use.

The FDA regulates the use of nitrites in smoked-fish products and in meat-curing mixes for home curing under 21 CFR 172.175. The USDA, which has jurisdiction over meats, regulates its use solely by controlling the level allowed in various cured-meat products. Its use in foods other than the above is illegal. In 1972, the USDA was petitioned to ban the use of sodium nitrite, based on findings of nitrosamines in bacon. The petition was denied on the basis that there was not enough evidence to determine if the product was adulterated within the meaning of the Federal Meat Inspection Act (similar to the DES issue discussed previously). The USDA position was upheld in *Shuck vs. Butz* (500 F 2d 810 1974). Because of the complexity of the issue, the USDA formed an Expert Panel on Nitrites, Nitrates, and Nitrosamines at this time to review all aspects of meat curing. In 1974 the panel recommended that use of nitrate be eliminated and that the allowed level of nitrite be reduced to 156 ppm except for bacon and dry-cured meats pending further research.

In 1975 the USDA proposed to lower the limits in many products including bacon. The Department also initiated a program for analysis of bacon in 1978 and would not allow a plant to ship their product if it exceeded a certain nitrosamine level. The regulation (May 16, 1978, in 43 FR 20992) also required the use of ascorbic acid or its derivative, sodium erythrobate. These chemicals reduce the rate of nitrosamine formation. The monitoring program was upheld in court (*AMF vs. Bergland* 459 F.Supp. 1308, 1978).

On November 3, 1972, the FDA proposed deleting all nonessential uses of nitrite and nitrate such as in certain fish products and in canned meat and poultry products. It was stated in the Federal Register notice that nitrite was prior sanctioned for use as a curing agent for meat and poultry and was recognized as such by the USDA. This prior sanction was formalized in January 1983 (48 FR 1702, 21 CFR 182.33). In 1973 the FDA had banned the mixing of nitrite with certain curing-mix spices because of potential nitrosamine formation during storage. The FDA also sponsored an MIT study on the toxicity of nitrite beginning in 1971 under Dr. Paul Newberne. The final report (May 18, 1978) of this research concluded that nitrite appears more a promoter of the cancer-forming process than an initiator, but its effect is adverse and requires reconsideration. Thus nitrite itself was being questioned as a carcinogen. This prompted the FDA jointly with the USDA to announce on August 11, 1978, that nitrite would be phased out. A heated debate broke out in Congress on the issue. This resulted in questioning whether the study followed GLPs, and the House Agriculture Committee asked for the results to be reanalyzed. The FDA contracted the UAREP (Universities Associated for Research and Education in Pathology, Inc.) to reanalyze the data, which they did. They reported that the study did not prove that nitrite was a carcinogen (see Congressional Record, September 12, 1979 H7787). This points out the problem of interpretation of animal toxicity results. In August 1980 the FDA and the USDA dropped their proposed ban. In the interim, the FDA was petitioned after a court decision (*Public Citizen vs. Forman* 471 F.Supp. 586, 1979) to declare nitrite an illegal color additive because it imparts rather than fixes color (44 FR 75659; Dec. 21, 1979). The Court ruled otherwise, and stated that nitrite was intended solely for purposes other than color. The FDA did state at that time however that no prior sanction existed in the FDA's files for use in poultry products. They also notified the USDA that they had no such prior sanction in their files. Final action on this ruling however came in January 1983 when the FDA announced that in fact a prior sanction existed. This is most likely not the end of the story.

Caffeine

On October 21, 1980, in 45 FR 69817 the FDA proposed to delete caffeine from the GRAS list and to declare that no prior sanction existed for its use as a food ingredient. They also asked for more studies on its safety and promulgated an interim food additive status for the chemical. There were several causes for these actions. One was a study at the FDA by Dr. Thomas Collins that showed adverse effects on pregnant rats at fairly low level doses. Although the FDA concluded that there was no epidemiologic evidence to prove caffeine caused human birth defects, the March of Dimes advised pregnant women to limit soft drinks and cola beverages. Several scientists pointed out that the level used in the study was equivalent to consuming 44 cups of coffee a day, or 227 colas a day for a 110-pound woman. Because a subsequent study at the University of Florida did not show the same results, the toxic effect became debatable. However some studies with children showed a stimulant effect with single low doses (10 mg./kg.). High users of coffee consume about 11–12 mg./kg./day while low users consume about 1 mg./kg./day. Total food use amounts to about 206 mg. per person per day on the average. Caffeine in coffee ranges from 50–85 mg. per cup, in tea about 5 mg. per cup, and in cola beverages about 48 mg. per 12 ounces. It is also present in many cold tablets, allergy tablets, aspirin-like products, and stay-awake pills. It is used in these over-the-counter drugs as a central nervous system stimulant.

The history of caffeine is interesting. It was originally used in secret formulas for cola and pepper type beverages. In 1916 the U.S. government seized some cola beverage and charged the company that the food was adulterated as it contained an added poisonous and deleterious substance. The trial court felt otherwise, but the decision was reversed on appeal to the U.S. Supreme Court and remanded for retrial (*U.S. vs. 40 Barrels and 20 Kegs of Coca Cola* 24 US 265; 1916). The case was never retried, but cola companies reduced the level of caffeine substantially. Remember that in 1916 the USDA had jurisdiction and would have had to prove that caffeine could render the food injurious to health. Since that case, nothing was done until the FDA notice in 1980 to amend the carbonated beverage standards of identity to allow the product to meet the standard without the need to add caffeine or kola nut extract, that is, the addition of caffeine was optional. The order would set a maximum of 0.02% and require labeling of it. Many consumer groups would like to see caffeine banned outright while others agree that the level should be set at 0.01%. What will happen is not known at this time. Japanese evidence in 1981 showed caffeine to be carcinogenic but other data refutes this.

Other Problem Additives

We could fill a whole book with stories about additives or environmental chemicals contaminating food. The case of selenium is an interesting one. Selenium is required by cattle, and probably by humans, in very low doses. It is added to animal feed in areas where it is poor in the natural forage to prevent a nutritional deficiency. Animal tests for toxicity indicate that it might be a carcinogen at very high levels. However the dose determines the effect of a chemical and makes risk/benefit analysis difficult.

From 1970 through 1978 much was published about artificial colors, especially Yellow No. 5, causing hyperkinesis in children. This symptom is associated with a learning disability and estimates of afflicted children range from a low of several hundred thousand to a high of 12 million. Unfortunately, uncontrolled studies have been highly publicized. It is known that difficulties during labor resulting in oxygen deprivation during birth is one cause of hyperkinesis. Exposure to lead or carbon monoxide at low levels has also been implicated. Dr. Ben Feingold of California claimed that processed foods containing additives were the primary cause. He had only clinical observations with no controls, yet he recommended the use of a strict exclusion diet for children. What is not thoroughly understood by the public is that he recommended excluding over 21 fruits and vegetables from the child's diet. A study at the University of Wisconsin has shown that there is probably no benefit to the Feingold diet for most hyperkinetic children of age 6 through 12. However, more work is being done in this area to obtain better evidence either pro or con, especially for younger children. In the meantime the FDA now requires that all foods with Yellow No. 5 identify it by name on the ingredient list rather than just listing it as "artificial color."

MSG, a flavor enhancer, has caused tissue damage to the brain when injected in large doses into the base of the skull of immature rats. Unfortunately, the infant animal does not have full brain development as the infant human does, so some effect might be expected. MSG was used in baby food, but has been removed because of pressure by the media and consumer groups. Since the original purpose of using MSG in baby food was to make the baby food appeal to parents rather than to babies, its removal was justified from that standpoint.

Some people may also be sensitive to MSG. A condition known as the Chinese Restaurant Syndrome (CRS) occurs if these people eat soup or other Chinese foods with high levels of MSG, especially after not having had food all day. A severe headache and dizziness occurs. MSG is essentially the salt of the natural amino acid, glutamic acid. It has not been found to be toxic by regular test procedures and thus is allowed as a GRAS substance. Many toxicologists question the validity of the injection procedure and the CRS syndrome.

BHA and BHT have been implicated several times in the press as being dangerous. These are two food additives that have actually been studied with primates (monkeys), which should give the best evaluation with respect to humans. The studies showed no clinical problems at up to 500 mg./kg. of body weight per day. Many foods fabricated with unsaturated fats contain only 100 to 200 parts per million, so you would need to consume 500 kg. of fat a day to reach the test levels. In 1982, one flawed Japanese study with BHA caused the Japanese government to propose a ban. Because we are now an international community and because of the Delaney Clause, pressure was put on the FDA and the Health Protection Branch in Canada to follow suit. As of 1983, BHA was still being used, even in Japan although they insist that the study shows BHA to be a cancer promoter. Perhaps this chemical will lead to a true test of risk/benefit.

NATURAL TOXICANTS IN FOODS

Many foods contain natural toxicants that can make them inedible or at least cause the foods to be first processed to remove the toxic factor. Other foods can be toxic if too much is consumed at one time.

The Amanita species of mushroom is the best example of a highly toxic natural plant. Death occurs rapidly after eating this plant. Those who pick wild mushrooms should learn what kind of species to avoid and should be able to identify them.

Alcohol, which is common in the diet of some people, can also be dangerous if consumed in excess. The problem comes partially from addiction, which results in very poor dietary habits. Moderation is the answer. It is also absolutely essential that pregnant women either severely limit or abstain from alcohol.

Unrefined oil seeds naturally contain a gastric cancer-causing chemical, 3,4-dibenzepyrene. It is removed in the normal refining process used by the food industry. The level is initially 10 mg./kg. It is interesting to note that raw cabbage contains about 13 mg./kg. of this chemical. Lettuce and spinach also have some naturally. When one barbecues food over charcoal or wood, the burning fat deposits benzepyrene on the surface of the meat at up to 23 mg./kg. Epidemiological evidence shows high gastric cancer rates in places around the world where a lot of barbecued foods or smoked foods are consumed. In Iceland for example, 35% of all deaths are from gastric cancer and may be due to this or to nitrosamine from cured meats.

Cabbage, cauliflower, and brussels sprouts, when consumed in large quantities, can suppress the uptake of iodine by the thyroid gland because of a chemical they contain. These same foods contain oxalic acid that prevents calcium and iron absorption. Rhubarb leaves, some cereals, and spinach also fall into this class. Honey can also be toxic when manufactured by bees that extract pollen from certain plants that grow in southern Greece, Italy, and parts of the West Coast.

Various kinds of legumes can cause diseases. Many of the diseases are found among poor desert populations. For example, in parts of Africa during a drought, plants such as chickpeas are the only ones able to survive. Being available, these plants may be consumed in large quantities. But chickpeas contain a chemical that causes muscular weakness and can lead to death if overconsumed. Uncooked soybeans contain chemicals that prevent protein digestion (antitrypsin factor) and can destroy red blood cells. Heat processing in steam, however, can destroy these factors.

Nutmeg can also be lethal in a quantity as small as one tablespoon. The same is true of green potatoes. The green color indicates the presence of an alkaloid called solanine, which affects the central nervous system. It has been responsible for the death of several people consuming an excess of green potatoes or making potato sprout soup. The normal potato contains 5–8 mg. of solanine per 100 grams. The LD_{50} in rabbits for solanine is 20 mg./kg. of body weight. For a 50-kg. person the LD_{50} would be about 1,000 mg. Thus the safety factor is at least 100 to 1. If we combine all the potatoes we eat in one year we would total at least 5,000 mg. of solanine, possibly more. This is obviously enough to kill one by over five times. Potatoes are not dangerous under normal consumption patterns; the dose is the important factor.

Manioca or cassava is a plant that is the seventh largest consumed food in the world. We know it in its refined form as tapioca. It is used by many people in developing tropical countries. Manioca is a root type food that contains a chemical that breaks down into hydrogen cyanide in the stomach. It would be fatal if cooked and eaten directly. However, preparation procedures have been developed to make it safe for consumption by washing and extracting. Normal cassava contains about 245 mg. of cyanide in 100 grams. Since the LD_{50} is 0.5 mg./kg. of body weight, a normal 70-kg. person consuming an average serving is taking seven to ten times the lethal dose if it is not removed.

Alfalfa sprouts, eaten by many vegetarians, contain a steroid that depresses chick growth at only 0.2% in the diet. It does not affect rats however. It is not clear whether it affects humans, but this points out again the problem with animal studies.

One area that we are learning more about is the interaction of drugs with the diet. For example, there are some tranquilizers that can produce deleterious effects if taken simultaneously with certain foods. They suppress an enzyme in the liver that detoxifies tyramine, a natural chemical that is found in bananas, wine, beer, yogurt, and certain cheeses. Camembert cheese, for example, contains 200 mg. of tyramine in about 3.5 ounces. Normally our liver converts it to tyrosine, a natural amino acid. The monoamine oxidase inhibitor (MAOI) tranquilizers suppress this reaction and thus lead to the adverse toxic effect. It is interesting to note that if we extracted the tyramine from about three ounces of cheese and injected it into the blood stream, death would occur very rapidly. The mode of action of tyramine is in the brain. Many doctors are aware of this but sometimes fail to notify their patients of the problem.

Antacids will irreversibly bind calcium and iron, cutting down on the absorption of these important nutrients from the small intestine. The extent of the problem this creates is not known.

SUMMARY

Anything consumed in excess can be harmful; it is not always the chemical but sometimes the dose ingested that causes the harm. We must understand the risks involved in consuming certain additives and the benefits they give us. For example, much bread produced centrally would mold rapidly if calcium propionate was not added. Calcium propionate is not a cancer-causing chemical but it is toxic to humans at some level; that is the risk. The benefit is increased shelf life and reduced waste. Bread would mold in three days without the mold inhibitor compared to ten days with it. This food lost to mold would be an economic loss to the country as a whole.

Cancer causation is sometimes hard to detect using animal experiments. The National Cancer Institute (NCI) routinely screens chemicals for carcinogenicity. The NCI evaluates chemicals based on the relative risk of the chemicals to society. The NCI's list of chemicals screened showed that pharmaceuticals and pesticides each accounted for 20% while food additives made up only 1.6% of the total screened. Interestingly, 5.7% of the screened compounds were from natural food products. Environmental and other synthetic chemicals made up the rest of the chemicals tested. The overreaction that has developed about food additives and cancer is amazing considering that the NCI holds the relationship to be relatively unimportant based on their relative screening rate. Obviously we don't have all the answers but we should at least learn more about the benefits versus the risks in our food supply.

It is also amazing that we have not banned cigarettes. There is about a one in seven chance of dying from smoking over one pack of cigarettes a day. An increasingly larger percent of young women smoke. Over 95% of all lung cancers are the result of smoking, and lung cancer is the only cancer disease still rising. The chance of dying in a car crash is only one in 4,000 over the year. Risk versus benefit must always be considered but the risk is sometimes blown out of proportion.

This chapter has pointed out the risk versus benefit controversy in regard to some food and feed additives. Some decisions were arbitrary and not based on scientific fact. If some natural foods were tested and examined in the same way, they would also have to be banned. We don't have all the answers, but the public should be assured that the FDA does the best job possible in keeping the food supply safe.

Multiple Choice Study Questions

1. Which additive did the FDA try to ban based on the Delaney Clause?

   A. cyclamates
   B. Red No. 2
   C. DES
   D. Violet No. 1
   E. saccharin

2. Which substance occurs naturally in plants and may be carcinogenic?

   A. caffeine
   B. solanine
   C. DES
   D. allergens
   E. Red No. 2

3. Barbecued foods can be related to

   A. intestinal cancer because of nitrosamines
   B. esophageal cancer because of benze-pyrene
   C. liver cancer because of aflatoxin
   D. nothing and are safe to eat in any quantity
   E. nutritional disease because all vitamins are destroyed

4. Which food coloring used in fresh meat was banned?

   A. Red # 4
   B. Red # 2
   C. Orange # 40
   D. Violet # 1
   E. Yellow # 5

5. Nitrite is a problem because

   A. of the color it forms
   B. it destroys botulinum organisms
   C. it causes cancer
   D. it forms nitrosamines in alkaline conditions
   E. it forms nitrosamines under heat

6. Which food containing natural toxicants causes the most problems in the U.S.?

A. coffee
B. alcohol
C. yogurt
D. nugmeg
E. unrefined oils

7. An example of the toxicity condition under the category of an abnormal sensitivity is

A. phenylketonuria (PKU)
B. obesity
C. cholesterol and heart disease
D. eating amanita mushrooms
E. eating swordfish

Essay Study Questions

1. List the three categories of toxicity and give an example of each.

2. Relate the toxicological and regulatory status of DES.

3. What are the risks and benefits of using artificial sweeteners?

4. What problems have occurred with artificial food colors? Should they and/or natural colors be used?

5. What are the problems in using nitrite to cure meat?

6. List some natural foods that contain natural toxicants.

7. What is the problem with caffeine?

Things to Do

1. Read some controversial books on food additives such as: *The Poisons In Your Food,* William Longgood (1960), Grove Press, NY 60¢; *Consumer Beware,* Beatrice Trum Hunter (1972), Bantam, NY $1.95; *Eaters' Digest,* Michael Jacobson (1972), Doubleday, $1.95. Discuss their points on the use of food additives and the effectiveness of the FDA.

2. Interview people with respect to their feelings on: smoking vs. saccharin; red dye no. 2; DES; yellow # 5. Discuss in class.

Chapter 26. Answers to Multiple-Choice Study Questions: 1, E; 2, A; 3, B; 4, D; 5, E; 6, B; 7, A.

BIBLIOGRAPHY

In this book we have attempted to examine the nature of the relationship of food to humans and their well-being. We have learned about the chemicals that compose food and their functions in the body. We have also discussed the nutritional requirements of the human body in relationship to these chemicals and how they affect growth, maintenance, and repair. This book has covered the why's and how's of processed food, as well as the way government regulates the food industry, something many of us know little about. This information should help create a better understanding of the value and safety of our food supply. The nutritional problems of coronary heart disease, obesity, and fad diets in the United States were also examined. An overall picture of nutrition and food has been given to furnish a basis for making wise and reasonable choices about your diet. Facts have been presented to help counter the many fallacious claims made by faddists, dieters, and others in general conversations. For those who wish to do more reading, this section lists some other recommended texts.

* Arlin, M.T. 1972. *The science of nutrition.* New York: Macmillan Press.

   Bernarde, M.A. 1970. *The chemicals we eat.* New York: American Heritage Press.

   Carter, R. 1964. *Your food and your health.* New York: Harper and Row.

   Chaney, M.S., and Ross, M.L. 1966. *Nutrition.* 7th ed. Boston: Houghton & Co.

* Clydesdale, F.M. and F.J. Francis. 1977. *Food and nutrition and you.* New York: Prentice Hall.

   Crampton, E., and Lloyd, L. 1959. *Fundamentals of nutrition.* San Francisco: W.H. Freeman & Co.

* Davidson, S.; Passmore, R.; and Brock, J.F. 1972. *Human nutrition and dietetics.* 5th ed. Baltimore: Williams & Wilkins Co.

   Deutsch, R. 1976. *The realities of nutrition.* Palo Alto: Bull Pub. Co.

* Deutsch, R. 1962. *The nuts among the berries.* New York: Ballentine Books.

* Deutsch, R.M.   1977.   *The new nuts among the berries.*   Palo Alto: Bull Pub. Co.

* Deutsch R.   1971.   *The family guide to better food and better health.*   New York: Bantam Books, Inc.

* Gerard, R.W.   1965.   *Food for life.*   Chicago: Univ. of Chicago Press.

Harris, R.S., and Karmas, E.   1975.   *Nutritional evaluation of food processing.*   Westport, Conn.: AVI Publishing Co.

* Herbert, V.   1980.   *Nutrition cultism facts and fiction.*   Philadelphia: G. Stuckley Co.

Hofman, L.   1978.   *The great American nutrition hassle.*   Palo Alto: Mayfield Publishing Co.

Hutchinson, R.C.   1958.   *Food for better living.*   New York: Cambridge Univ.

Jacobson, M.   1973.   *Eater's digest.*   New York: Ballentine Press.

* Labuza, T.P., and A.E. Sloan,   1979.   *Contemporary nutrition controversies.*   St. Paul: West Publishing Co.

Lamb, M.W., and Harden, M.   1973.   *The meaning of human nutrition.*   New York: Pergamon Press, Inc.

* Leverton, R.M.   1965.   *Food becomes you.*   3rd ed. Ames, Iowa: Iowa State Univ. Press.

* McHenry, E.E.   1960.   *Foods without fads.*   Philadelphia: J.B. Lippincott Co.

MFG. Chemists Assoc.   *Food additives: What they are, how they are used.*   Washington, D.C.

Nasset, E.S.   1962.   *Your diet, digestion and health.*   2nd ed. New York: Barnes and Noble.

* Potter, N.N.   1973.   *Food science.*   2nd ed. Westport, Conn.: AVI Publishing Co.

Robinson, C.H.   1965.   *Basic nutrition and diet therapy.*   New York: The Macmillan Co.

* Runyon, Thora.   1976.   *Nutrition for today.*   New York: Harper and Row.

Salmon, M.B.   1965.   *Food facts for teenagers.*   Springfield, Ill: C.C. Thomas Co.

Sebrell, W.H., Jr.; Haggerty, J.J.; and the editors of Life.   1967.   *Food and nutrition.*   Chicago: TIME–LIFE Books.

* Smith, N.   1976.   *Food for sport.*   Palo Alto, Calif: Bull Pub. Co.

Spock, D., and Lowenberg, M.   1956.   *Feeding your baby and child.*   New York: Pocket Books.

* Stewart, G., and Amerine, M.A. 1973. *Introduction to food science.* New York: Academic Press.

Tatkon, M.D. 1968. *The great vitamin hoax.* New York: The Macmillan Co.

Turner, J. 1970. *The chemical feast.* New York: Grossman Publishing Co.

U.S. Dept. of Agriculture Handbook # 456. *Nutritional Value of American Foods in Common Units.* U.S. Government Printing Office, Washington, D.C.

Wayler, T.J., and Klein, R.S. 1965. *Applied nutrition.* New York: The Macmillan Co.

Whelan, E. and F. Stare. 1975. *Panic in the pantry.* New York: Atheneum Press.

* White, P.L. 1974. *Let's talk about food.* Chicago: The American Medical Association.

* Whitney E., and M. Hamilton. 1977. *Understanding nutrition.* St. Paul: West Publishing Co.

* Wilson, E.D.; Fisher, K.H.; and Fuqua, M.E. 1974. *Principles of nutrition.* 3rd ed. New York: John Wiley & Sons.

* Young, J.H. 1967. *The medical messiahs.* Princeton, N.J.: Princeton Univ. Press.

* Highly recommended.

GLOSSARY

Absorption The process by which nutrients are transported from the intestinal tract into the circulatory system of the body.

Acute toxicity test Procedure for determining LD_{50} of a chemical or drug.

ADI (acceptable daily intake) The no effect dose divided by 100—determines the maximum level allowed for a regulated additive.

Adulteration Part of 1938 FD & C Act; defines violations with respect to foods containing harmful or undesirable substances.

Aerobes Microorganisms that need oxygen for growth, for example, molds.

Aflatoxin A chemical produced by a mold that can cause liver cancer.

Amino acids The building blocks of proteins.

Amygdalin A chemical naturally found in some foods that breaks down into cyanide in the body.

Anaerobes Microbes that can grow only in the absence of oxygen. *Clostridium botulinum* is a good example. Facultative anaerobes can grow with or without oxygen.

Anemia A disease caused by the lack of certain nutrients such as iron deficiency anemia (iron) or pernicious anemia (B_{12}).

Anorexia nervosa A disease in which extreme loss of appetite occurs with the result of body wasting.

Antioxidants Chemicals added to foods to prevent rancidity by combining with free radicals. BHA and BHT are the most common.

Appertizing Heat processing of food for sterilization purposes.

Asceptic processing Processing foods at high temperature and then filling into sterile pouches or cans and sealing.

Atherosclerosis A hardening of the arteries bringing blood to the heart muscles. Can lead to a heart attack.

ATP (adenosine tri-phosphate) An energy-rich chemical released in the utilization of carbohydrates, fats, and proteins. It is used to supply energy to many other reactions.

Basic Four Food Guide   A method to help attain a diet containing the necessary nutrients.

BATF   Bureau of Alcohol, Tobacco, and Firearms.

Behavior modification   A psychological technique that can be used to help in obesity treatment.

Beriberi   A disease caused by lack of vitamin B_1, in the diet, also called *polyneuritis*.

Bile salts   Chemicals produced in the liver; help to decrease the acidity of the food from the stomach and emulsifies the fat.

Bioavailability   Biological utilization of chemically-present nutrients in a food.

Biochemical pathway   The route by which a chemical is converted into other entities in the body.

Biochemistry   The science of chemical reactions that occur in a living organism.

BMR (basal metabolic rate)   The energy in calories/day needed by the human body for maintaining involuntary functions. Determined under specific conditions.

Browning   A general term for reactions that lead to darkening of the food during storage. Enzymatic browning is caused by enzymes, is rapid, and is most prevalent in fruits and vegetables.

Calcium/phosphorus ratio   Important relationship of these two minerals in the diet in terms of the effect on bone depletion.

Calorie/Cal   One thousand small calories where a small calorie is the energy needed to raise 1 g. water (1/454 of a pound) by 1° C (from 15 to 16° C).

Carbohydrate loading   A technique to increase the storage energy in the muscle tissues.

Carbohydrates   Simple and complex sugars.

Carcinogen   A chemical that causes cancer.

Celiac disease   A disease in which the protein in some cereals irritates the intestinal lining causing malabsorption of nutrients.

Cellulite   A French-derived word used to describe excess fat cells.

CHD (coronary heart disease)   A disease in which blood vessels leading to the heart may become blocked or weakened, thus starving the heart muscles and leading to a heart attack.

Chelating agents   Compounds such as citric acid and EDTA that tie up trace metals and thus prevent or slow the development of rancidity.

Chemical score A method to rate protein quality as compared to egg protein.

Cholesterol A sterol found in foods as well as produced in the body. Used in many body functions, but also implicated in heart disease.

Chronic toxicity test Three-year test procedure for determining long-range and cancer effects of a chemical or drug.

Codex Alimentarius International body set up to establish guidelines for foods that will be in international commerce.

Colon The lower part of the large intestine.

Commercial sterility The heat process given canned foods that insures safety from botulism and no spoilage if the cans are held at room temperature. Thermophilic spores may still be present but do not grow.

Common or usual name FDA regulation controlling the name of a food product.

Correlation A positive relationship between two factors such as diet and heart disease.

Curds The coagulated proteins produced in cheese making.

D value Time necessary to reduce the number of microorganisms by 90% at a constant temperature.

Delaney Clause Refers to 1958 food additive amendment to 1938 [FD & C Act that prevents addition of cancer-causing chemicals to foods (zero tolerance)].

DES (diethylstilbestrol) A growth-promoting synthetic hormone.

Diabetes A malfunction of glucose metabolism.

Diet The food we consume or use in animal tests.

Diglyceride A fat type molecule with a glycerol backbone and two fatty acids.

Disaccharide Two simple sugars combined chemically.

Diverticulosis A physiological problem in which the large intestinal wall weakens and balloons out. Fecal matter can be entrapped in these areas and cause infection.

Drip The loss of tissue water from frozen foods during thawing.

Drum drying A process in which slurried foods such as mashed potatoes are dried.

Duodenum The initial section of the small intestine in which many enzymes break down food constituents into smaller units.

Efficacy test   Test procedure to determine level of use of a food additive.

Emulsifier   A chemical that can be used to prevent separation of oil and water such as in a salad dressing.

Enrichment   The addition of nutrients to specific foods as required by law for specific purposes. Bread is enriched with thiamine, riboflavin, niacin, and iron.

Enzyme   A chemical compound formed from proteins and other molecules that helps induce chemical reactions to proceed faster at body temperature than without the enzyme. These are also called biological catalysts.

EPA   Environmental Protection Agency.

Epidemiology   The study of the relationship between population characteristics and certain factors such as diseases. For example, many people in countries with high fiber consumption have less coronary heart disease.

Esophagus   The connection of the dietary tract between the mouth and stomach.

Essential nutrient   A chemical compound that the body cannot manufacture itself. Required for growth maintenance and repair.

Ethylene   A gas that is a normal growth hormone produced by fruits and vegetables that controls ripening; used artificially to bring produce to a certain state of ripeness.

Exogenous   Refers to a nutrient available in the food we eat.

FDA (Food and Drug Administration)   Administers laws regulating interstate production of foods.

FD & C Color   An approved synthetic coloring additive allowed for use in foods under the 1960 Food, Drug, and Cosmetic Act, Color Additives Amendment (FD & C No. 40 is an example).

Federal, Food, Drug, and Cosmetic Act   Passed in 1938; basic laws pertaining to foods that protect the public.

Fiber   Polymers of simple carbohydrates that are undigestable by humans and thus do not supply calories. Crude fiber is that fiber measured by chemical methods. Dietary fiber is that fiber undigested by humans.

Filth tolerances   Amounts of filth allowed in processed foods if good manufacturing practices are used.

FOI   1971 Freedom of Information Act.

Food Additive Amendment   Passed in 1958; defines regulated and GRAS list chemicals.

Food disappearance Data on the production of foods in the United States plus imports less exports. If an amount of food is divided by the number of people in the population this gives a value of pounds per person per year, sometimes used as a consumption value.

Fortification The addition of nutrients to foods for special dietary purposes. For example, many cereals are fortified to provide about 25% of the RDA in a serving.

FPLA (1966 Fair Packaging and Labeling Act) Defines what can be put on a package and what can be advertised about foods.

Free radicals Very reactive compounds produced during rancidity.

Freeze drying A very expensive process for drying foods in the frozen state under vacuum. Very little nutrient or quality loss takes place.

Freezer burn Dark spots that form on frozen foods, especially meats, due to evaporation of ice during frozen storage. The spot forms because of chemical reactions that occur in the place where the water evaporates.

FSIS (Food Safety and Inspection Service) Part of the USDA that controls meat slaughter and processing.

FTC (Federal Trade Commission) Regulates the advertising of food in the media.

Functional ingredient A food additive that performs some specific effect in foods, usually with respect to textural characteristics.

Gas chromatograph An analytical instrument used to separate and identify food flavor compounds.

Glycogen A polymer of glucose, serves as a storage of carbohydrates in the body.

GMP (good manufacturing practices) Guidelines for insurance of quality and safety in the processing of foods.

Goiter A disease of iodine deficiency resulting in an enlarged thyroid gland.

Gout A disease that can lead to deposits of crystalline materials in joints and in the kidneys.

HACCP (Hazard Analysis and Critical Control Point Procedures) Methods for control and inspection during food processing to insure against food poisoning.

Hemochromatosis An iron storage disease.

Hemoglobin An iron-containing protein molecule found in the blood that carries oxygen to cells.

HHS Department of Health and Human Services—department in which FDA is located.

HMA (host mediated assay) An animal test procedure for determining the possible mutagenic effect of a chemical.

Hormones Special chemicals in the body that are used to control specific reactions. For example, insulin controls the utilization of glucose by the cells.

HTST High temperature short time canning processes.

Humectants Chemical agents added to food to bind water; sugar and salt are examples.

Hyperplasia Increase in numbers of tissue cells.

Hypertension A disease of high blood pressure. Excess salt intake may exacerbate the condition.

Hypertrophy Increase in cell size.

Hypoglycemia A disease of carbohydrate metabolism in which the level of glucose falls so rapidly in the bloodstream that not enough energy is supplied to the brain or central nervous system.

Ileum The third section of the small intestine. Absorption of nutrients, especially cholesterol, occurs here.

Imitation food Food that resembles, substitutes for, and is nutritionally inferior to the regular product.

Indogenous A chemical (nutrient) produced in the body.

Ingredient list List of components of a food in order of predominance by weight. Must be on food package, right side of label.

Inhibitor A chemical used to prevent growth of microorganisms.

Insulin resistance A condition commonly occurring with obesity that results in the need for higher levels of insulin in the bloodstream so that the body can utilize carbohydrates as a source of energy.

International unit Defined as an equivalent for vitamins that may have several different chemical forms. For example, vitamin A can be defined in terms of carotene or retinol equivalents.

Intoxication A food-borne disease caused by a harmful chemical in the food. This toxin may be produced by a microorganism.

Jejunal-ileal bypass A dangerous surgical procedure used in obesity treatment.

Jejunum The second part of the small intestinal tract. Absorption of nutrients occurs here, especially glucose, protein, iron, calcium, and vitamin A.

Ketosis A condition resulting from the utilization of fats as the major source of energy. When this occurs chemical compounds (acids and ketones) build up in the bloodstream and can have an adverse health effect.

Kjeldahl apparatus Device for measuring nitrogen content of a food.

Krebs Cycle A chemical process in the body by which glucose is maximally utilized and ATP is produced.

Kwashiorkor A disease caused by lack of protein in the diet. If calories are also lacking the disease is called Marasmus.

Lactose deficiency The inability to digest milk sugar.

LD_{50} Dose of a chemical in mg./kg. body weight at which 50% of the population consuming it would die.

Linoleic acid A polyunsaturated fatty acid that is an essential nutrient.

Lipase An enzyme that splits fatty acids off of triglycerides.

Lipid A fat molecule.

Log scale A special way to plot data graphically so that a straight line is obtained.

Low-calorie food Food with less than 40 calories per serving.

Lysine A very important essential amino acid that is low in many cereal proteins.

Malignant A cancerous cell.

Malnutrition An improper health state due to an imbalance in nutrient intake.

Maturity-onset obesity A condition of excess weight gain that occurs after young adulthood.

MDR Minimum daily requirement of a nutrient.

Mesophiles Microorganisms that grow optimally in the range of 15 to 40° C.

Metabolism The utilization of chemical nutrients from the diet by the body.

Microorganism A microscopic organism such as a bacteria, yeast, or mold.

Misbranding Part of 1938 FD & C Act. Defines labeling and ingredient violations with respect to foods.

Monoglyceride A fat type molecule with a glycerol backbone and one fatty acid.

Mono-saccharide A simple sugar based on 5 or 6 carbons.

MTD Maximum tolerated dose of a chemical at which no toxic effect occurs.

Mutagen A chemical that can cause a mutation in a cell.

NAS/NRC (National Academy of Science/National Research Council) A scientific body appointed to review and establish certain facts of science.

Natural foods Unprocessed or minimally processed foods.

NED (no effect dose) Level of consumption of a chemical or food additive in mg./kg. body weight at which no adverse biological effect occurs.

Net weight The amount of food in a package.

Nitrosamine A carcinogenic chemical formed between the reaction of nitrite and certain amine chemicals.

NOEL No observed effect level in subacute toxicity testing.

Nonenzymatic browning (NEB) A reaction between certain sugars with amino acids or proteins leading to darkening, off-flavors, toughening, and loss of protein quality.

Nonessential nutrient A chemical compound used by the body for various functions. It can either be supplied in the diet or manufactured in the body by various mechanisms if not supplied.

Nutrient density The ratio of nutrients to calories in a food.

Nutrients The chemical constituents of foods that are utilized in the body.

Nutrification The addition of essential nutrients to a fabricated food that serves as a substitute for a normal food in the diet.

Nutrition The sum total of all the biochemical processes that utilize foods in the body for the processes of growth, repair, and maintenance.

Nutritional adequacy The state of well-being resulting from the consumption of nutrients.

Obesity Fifteen percent or more over the normal weight.

Oncology The study of cancerous tumors caused by chemicals.

Open dating Date on package to give consumers some idea of shelf life.

Organic chemistry The study of chemical compounds in which carbon serves as a basis.

Organic foods Fruits and vegetables produced on land without the use of synthetic fertilizers, pesticides, and so on.

OSHA Occupational Safety and Health Administration.

Osteoporosis A disease primarily found in older women in which calcium is depleted from the bones.

Overweight Up to 15% over the normal weight.

Oxidative phosphorylation The process by which ATP is released during the utilization of calorie sources.

Package ice The ice crystals that form inside a frozen food package during storage. Usually due to temperature fluctuations.

Pasteurization The reduction in the number of microorganisms in foods by heat treatment to increase shelf life.

Pathogen A microorganism that can cause a disease in humans.

Pellegra The disease caused by niacin deficiency. Leads to the 3Ds: dementia, diarrhea, dermatitis.

PER A method to rank protein quality through the measurement of weight gain of rats.

ERH An equilibrium relative humidity, that is, the relative humidity at which a food of a certain water content will neither lose nor gain moisture.

pH A measure of the acidity of a system based on a scale from 0 to 14, with 0 being the highest acidity and 7 being neutral.

Phenylketonuria (PKU) A genetic disease in which an essential amino acid, phenylalanine, cannot be metabolized properly.

Phospholipid A fat molecule that contains phosphorus; lecithin is an example.

Plaque A build-up of fat, minerals, and proteins on arterial walls that can lead to weakening or blockage of a blood vessel.

Plasmid A ring of DNA found in bacteria that carries genetic material.

Polymer A long molecule made up of many single units that may or may not be different. Starch is a polymer of simple sugars.

Protein The major source of nitrogen in the diet. A large molecule made up of many smaller units called amino acids some of which are essential.

Psychrophiles Microorganisms that grow optimally in the range of 0 to 10° C.

Ptomaine poisoning A misnomer applied to all types of food poisoning.

PUFA (polyunsaturated fatty acid) A fatty acid with two or more double bonds between carbons.

Pull date Date after which food should not be sold but still may be edible.

Rancidity The reaction between oxygen and unsaturated fats causing undesirable flavors and odors as well as other deleterious reactions during storage of foods.

RDA Recommended daily allowance, that is, the recommended daily intakes for nutrients as established by the Food and Nutrition Board NAS/NRC that insures good health for 97% of the population.

Recall Procedure used by FDA to remove products from the marketplace that are in violation of the law.

Reduced Calorie Food Food with a caloric reduction of one-third as compared to the food it replaces.

Refined sugar Generally refers to white table sugar, which is sucrose. In refining, the dirt and nonedible part of the sugar cane or beet is removed.

Regulated additive A food additive for which a specific level of use is set based on animal testing.

Rennin An enzyme used to coagulate the protein for making cheese.

Restoration With respect to nutrient addition to foods, the addition to bring levels back to that prior to processing.

Retinol The biological equivalent of vitamin A

Rickets A vitamin D deficiency disease of children that leads to soft bones.

Risk/benefit A decision-making process for food additives in which the risk in its use is weighed against the benefits the additive provides the consumer.

Rules and regulations Procedures promulgated by the FDA to carry out the laws passed by Congress.

Ruminant An animal like the cow with a special stomach containing bacteria that can convert undigestible fiber materials into energy sources for the animal.

Saliva The juices produced in the mouth that help digest foods. Saliva contains amylase, which breaks down starches.

Scurvy   The disease caused by vitamin C (ascorbic acid) deficiency.

Senescence   The aging of fruits and vegetables once harvested.

Set point theory   A new theory related to internal control of body weight.

Single cell protein (SCP)   A fermentation process in which the desired end product is the microbe itself. The protein from this microbe can then be extracted and added to foods.

Skinner box   An intelligence testing device used especially for rats.

Solanine   A toxic chemical found naturally in potatoes.

Spore   A dormant state of a bacteria or mold.

Spray drying   A process by which liquid foods are sprayed into a chamber with hot air to remove the water. Instant coffee is made this way.

Staling   A physical change in bakery products such as bread leading to hardening.

Standard deviation   A statistical term used in estimating how different a given value (such as nutrient intake) is from the mean value of the population.

Standard of identity   Specific regulations for certain foods that stipulate their required contents.

Starter culture   The introduction into a food of a large number of microbes (inoculum) for fermentation.

Sterilization   The complete destruction of microorganisms in foods during heat processing.

Subacute toxicity test   Method for determining the no adverse biological effect level of a chemical.

Sulfite   A chemical used to retard browning.

Surfactant   Same effect as an emulsifier, also helps give a smoother texture to baked goods.

Teratogen   A chemical that causes a severe birth defect.

Thermophiles   Microorganisms that grow optimally in the range of 40–50° C.

Thyroxine   The hormone formed in the body that regulates metabolic rate. It has iodine as the base.

α-tocopherol   The international unit for vitamin E.

Triglyceride   A basic fat molecule with a glycerol base to which three fatty acids are attached. These fatty acids may be saturated or unsaturated (double bonds between carbons).

Trypsin   An enzyme that digests protein into polypeptides.

12D concept   Safety factor in food canning leading to about 1 in 10 billion chance of botulinum.

UPC (Universal Product Code) A set of numbers and lines used to electronically identify a product.

Urea The breakdown product of protein that is excreted in the urine.

Uremia A disease condition in which urea builds up in the bloodstream.

USDA United States Department of Agriculture; regulates meat slaughter and processing.

USRDA Set of nutrient standards for nutritional labeling based on 1968 RDAs.

Vegetative state The active growth phase of a microorganism.

Vitamin An essential organic molecule usually required by the body in minute amounts. Necessary for many different bodily functions.

Water activity % ERH ÷ 100 (see ERH).

APPENDIX I

Table of Food Composition

The table presented here is the standard table found in all nutrition textbooks and references. It presents the calorie content, energy-nutrient composition, and vitamin and mineral contents of 615 common foods by household measure.[1] It can be purchased from the U.S. Government Printing Office, The Superintendent of Documents, Washington, DC 20402, as a separate softcover booklet.

Of the minerals, only calcium and iron are included in this table. You might also be curious about zinc, but we have chosen not to present information here on the zinc contents of foods. A few references that do are available.[2]

Of the vitamins, vitamin A, thiamin, riboflavin, niacin, and ascorbic acid (vitamin C) are included. An expanded version of this table, presently being published in installments by the U.S. Department of Agriculture, Agricultural Research Service, includes folacin and other vitamin information, as well as the amino acid analyses of foods.

The nutrient content of brand-name products—cookies, snack foods, cookie mixes, canned fruit, TV dinners, condiments, and so on—not found in this table can be obtained from *Consumer Guide.*[3] The composition of foods used by various ethnic groups, also not found in this table, can be requested from the U.S. Department of Agriculture.[4]

Notes

1. U.S. Department of Agriculture, Nutritive values of the edible parts of foods, *Nutritive Value of Foods*, Home and Garden Bulletin no. 72 (Washington, D.C.: Government Printing Office, 1971), Table 1.

2. K. A. Haeflein and A. I. Rasmussen, Zinc content of selected foods, *Journal of the American Dietetic Association* 70 (1977): 610–616; E. W. Murphy, B. W. Willis, and B. K. Watt, Provisional tables on the zinc content of foods, *Journal of the American Dietetic Association* 66 (1975): 345–355; and J. H. Freeland and R. J. Cousins, Zinc content of selected foods, *Journal of the American Dietetic Association* 68 (1976): 526–529.

3. Food: *The Brand Name Game* (Skokie, Ill.: Consumer Guide, 1974).

4. *Composition of Foods Used by Ethnic Groups—Selected References to Sources of Data* can be requested from Dr. Louise Page, Food and Diet Appraisal Group, Consumer and Food Economics Institute, U.S. Department of Agriculture, Agricultural Research Service, Hyattsville MD 20782. For Japanese-American food equivalents, a reprint is available from the American Dietetic Association, 430 North Michigan Avenue, Chicago, IL 60611.

Appendix I   Table of Food Composition

Food, approximate measure, and weight (in grams)	Grams	Water Per-cent	Food energy kCalories	Pro-tein Grams	Fat Grams	Fatty acids Satu-rated (total) Grams	Unsaturated Oleic Grams	Lin-oleic Grams	Carbo-hy-drate Grams	Cal-cium Milli-grams	Iron Milli-grams	Vita-min A value Inter-national units	Thia-min Milli-grams	Ribo-flavin Milli-grams	Niacin Milli-grams	Ascor-bic acid Milli-grams
MILK, CHEESE, CREAM, IMITATION CREAM; RELATED PRODUCTS																
Milk:																
Fluid:																
1 Whole, 3.5% fat 1 cup	244	87	160	9	9	5	3	Trace	12	288	0.1	350	0.07	0.41	0.2	2
2 Nonfat (skim) 1 cup	245	90	90	9	Trace				12	296	.1	10	.09	.44	.2	2
3 Partly skimmed, 2% nonfat milk solids added 1 cup	246	87	145	10	5	3	2	Trace	15	352	.1	200	.10	.52	.2	2
Canned, concentrated, undiluted:																
4 Evaporated, un-sweetened 1 cup	252	74	345	18	20	11	7	1	24	635	.3	810	.10	.86	.5	3
5 Condensed, sweet-ened 1 cup	306	27	980	25	27	15	9	1	166	802	.3	1,100	.24	1.16	.6	3
Dry, nonfat instant:																
6 Low-density (1⅓ cups needed for re-constitution to 1 qt.) 1 cup	68	4	245	24	Trace				35	879	.4	¹20	.24	1.21	.6	5
7 High-density (⅞ cup needed for recon-stitution to 1 qt.) 1 cup	104	4	375	37	1				54	1,345	.6	¹30	.36	1.85	.9	7
Buttermilk:																
8 Fluid, cultured, made from skim milk 1 cup	245	90	90	9	Trace				12	296	.1	10	.10	.44	.2	2
9 Dried, packaged 1 cup	120	3	465	41	6	3	2	Trace	60	1,498	.7	260	.31	2.06	1.1	---
Cheese:																
Natural:																
Blue or Roquefort type:																
10 Ounce 1 oz.	28	40	105	6	9	5	3	Trace	1	89	.1	350	.01	.17	.3	0
11 Cubic inch 1 cu. in.	17	40	65	4	5	3	2	Trace	Trace	54	.1	210	.01	.11	.2	0

¹ Value applies to unfortified product; value for fortified low-density product would be 1500 I.U. and the fortified high-density product would be 2290 I.U.

Table of Food Composition (continued)

[Dashes in the columns for nutrients show that no suitable value could be found although there is reason to believe that a measurable amount of the nutrient may be present]

	Food, approximate measure, and weight (in grams)	Water	Food energy	Protein	Fat	Fatty acids Saturated (total)	Fatty acids Unsaturated Oleic	Fatty acids Unsaturated Linoleic	Carbohydrate	Calcium	Iron	Vitamin A value	Thiamin	Riboflavin	Niacin	Ascorbic acid
		Percent	kCalories	Grams	Grams	Grams	Grams	Grams	Grams	Milligrams	Milligrams	International units	Milligrams	Milligrams	Milligrams	Milligrams
	MILK, CHEESE, CREAM, IMITATION CREAM; RELATED PRODUCTS—Con.															
	Cheese—Continued															
	Natural—Continued															
12	Camembert, packaged in 4-oz. pkg. with 3 wedges per pkg. 1 wedge - - - 38	52	115	7	9	5	3	Trace	1	40	0.2	380	0.02	0.29	0.3	0
	Cheddar:															
13	Ounce - - - - 1 oz - - - 28	37	115	7	9	5	3	Trace	1	213	.3	370	.01	.13	Trace	0
14	Cubic inch - - - 1 cu. in. - - 17	37	70	4	6	3	2	Trace	Trace	129	.2	230	.01	.08	Trace	0
	Cottage, large or small curd:															
	Creamed:															
15	Package of 12-oz., net wt. 1 pkg - - - 340	78	360	46	14	8	5	Trace	10	320	1.0	580	.10	.85	.3	0
16	Cup, curd pressed down. 1 cup - - - 245	78	260	33	10	6	3	Trace	7	230	.7	420	.07	.61	.2	0
	Uncreamed:															
17	Package of 12-oz., net wt. 1 pkg - - - 340	79	290	58	1	1	Trace	Trace	9	306	1.4	30	.10	.95	.3	0
18	Cup, curd pressed down. 1 cup - - - 200	79	170	34	1	Trace	Trace	Trace	5	180	.8	20	.06	.56	.2	0
	Cream:															
19	Package of 8-oz., net wt. 1 pkg - - - 227	51	850	18	86	48	28	3	5	141	.5	3,500	.05	.54	.2	0
20	Package of 3-oz., net wt. 1 pkg - - - 85	51	320	7	32	18	11	1	2	53	.2	1,310	.02	.20	.1	0
21	Cubic inch - - - 1 cu. in. - - 16	51	60	1	6	3	2	Trace	Trace	10	Trace	250	Trace	.04	Trace	0
	Parmesan, grated:															
22	Cup, pressed down. 1 cup - - - 140	17	655	60	43	24	14	1	5	1,893	.7	1,760	.03	1.22	.3	0
23	Tablespoon - - - 1 tbsp. - - 5	17	25	2	2	1	Trace	Trace	Trace	68	Trace	60	Trace	.04	Trace	0
24	Ounce - - - - 1 oz. - - - 28	17	130	12	9	5	3	Trace	1	383	.1	360	.01	.25	.1	0
	Swiss:															
25	Ounce - - - - 1 oz. - - - 28	39	105	8	8	4	3	Trace	1	262	.3	320	Trace	.11	Trace	0
26	Cubic inch - - - 1 cu. in. - - 15	39	55	4	4	2	1	Trace	Trace	139	.1	170	Trace	.06	Trace	0

No.	Food, approximate measure	Grams	Water (%)	Food energy (cal)	Protein (g)	Fat (g)	Saturated fatty acids (total) (g)	Unsaturated — Oleic (g)	Unsaturated — Linoleic (g)	Carbohydrate (g)	Calcium (mg)	Iron (mg)	Vitamin A (I.U.)	Thiamin (mg)	Riboflavin (mg)	Niacin (mg)	Ascorbic acid (mg)
	Pasteurized processed cheese:																
	American:																
27	Ounce — 1 oz	28	40	105	7	9	5	3	Trace	1	198	.3	350	.01	.12	Trace	0
28	Cubic inch — 1 cu. in.	18	40	65	4	5	3	2	Trace	Trace	122	.2	210	Trace	.07	Trace	0
	Swiss:																
29	Ounce — 1 oz	28	40	100	8	8	4	3	Trace	1	251	.3	310	Trace	.11	Trace	0
30	Cubic inch — 1 cu. in.	18	40	65	5	5	3	2	Trace	Trace	159	.2	200	Trace	.07	Trace	0
	Pasteurized process cheese food, American:																
31	1 tbsp.	14	43	45	3	3	2	1	Trace	1	80	.1	140	Trace	.08	Trace	0
32	Cubic inch — 1 cu. in.	18	43	60	4	4	2	1	Trace	1	100	.1	170	Trace	.10	Trace	0
33	**Pasteurized process cheese spread, American.** — 1 oz	28	49	80	5	6	3	2	Trace	2	160	.2	250	Trace	.15	Trace	0
	Cream:																
34	Half-and-half (cream and milk) — 1 cup	242	80	325	8	28	15	9	1	11	261	.1	1,160	.07	.39	.1	2
35	1 tbsp.	15	80	20	1	2	1	1	Trace	1	16	Trace	70	Trace	.02	Trace	Trace
36	Light, coffee or table — 1 cup	240	72	505	7	49	27	16	1	10	245	.1	2,020	.07	.36	.1	2
37	1 tbsp.	15	72	30	1	3	2	1	Trace	1	15	Trace	130	Trace	.02	Trace	Trace
38	Sour — 1 cup	230	72	485	7	47	26	16	1	10	235	.1	1,930	.07	.35	.1	2
39	1 tbsp.	12	72	25	Trace	2	1	1	Trace	1	12	Trace	100	Trace	.02	Trace	Trace
40	Whipped topping (pressurized). — 1 cup	60	62	155	2	14	8	5	Trace	6	67	---	570	---	.04	---	---
41	1 tbsp.	3	62	10	Trace	1	Trace	Trace	Trace	Trace	3	Trace	30	Trace	Trace	---	---
	Whipping, unwhipped (volume about double when whipped):																
42	Light — 1 cup	239	62	715	6	75	41	25	2	9	203	.1	3,060	.05	.29	.1	2
43	1 tbsp.	15	62	45	Trace	5	3	2	Trace	1	13	Trace	190	Trace	.02	Trace	Trace
44	Heavy — 1 cup	238	57	840	5	90	50	30	3	7	179	.1	3,670	.05	.26	.1	2
45	1 tbsp.	15	57	55	Trace	6	3	2	Trace	1	11	Trace	230	Trace	.02	Trace	Trace
	Imitation cream products (made with vegetable fat):																
	Creamers:																
46	Powdered — 1 cup	94	2	505	4	33	31	1	0	52	21	.6	²200	0	Trace	Trace	---
47	1 tsp.	2	2	10	Trace	1	Trace	Trace	0	1	1	Trace	²Trace	0	Trace	Trace	---
48	Liquid (frozen) — 1 cup	245	77	345	3	27	25	1	0	25	29	---	²100	0	0	---	---
49	1 tbsp.	15	77	20	Trace	2	1	Trace	0	2	2	---	²10	0	0	---	---
50	**Sour dressing (imitation sour cream) made with nonfat dry milk.** — 1 cup	235	72	440	9	38	35	1	Trace	17	277	.1	10	.09	.38	.2	2
51	1 tbsp.	12	72	20	Trace	2	2	Trace	Trace	1	14	Trace	Trace	Trace	Trace	Trace	Trace
	Whipped topping:																
52	Pressurized — 1 cup	70	61	190	1	17	15	1	0	9	5	---	²340	0	0	Trace	1
53	1 tbsp.	4	61	10	Trace	1	1	Trace	0	Trace	Trace	---	²20	0	0	Trace	---

² Contributed largely from beta-carotene used for coloring.

Table of Food Composition (continued)

[Dashes in the columns for nutrients show that no suitable value could be found although there is reason to believe that a measurable amount of the nutrient may be present]

	Food, approximate measure, and weight (in grams)		Water	Food energy	Protein	Fat	Fatty acids			Carbohydrate	Calcium	Iron	Vitamin A value	Thiamin	Riboflavin	Niacin	Ascorbic acid
							Saturated (total)	Unsaturated Oleic	Linoleic								
		Grams	Percent	kCalories	Grams	Grams	Grams	Grams	Grams	Grams	Milligrams	Milligrams	International units	Milligrams	Milligrams	Milligrams	Milligrams
	MILK, CHEESE, CREAM, IMITATION CREAM; RELATED PRODUCTS—Con.																
	Whipped topping—Continued																
54	Frozen — 1 cup	75	52	230	1	20	18	Trace	0	15	5	---	²560	---	0	---	---
55	1 tbsp	4	52	10	Trace	1	1	Trace	0	1	Trace	Trace	²30	---	0	---	---
56	Powdered, made with 1 cup whole milk. — 1 cup	75	58	175	3	12	10	1	Trace	15	62	Trace	²330	.02	.08	.1	Trace
57	1 tbsp	4	58	10	Trace	1	1	Trace	Trace	1	3	Trace	²20	Trace	Trace	Trace	Trace
	Milk beverages:																
58	Cocoa, homemade — 1 cup	250	79	245	10	12	7	4	Trace	27	295	1.0	400	.10	.45	.5	3
59	Chocolate-flavored drink made with skim milk and 2% added butterfat. — 1 cup	250	83	190	8	6	3	2	Trace	27	270	.5	210	.10	.40	.3	3
	Malted milk:																
60	Dry powder, approx. 3 heaping teaspoons per ounce. — 1 oz	28	3	115	4	2	---	---	---	20	82	.6	290	.09	.15	.1	0
61	Beverage — 1 cup	235	78	245	11	10	7	5	1	28	317	.7	590	.14	.49	.2	2
	Milk desserts:																
62	Custard, baked — 1 cup	265	77	305	14	15	7	5	3	29	297	1.1	930	.11	.50	.3	1
	Ice cream:																
63	Regular (approx. 10% fat). — ½ gal.	1,064	63	2,055	48	113	62	37	3	221	1,553	.5	4,680	.43	2.23	1.1	11
64	1 cup	133	63	255	6	14	8	5	Trace	28	194	.1	590	.05	.28	.1	1
65	3 fl. oz. cup	50	63	95	2	5	3	2	Trace	10	73	Trace	220	.02	.11	.1	1
66	Rich (approx. 16% fat). — ½ gal.	1,188	63	2,635	31	191	105	63	6	214	927	.2	7,840	.24	1.31	1.2	12
67	1 cup	148	63	330	4	24	13	8	1	27	115	Trace	980	.03	.16	.1	1
	Ice milk:																
68	Hardened — ½ gal.	1,048	67	1,595	50	53	29	17	2	235	1,635	1.0	2,200	.52	2.31	1.0	10
69	1 cup	131	67	200	6	7	4	2	Trace	29	204	.1	280	.07	.29	.1	1
70	Soft-serve — 1 cup	175	67	265	8	9	5	3	Trace	39	273	.2	370	.09	.39	.2	2

No.	Food and description	Measure	Grams	Water (%)	Food energy (Cal.)	Protein (g)	Fat (g)	Saturated (g)	Oleic (g)	Linoleic (g)	Carbohydrate (g)	Calcium (mg)	Iron (mg)	Vitamin A (I.U.)	Thiamine (mg)	Riboflavin (mg)	Niacin (mg)	Ascorbic acid (mg)
	Yoghurt:																	
71	Made from partially skimmed milk.	1 cup	245	89	125	8	4	2	1	Trace	13	294	.1	170	.10	.44	.2	2
72	Made from whole milk.	1 cup	245	88	150	7	8	5	3	Trace	12	272	.1	340	.07	.39	.2	2
	EGGS																	
	Eggs, large, 24 ounces per dozen:																	
	Raw or cooked in shell or with nothing added:																	
73	Whole, without shell.	1 egg	50	74	80	6	6	2	3	Trace	Trace	27	1.1	590	.05	.15	Trace	0
74	White of egg.	1 white	33	88	15	4	Trace	—	—	—	Trace	3	Trace	0	Trace	.09	Trace	0
75	Yolk of egg.	1 yolk	17	51	60	3	5	2	2	Trace	Trace	24	.9	580	.04	.07	Trace	0
76	Scrambled with milk and fat.	1 egg	64	72	110	7	8	3	3	Trace	1	51	1.1	690	.05	.18	Trace	0
	MEAT, POULTRY, FISH, SHELLFISH; RELATED PRODUCTS																	
77	Bacon, (20 slices per lb. raw), broiled or fried, crisp.	2 slices	15	8	90	5	8	3	4	1	1	2	.5	0	.08	.05	.8	—
	Beef,[3] cooked:																	
	Cuts braised, simmered, or pot-roasted:																	
78	Lean and fat.	3 ounces	85	53	245	23	16	8	7	Trace	0	10	2.9	30	.04	.18	3.5	—
79	Lean only.	2.5 ounces	72	62	140	22	5	2	2	Trace	0	10	2.7	10	.04	.16	3.3	—
	Hamburger (ground beef), broiled:																	
80	Lean.	3 ounces	85	60	185	23	10	5	4	Trace	0	10	3.0	20	.08	.20	5.1	—
81	Regular.	3 ounces	85	54	245	21	17	8	8	Trace	0	9	2.7	30	.07	.18	4.6	—
	Roast, oven-cooked, no liquid added:																	
	Relatively fat, such as rib:																	
82	Lean and fat.	3 ounces	85	40	375	17	34	16	15	1	0	8	2.2	70	.05	.13	3.1	—
83	Lean only.	1.8 ounces	51	57	125	14	7	3	3	Trace	0	6	1.8	10	.04	.11	2.6	—
	Relatively lean, such as heel of round:																	
84	Lean and fat.	3 ounces	85	62	165	25	7	3	3	Trace	0	11	3.2	10	.06	.19	4.5	—
85	Lean only.	2.7 ounces	78	65	125	24	3	1	1	Trace	0	10	3.0	Trace	.06	.18	4.3	—
	Steak, broiled:																	
	Relatively fat, such as sirloin:																	
86	Lean and fat.	3 ounces	85	44	330	20	27	13	12	1	0	9	2.5	50	.05	.16	4.0	—
87	Lean only.	2.0 ounces	56	59	115	18	4	2	2	Trace	0	7	2.2	10	.05	.14	3.6	—
	Relatively lean, such as round:																	
88	Lean and fat.	3 ounces	85	55	220	24	13	6	6	Trace	0	10	3.0	20	.07	.19	4.8	—
89	Lean only.	2.4 ounces	68	61	130	21	4	2	2	Trace	0	9	2.5	10	.06	.16	4.1	—
	Beef, canned:																	
90	Corned beef.	3 ounces	85	59	185	22	10	5	4	Trace	0	17	3.7	20	.01	.20	2.9	—
91	Corned beef hash.	3 ounces	85	67	155	7	10	5	4	Trace	9	11	1.7	—	.01	.08	1.8	—
92	Beef, dried or chipped.	2 ounces	57	48	115	19	4	2	2	Trace	0	11	2.9	—	.04	.18	2.2	—
93	Beef and vegetable stew.	1 cup	235	82	210	15	10	5	4	Trace	15	28	2.8	2,310[2]	.13	.17	4.4	15

[2] Contributed largely from beta-carotene used for coloring.

[3] Outer layer of fat on the cut was removed to within approximately ½-inch of the lean. Deposits of fat within the cut were not removed.

Table of Food Composition (continued)

[Dashes in the columns for nutrients show that no suitable value could be found although there is reason to believe that a measurable amount of the nutrient may be present]

	Food, approximate measure, and weight (in grams)	Water	Food energy	Protein	Fat	Fatty acids — Saturated (total)	Fatty acids — Unsaturated Oleic	Fatty acids — Unsaturated Linoleic	Carbohydrate	Calcium	Iron	Vitamin A value	Thiamin	Riboflavin	Niacin	Ascorbic acid
	Grams	Percent	kCalories	Grams	Grams	Grams	Grams	Grams	Grams	Milligrams	Milligrams	International units	Milligrams	Milligrams	Milligrams	Milligrams
	MEAT, POULTRY, FISH, SHELLFISH; RELATED PRODUCTS—Continued															
94	Beef potpie, baked, 4¼-inch diam., weight before baking about 8 ounces. 1 pie — 227	55	560	23	33	9	20	2	43	32	4.1	1,860	0.25	0.27	4.5	7
	Chicken, cooked:															
95	Flesh only, broiled — 3 ounces — 85	71	115	20	3	1	1	1	0	8	1.4	80	.05	.16	7.4	---
	Breast, fried, ½ breast:															
96	With bone — 3.3 ounces — 94	58	155	25	5	1	2	1	1	9	1.3	70	.04	.17	11.2	---
97	Flesh and skin only — 2.7 ounces — 76	58	155	25	5	1	2	1	1	9	1.3	70	.04	.17	11.2	---
	Drumstick, fried:															
98	With bone — 2.1 ounces — 59	55	90	12	4	1	2	1	Trace	6	.9	50	.03	.15	2.7	---
99	Flesh and skin only — 1.3 ounces — 38	55	90	12	4	1	2	1	Trace	6	.9	50	.03	.15	2.7	---
100	Chicken, canned, boneless 3 ounces — 85	65	170	18	10	3	4	2	0	18	1.3	200	.03	.11	3.7	3
101	Chicken potpie, baked 4¼-inch diam., weight before baking about 8 ounces. 1 pie — 227	57	535	23	31	10	15	3	42	68	3.0	3,020	.25	.26	4.1	5
	Chili con carne, canned:															
102	With beans 1 cup — 250	72	335	19	15	7	7	Trace	30	80	4.2	150	.08	.18	3.2	---
103	Without beans 1 cup — 255	67	510	26	38	18	17	1	15	97	3.6	380	.05	.31	5.6	---
104	Heart, beef, lean, braised 3 ounces — 85	61	160	27	5	---	---	---	1	5	5.0	20	.21	1.04	6.5	1
	Lamb, cooked:															
105	Chop, thick, with bone, 1 chop, broiled. 4.8 ounces. — 137	47	400	25	33	18	12	1	0	10	1.5	---	.14	.25	5.6	---
106	Lean and fat — 4.0 ounces — 112	47	400	25	33	18	12	1	0	10	1.5	---	.14	.25	5.6	---
107	Lean only — 2.6 ounces — 74	62	140	21	6	3	2	Trace	0	9	1.5	---	.11	.20	4.5	---
	Leg, roasted:															
108	Lean and fat — 3 ounces — 85	54	235	22	16	9	6	Trace	0	9	1.4	---	.13	.23	4.7	---
109	Lean only — 2.5 ounces — 71	62	130	20	5	3	2	Trace	0	9	1.4	---	.12	.21	4.4	---
	Shoulder, roasted:															
110	Lean and fat — 3 ounces — 85	50	285	18	23	13	8	1	0	9	1.0	---	.11	.20	4.0	---
111	Lean only — 2.3 ounces — 64	61	130	17	6	3	2	Trace	0	8	1.0	---	.10	.18	3.7	---

No.	Food	Measure	Grams	Water (%)	Food energy	Protein (g)	Fat (g)	Saturated (g)	Oleic (g)	Linoleic (g)	Carbohydrate (g)	Calcium (mg)	Iron (mg)	Vitamin A (I.U.)	Thiamine (mg)	Riboflavin (mg)	Niacin (mg)	Ascorbic acid (mg)
112	Liver, beef, fried	2 ounces	57	57	130	15	6	—	—	—	3	6	5.0	30,280	.15	2.37	9.4	15
113	Pork, cured, cooked: Ham, light cure, lean and fat, roasted.	3 ounces	85	54	245	18	19	7	8	2	0	8	2.2	0	.40	.16	3.1	—
114	Luncheon meat: Boiled ham, sliced	2 ounces	57	59	135	11	10	4	4	1	0	6	1.6	0	.25	.09	1.5	—
115	Canned, spiced or unspiced.	2 ounces	57	55	165	8	14	5	6	1	1	5	1.2	0	.18	.12	1.6	—
116	Pork, fresh,³ cooked: Chop, thick, with bone.	1 chop, 3.5 ounces	98	42	260	16	21	8	9	2	0	8	2.2	0	.63	.18	3.8	—
117	Lean and fat	2.3 ounces	66	42	260	16	21	8	9	2	0	8	2.2	0	.63	.18	3.8	—
118	Lean only	1.7 ounces	48	53	130	15	7	2	3	1	0	7	1.9	0	.54	.16	3.3	—
119	Roast, oven-cooked, no liquid added: Lean and fat	3 ounces	85	46	310	21	24	9	10	2	0	9	2.7	0	.78	.22	4.7	—
120	Lean only	2.4 ounces	68	55	175	20	10	3	4	1	0	9	2.6	0	.73	.21	4.4	—
121	Cuts, simmered: Lean and fat	3 ounces	85	46	320	20	26	9	11	2	0	8	2.5	0	.46	.21	4.1	—
122	Lean only	2.2 ounces	63	60	135	18	6	2	3	1	0	8	2.3	0	.42	.19	3.7	—
123	Sausage: Bologna, slice, 3-in. diam. by ⅛ inch.	2 slices	26	56	80	3	7	—	—	—	Trace	2	.5	—	.04	.06	.7	—
124	Braunschweiger, slice 2-in. diam. by ¼ inch.	2 slices	20	53	65	3	5	—	—	—	Trace	2	1.2	1,310	.03	.29	1.6	—
125	Deviled ham, canned	1 tbsp.	13	51	45	2	4	2	2	Trace	0	1	.3	—	.02	.01	.2	—
126	Frankfurter, heated (8 per lb. purchased pkg.).	1 frank.	56	57	170	7	15	—	—	—	1	3	.8	—	.08	.11	1.4	—
127	Pork links, cooked (16 links per lb. raw).	2 links	26	35	125	5	11	4	5	1	Trace	2	.6	0	.21	.09	1.0	—
128	Salami, dry type	1 oz.	28	30	130	7	11	—	—	—	Trace	4	1.0	—	.10	.07	1.5	—
129	Salami, cooked	1 oz.	28	51	90	5	7	—	—	—	Trace	3	.7	—	.07	.07	1.2	—
130	Vienna, canned (7 sausages per 5-oz. can).	1 sausage	16	63	40	2	3	—	—	—	Trace	1	.3	—	.01	.02	.4	—
131	Veal, medium fat, cooked, bone removed: Cutlet	3 oz.	85	60	185	23	9	5	4	Trace	0	9	2.7	—	.06	.21	4.6	—
132	Roast	3 oz.	85	55	230	23	14	7	6	Trace	0	10	2.9	—	.11	.26	6.6	—
133	Fish and shellfish: Bluefish, baked with table fat.	3 oz.	85	68	135	22	4	—	—	—	0	25	.6	40	.09	.08	1.6	—
134	Clams: Raw, meat only	3 oz.	85	82	65	11	1	—	—	—	2	59	5.2	90	.08	.15	1.1	8
135	Canned, solids and liquid.	3 oz.	85	86	45	7	1	—	—	—	2	47	3.5	—	.01	.09	.9	—
136	Crabmeat, canned	3 oz.	85	77	85	15	2	—	—	—	1	38	.7	—	.07	.07	1.6	—

³ Outer layer of fat on the cut was removed to within approximately ½-inch of the lean. Deposits of fat within the cut were not removed.

Table of Food Composition (continued)

[Dashes in the columns for nutrients show that no suitable value could be found although there is reason to believe that a measurable amount of the nutrient may be present]

No.	Food, approximate measure, and weight (in grams)	Weight (Grams)	Water (Percent)	Food energy (kCalories)	Protein (Grams)	Fat (Grams)	Saturated (total) (Grams)	Unsaturated Oleic (Grams)	Unsaturated Linoleic (Grams)	Carbohydrate (Grams)	Calcium (Milligrams)	Iron (Milligrams)	Vitamin A value (International units)	Thiamin (Milligrams)	Riboflavin (Milligrams)	Niacin (Milligrams)	Ascorbic acid (Milligrams)
	MEAT, POULTRY, FISH, SHELLFISH; RELATED PRODUCTS—Continued																
	Fish and shellfish—Continued																
137	Fish sticks, breaded, cooked, frozen; stick 3¾ by 1 by ½ inch. 10 sticks or 8 oz. pkg.	227	66	400	38	20	5	4	10	15	25	0.9	---	0.09	0.16	3.6	---
138	Haddock, breaded, fried 3 oz.	85	66	140	17	5	1	3	Trace	5	34	1.0	---	.03	.06	2.7	---
139	Ocean perch, breaded, fried. 3 oz.	85	59	195	16	11	---	---	---	6	28	1.1	---	.08	.09	1.5	2
140	Oysters, raw, meat only (13–19 med. selects). 1 cup	240	85	160	20	4	---	---	---	8	226	13.2	740	.33	.43	6.0	---
141	Salmon, pink, canned. 3 oz.	85	71	120	17	5	1	1	Trace	0	¹167	.7	60	.03	.16	6.8	---
142	Sardines, Atlantic, canned in oil, drained solids. 3 oz.	85	62	175	20	9	---	---	---	0	372	2.5	190	.02	.17	4.6	---
143	Shad, baked with table fat and bacon. 3 oz.	85	64	170	20	10	---	---	---	0	20	.5	20	.11	.22	7.3	---
144	Shrimp, canned, meat. 3 oz.	85	70	100	21	1	---	---	---	1	98	2.6	50	.01	.03	1.5	---
145	Swordfish, broiled with butter or margarine. 3 oz.	85	65	150	24	5	---	---	---	0	23	1.1	1,750	.03	.04	9.3	---
146	Tuna, canned in oil, drained solids. 3 oz.	85	61	170	24	7	2	1	1	0	7	1.6	70	.04	.10	10.1	---
	MATURE DRY BEANS AND PEAS, NUTS, PEANUTS; RELATED PRODUCTS																
147	Almonds, shelled, whole kernels. 1 cup	142	5	850	26	77	6	52	15	28	332	6.7	0	.34	1.31	5.0	Trace
	Beans, dry: Common varieties as Great Northern, navy, and others: Cooked, drained:																
148	Great Northern. 1 cup	180	69	210	14	1	---	---	---	38	90	4.9	0	.25	.13	1.3	0

#	Food	Measure																
149	Navy (pea)	1 cup	190	69	225	15	1	—	—	—	40	95	5.1	0	.27	.13	1.3	0
	Canned, solids and liquid: White with—																	
150	Frankfurters (sliced).	1 cup	255	71	365	19	18	—	3	1	32	94	4.8	330	.18	.15	3.3	Trace
151	Pork and tomato sauce.	1 cup	255	71	310	16	7	2	3	—	49	138	4.6	330	.20	.08	1.5	5
152	Pork and sweet sauce.	1 cup	255	66	385	12	12	4	5	1	54	161	5.9	—	.15	.10	1.3	—
153	Red kidney	1 cup	255	76	230	15	1	—	—	—	42	74	4.6	10	.13	.10	1.5	—
154	Lima, cooked, drained.	1 cup	190	64	260	16	1	—	—	—	49	55	5.9	—	.25	.11	1.3	—
155	Cashew nuts, roasted	1 cup	140	5	785	24	64	11	45	4	41	53	5.3	140	.60	.35	2.5	—
	Coconut, fresh, meat only:																	
156	Pieces, approx. 2 by 2 by ½ inch.	1 piece	45	51	155	2	16	14	1	Trace	4	6	.8	0	.02	.01	.2	1
157	Shredded or grated, firmly packed.	1 cup	130	51	450	5	46	39	3	Trace	12	17	2.2	0	.07	.03	.7	4
158	Cowpeas or blackeye peas, dry, cooked.	1 cup	248	80	190	13	1	—	—	—	34	42	3.2	20	.41	.11	1.1	Trace
159	Peanuts, roasted, salted, halves.	1 cup	144	2	840	37	72	16	31	21	27	107	3.0	—	.46	.19	24.7	0
160	Peanut butter	1 tbsp.	16	2	95	4	8	2	4	2	3	9	.3	—	.02	.02	2.4	0
161	Peas, split, dry, cooked	1 cup	250	70	290	20	1	—	—	—	52	28	4.2	100	.37	.22	2.2	—
162	Pecans, halves	1 cup	108	3	740	10	77	5	48	15	16	79	2.6	140	.93	.14	1.0	2
163	Walnuts, black or native, chopped.	1 cup	126	3	790	26	75	4	26	36	19	Trace	7.6	380	.28	.14	.9	—

VEGETABLES AND VEGETABLE PRODUCTS

#	Food	Measure																
	Asparagus, green: Cooked, drained:																	
164	Spears, ½-in. diam. at base.	4 spears	60	94	10	1	Trace	—	—	—	2	13	.4	540	.10	.11	.8	16
165	Pieces, 1½ to 2-in. lengths.	1 cup	145	94	30	3	Trace	—	—	—	5	30	.9	1,310	.23	.26	2.0	38
166	Canned, solids and liquid	1 cup	244	94	45	5	1	—	—	—	7	44	4.1	1,240	.15	.22	2.0	37
	Beans:																	
167	Lima, immature seeds, cooked, drained.	1 cup	170	71	190	13	1	—	—	—	34	80	4.3	480	.31	.17	2.2	29
	Snap: Green:																	
168	Cooked, drained	1 cup	125	92	30	2	Trace	—	—	—	7	63	.8	680	.09	.11	.6	15
169	Canned, solids and liquid.	1 cup	239	94	45	2	Trace	—	—	—	10	81	2.9	690	.07	.10	.7	10

¹ If bones are discarded, value will be greatly reduced.

Table of Food Composition (continued)

[Dashes in the columns for nutrients show that no suitable value could be found although there is reason to believe that a measurable amount of the nutrient may be present]

	Food, approximate measure, and weight (in grams)		Water	Food energy	Protein	Fat	Fatty acids			Carbohydrate	Calcium	Iron	Vitamin A value	Thiamin	Riboflavin	Niacin	Ascorbic acid
							Saturated (total)	Unsaturated Oleic	Linoleic								
		Grams	Per cent	kCalories	Grams	Grams	Grams	Grams	Grams	Grams	Milligrams	Milligrams	International units	Milligrams	Milligrams	Milligrams	Milligrams
	VEGETABLES AND VEGETABLE PRODUCTS—Continued																
	Beans—Continued																
	Snap—Continued																
	Yellow or wax:																
170	Cooked, drained-- 1 cup	125	93	30	2	Trace	---	---	---	6	63	0.8	290	0.09	0.11	0.6	16
171	Canned, solids and liquid. 1 cup	239	94	45	2	1	---	---	---	10	81	2.9	140	.07	.10	.7	12
172	Sprouted mung beans, cooked, drained. 1 cup	125	91	35	4	Trace	---	---	---	7	21	1.1	30	.11	.13	.9	8
	Beets:																
	Cooked, drained, peeled:																
173	Whole beets, 2-in. diam. 2 beets	100	91	30	1	Trace				7	14	.5	20	.03	.04	.3	6
174	Diced or sliced 1 cup	170	91	55	2	Trace	---	---	---	12	24	.9	30	.05	.07	.5	10
175	Canned, solids and liquid. 1 cup	246	90	85	2	Trace	---	---	---	19	34	1.5	20	.02	.05	.2	7
176	Beet greens, leaves and stems, cooked, drained. 1 cup	145	94	25	3	Trace	---	---	---	5	144	2.8	7,400	.10	.22	.4	22
	Blackeye peas. See Cowpeas.																
	Broccoli, cooked, drained:																
177	Whole stalks, medium size. 1 stalk	180	91	45	6	1	---	---	---	8	158	1.4	4,500	.16	.36	1.4	162
178	Stalks cut into ½-in. pieces. 1 cup	155	91	40	5	1	---	---	---	7	136	1.2	3,880	.14	.31	1.2	140
179	Chopped, yield from 10-oz. frozen pkg. 1⅜ cups	250	92	65	7	1	---	---	---	12	135	1.8	6,500	.15	.30	1.3	143
180	Brussels sprouts, 7-8 sprouts (1¼ to 1½ in. diam.) per cup, cooked. 1 cup	155	88	55	7	1	---	---	---	10	50	1.7	810	.12	.22	1.2	135
	Cabbage:																
	Common varieties:																

No.	Food	Measure	Grams	Water (%)	Food energy	Protein (g)	Fat (g)	Fatty acids			Carbohydrate (g)	Calcium (mg)	Iron (mg)	Vitamin A (I.U.)	Thiamin (mg)	Riboflavin (mg)	Niacin (mg)	Ascorbic acid (mg)
	Raw:																	
181	Coarsely shredded or sliced.	1 cup	70	92	15	1	Trace	---	---	---	4	34	.3	90	.04	.04	.2	33
182	Finely shredded or chopped.	1 cup	90	92	20	1	Trace	---	---	---	5	44	.4	120	.05	.05	.3	42
183	Cooked.	1 cup	145	94	30	2	Trace	---	---	---	6	64	.4	190	.06	.06	.4	48
184	Red, raw, coarsely shredded.	1 cup	70	90	20	1	Trace	---	---	---	5	29	.6	30	.06	.04	.3	43
185	Savoy, raw, coarsely shredded.	1 cup	70	92	15	2	Trace	---	---	---	3	47	.6	140	.04	.06	.2	39
186	Cabbage, celery or Chinese, raw, cut in 1-in. pieces.	1 cup	75	95	10	1	Trace	---	---	---	2	32	.5	110	.04	.03	.5	19
187	Cabbage, spoon (or pakchoy), cooked.	1 cup	170	95	25	2	Trace	---	---	---	4	252	1.0	5,270	.07	.14	1.2	26
	Carrots:																	
	Raw:																	
188	Whole, 5½ by 1 inch, 1 carrot (25 thin strips).	1 carrot	50	88	20	1	Trace	---	---	---	5	18	.4	5,500	.03	.03	.3	4
189	Grated.	1 cup	110	88	45	1	Trace	---	---	---	11	41	.8	12,100	.06	.06	.7	9
190	Cooked, diced.	1 cup	145	91	45	1	Trace	---	---	---	10	48	.9	15,220	.08	.07	.7	9
191	Canned, strained or chopped (baby food).	1 ounce	28	92	10	Trace	Trace	---	---	---	2	7	.1	3,690	.01	.01	.1	1
192	Cauliflower, cooked, flowerbuds.	1 cup	120	93	25	3	Trace	---	---	---	5	25	.8	70	.11	.10	.7	66
	Celery, raw:																	
193	Stalk, large outer, 8 by about 1½ inches, at root end.	1 stalk	40	94	5	Trace	Trace	---	---	---	2	16	.1	100	.01	.01	.1	4
194	Pieces, diced.	1 cup	100	94	15	1	Trace	---	---	---	4	39	.3	240	.03	.03	.3	9
195	Collards, cooked.	1 cup	190	91	55	5	1	---	---	---	9	289	1.1	10,260	.27	.37	2.4	87
	Corn, sweet:																	
196	Cooked, ear 5 by 1¾ inches.[5]	1 ear	140	74	70	3	1	---	---	---	16	2	.5	310[*]	.09	.08	1.0	7
197	Canned, solids and liquid.	1 cup	256	81	170	5	2	---	---	---	40	10	1.0	690[*]	.07	.12	2.3	13
198	Cowpeas, cooked, immature seeds.	1 cup	160	72	175	13	1	---	---	---	29	38	3.4	560	.49	.18	2.3	28
	Cucumbers, 10-ounce; 7½ by about 2 inches:																	
199	Raw, pared.	1 cucumber	207	96	30	1	Trace	---	---	---	7	35	.6	Trace	.07	.09	.4	23
200	Raw, pared, center slice ⅛-inch thick.	6 slices	50	96	5	Trace	Trace	---	---	---	2	8	.2	Trace	.02	.02	.1	6
201	Dandelion greens, cooked.	1 cup	180	90	60	4	1	---	---	---	12	252	3.2	21,060	.24	.29		32

* Measure and weight apply to entire vegetable or fruit including parts not usually eaten.

* Based on yellow varieties; white varieties contain only a trace of cryptoxanthin and carotenes, the pigments in corn that have biological activity.

Table of Food Composition (continued)

[Dashes in the columns for nutrients show that no suitable value could be found although there is reason to believe that a measurable amount of the nutrient may be present]

	Food, approximate measure, and weight (in grams)	Water	Food energy	Pro-tein	Fat	Fatty acids Satu-rated (total)	Fatty acids Unsaturated Oleic	Fatty acids Unsaturated Lin-oleic	Carbo-hy-drate	Cal-cium	Iron	Vita-min A value	Thia-min	Ribo-flavin	Niacin	Ascor-bic acid
		Per-cent	*kCalo-ries*	*Grams*	*Grams*	*Grams*	*Grams*	*Grams*	*Grams*	*Milli-grams*	*Milli-grams*	*Inter-national units*	*Milli-grams*	*Milli-grams*	*Milli-grams*	*Milli-grams*
	VEGETABLES AND VEGETABLE PRODUCTS—Continued															
202	Endive, curly (including escarole). 2 ounces — 57	93	10	1	Trace				2	46	1.0	1,870	0.04	0.08	0.3	6
203	Kale, leaves including stems, cooked. 1 cup — 110	91	30	4	1				4	147	1.3	8,140	—	—	—	68
	Lettuce, raw:															
204	Butterhead, as Boston types; head, 4-inch diameter. 1 head — 220	95	30	3	Trace				6	77	4.4	2,130	.14	.13	.6	18
205	Crisphead, as Iceberg; 1 head, 4¾-inch diameter. 1 head — 454	96	60	4	Trace				13	91	2.3	1,500	.29	.27	1.3	29
206	Looseleaf, or bunching varieties, leaves. 2 large — 50	94	10	1	Trace				2	34	.7	950	.03	.04	.2	9
207	Mushrooms, canned, solids and liquid. 1 cup — 244	93	40	5	Trace				6	15	1.2	Trace	.04	.60	4.8	4
208	Mustard greens, cooked. 1 cup — 140	93	35	3	1				6	193	2.5	8,120	.11	.19	.9	68
209	Okra, cooked, pod 3 by ⅝ inch. 8 pods — 85	91	25	2	Trace				5	78	.4	420	.11	.15	.8	17
	Onions:															
	Mature:															
210	Raw, onion 2½-inch diameter. 1 onion — 110	89	40	2	Trace				10	30	.6	40	.04	.04	.2	11
211	Cooked. 1 cup — 210	92	60	3	Trace				14	50	.8	80	.06	.06	.4	14
212	Young green, small, without tops. 6 onions — 50	88	20	1	Trace				5	20	.3	Trace	.02	.02	.2	12
213	Parsley, raw, chopped. 1 tablespoon — 4	85	Trace	Trace	Trace				Trace	8	.2	340	Trace	.01	Trace	7
214	Parsnips, cooked. 1 cup — 155	82	100	2	1				23	70	.9	50	.11	.12	.2	16
	Peas, green:															
215	Cooked. 1 cup — 160	82	115	9	1				19	37	2.9	860	.44	.17	3.7	33
216	Canned, solids and liquid. 1 cup — 249	83	165	9	1				31	50	4.2	1,120	.23	.13	2.2	22

No.	Food, approximate measure, and weight	Grams	Water (%)	Food energy (cal.)	Protein (g)	Fat (g)	Saturated	Oleic	Linoleic	Carbohydrate (g)	Calcium (mg)	Iron (mg)	Vitamin A (I.U.)	Thiamine (mg)	Riboflavin (mg)	Niacin (mg)	Ascorbic acid (mg)
217	Canned, strained (baby food). 1 ounce	28	86	15	1	Trace	---	---	---	3	3	.4	140	.02	.02	.4	3
218	Peppers, hot, red, without seeds, dried (ground chili powder, added seasonings). 1 tablespoon	15	8	50	2	2	---	---	---	8	40	2.3	9,750	.03	.17	1.3	2
	Peppers, sweet:																
219	Raw, about 5 per pound: Green pod without stem and seeds. 1 pod	74	93	15	1	Trace	---	---	---	4	7	.5	310	.06	.06	.4	94
220	Cooked, boiled, drained 1 pod	73	95	15	1	Trace	---	---	---	3	7	.4	310	.05	.05	.4	70
	Potatoes, medium (about 3 per pound raw):																
221	Baked, peeled after baking. 1 potato	99	75	90	3	Trace	---	---	---	21	9	.7	Trace	.10	.04	1.7	20
	Boiled:																
222	Peeled after boiling 1 potato	136	80	105	3	Trace	---	---	---	23	10	.8	Trace	.13	.05	2.0	22
223	Peeled before boiling 1 potato	122	83	80	2	Trace	---	---	---	18	7	.6	Trace	.11	.04	1.4	20
	French-fried, piece 2 by ½ by ½ inch:																
224	Cooked in deep fat 10 pieces	57	45	155	2	7	2	2	4	20	9	.7	Trace	.07	.04	1.8	12
225	Frozen, heated 10 pieces	57	53	125	2	5	1	1	2	19	5	1.0	Trace	.08	.01	1.5	12
	Mashed:																
226	Milk added 1 cup	195	83	125	4	1	---	---	---	25	47	.8	50	.16	.10	2.0	19
227	Milk and butter added. 1 cup	195	80	185	4	8	4	3	Trace	24	47	.8	330	.16	.10	1.9	18
228	Potato chips, medium, 2-inch diameter. 10 chips	20	2	115	1	8	2	2	4	10	8	.4	Trace	.04	.01	1.0	3
229	Pumpkin, canned 1 cup	228	90	75	2	1	---	---	---	18	57	.9	14,590	.07	.12	1.3	12
230	Radishes, raw, small, without tops. 4 radishes	40	94	5	Trace	Trace	---	---	---	1	12	.4	Trace	.01	.01	.1	10
231	Sauerkraut, canned, solids and liquid. 1 cup	235	93	45	2	Trace	---	---	---	9	85	1.2	120	.07	.09	.4	33
	Spinach:																
232	Cooked 1 cup	180	92	40	5	1	---	---	---	6	167	4.0	14,580	.13	.25	1.0	50
233	Canned, drained solids 1 cup	180	91	45	5	1	---	---	---	6	212	4.7	14,400	.03	.21	.6	24
	Squash: Cooked:																
234	Summer, diced 1 cup	210	96	30	2	Trace	---	---	---	7	52	.8	820	.10	.16	1.6	21
235	Winter, baked, mashed. 1 cup	205	81	130	4	1	---	---	---	32	57	1.6	8,610	.10	.27	1.4	27
	Sweetpotatoes: Cooked, medium, 5 by 2 inches, weight raw about 6 ounces:																
236	Baked, peeled after baking. 1 sweetpotato	110	64	155	2	1	---	---	---	36	44	1.0	8,910	.10	.07	.7	24
237	Boiled, peeled after boiling. 1 sweetpotato	147	71	170	2	1	---	---	---	39	47	1.0	11,610	.13	.09	.9	25

Table of Food Composition (continued)

[Dashes in the columns for nutrients show that no suitable value could be found although there is reason to believe that a measurable amount of the nutrient may be present]

	Food, approximate measure, and weight (in grams)		Water	Food energy	Protein	Fat	Fatty acids			Carbo-hydrate	Calcium	Iron	Vitamin A value	Thiamin	Ribo-flavin	Niacin	Ascorbic acid
							Satu-rated (total)	Unsaturated Oleic	Unsaturated Lin-oleic								
		Grams	Per cent	kCalo-ries	Grams	Grams	Grams	Grams	Grams	Grams	Milli-grams	Milli-grams	Inter-national units	Milli-grams	Milli-grams	Milli-grams	Milli-grams
	VEGETABLES AND VEGETABLE PRODUCTS—Continued																
	Sweetpotatoes—Continued																
238	Candied, 3½ by 2¼ inches.	1 sweet-potato. 175	60	295	2	6	2	3	1	60	65	1.6	11,030	0.10	0.08	0.8	17
239	Canned, vacuum or solid pack.	1 cup 218	72	235	4	Trace				54	54	1.7	17,000	.10	.10	1.4	30
	Tomatoes:																
240	Raw, approx. 3-in. diam. 2⅛ in. high; wt., 7 oz.	1 tomato 200	94	40	2	Trace				9	24	.9	1,640	.11	.07	1.3	⁷42
241	Canned, solids and liquid.	1 cup 241	94	50	2	1				10	14	1.2	2,170	.12	.07	1.7	41
	Tomato catsup:																
242	Cup	1 cup 273	69	290	6	1				69	60	2.2	3,820	.25	.19	4.4	41
243	Tablespoon	1 tbsp. 15	69	15	Trace	Trace				4	3	.1	210	.01	.01	.2	2
	Tomato juice, canned:																
244	Cup	1 cup 243	94	45	2	Trace				10	17	2.2	1,940	.12	.07	1.9	39
245	Glass (6 fl. oz.)	1 glass 182	94	35	2	Trace				8	13	1.6	1,460	.09	.05	1.5	29
246	Turnips, cooked, diced	1 cup 155	94	35	1	Trace				8	54	.6	Trace	.06	.08	.5	34
247	Turnip greens, cooked	1 cup 145	94	30	3	Trace				5	252	1.5	8,270	.15	.33	.7	68
	FRUITS AND FRUIT PRODUCTS																
248	Apples, raw (about 3 per lb.).⁵	1 apple 150	85	70	Trace	Trace				18	8	.4	50	.04	.02	.1	3
249	Apple juice, bottled or canned.	1 cup 248	88	120	Trace	Trace				30	15	1.5	---	.02	.05	.2	2
	Applesauce, canned:																
250	Sweetened	1 cup 255	76	230	1	Trace				61	10	1.3	100	.05	.03	.1	⁸3
251	Unsweetened or artificially sweetened.	1 cup 244	88	100	1	Trace				26	10	1.2	100	.05	.02	.1	⁸2

No.	Food, approximate measure	Weight (g)	Water (%)	Food energy (Cal.)	Protein (g)	Fat (g)	Saturated fatty acids (total) (g)	Unsaturated oleic (g)	Unsaturated linoleic (g)	Carbohydrate (g)	Calcium (mg)	Iron (mg)	Vitamin A (I.U.)	Thiamine (mg)	Riboflavin (mg)	Niacin (mg)	Ascorbic acid (mg)
	Apricots:																
252	Raw (about 12 per lb.) [5] 3 apricots	114	85	55	1	Trace	---	---	---	14	18	.5	2,890	.03	.04	.7	10
253	Canned in heavy sirup 1 cup	259	77	220	2	Trace	---	---	---	57	28	.8	4,510	.05	.06	.9	10
254	Dried, uncooked (40 halves per cup) 1 cup	150	25	390	8	1	---	---	---	100	100	8.2	16,350	.02	.23	4.9	19
255	Cooked, unsweetened, fruit and liquid 1 cup	285	76	240	5	1	---	---	---	62	63	5.1	8,550	.01	.13	2.8	8
256	Apricot nectar, canned 1 cup	251	85	140	1	Trace	---	---	---	37	23	.5	2,380	.03	.03	.5	[8] 8
257	Avocados, whole fruit, raw: [5] California (mid- and late-winter; diam. 3⅛ in.) 1 avocado	284	74	370	5	37	7	17	5	13	22	1.3	630	.24	.43	3.5	30
258	Florida (late summer, fall; diam. 3⅝ in.) 1 avocado	454	78	390	4	33	7	15	4	27	30	1.8	880	.33	.61	4.9	43
259	Bananas, raw, medium size. [5] 1 banana	175	76	100	1	Trace	---	---	---	26	10	.8	230	.06	.07	.8	12
260	Banana flakes 1 cup	100	3	340	4	1	---	---	---	89	32	2.8	760	.18	.24	2.8	7
261	Blackberries, raw 1 cup	144	84	85	2	1	---	---	---	19	46	1.3	290	.05	.06	.5	30
262	Blueberries, raw 1 cup	140	83	85	1	1	---	---	---	21	21	1.4	140	.04	.08	.6	20
263	Cantaloups, raw; medium; 5-inch diameter about 1⅔ pounds. [5] ½ melon	385	91	60	1	Trace	---	---	---	14	27	.8	[9] 6,540	.08	.06	1.2	63
264	Cherries, canned, red, sour, pitted, water pack 1 cup	244	88	105	2	Trace	---	---	---	26	37	.7	1,660	.07	.05	.5	12
265	Cranberry juice cocktail, canned. 1 cup	250	83	165	Trace	Trace	---	---	---	42	13	.8	Trace	.03	.03	.1	[10] 40
266	Cranberry sauce, sweetened, canned, strained. 1 cup	277	62	405	Trace	1	---	---	---	104	17	.6	60	.03	.03	.1	6
267	Dates, pitted, cut 1 cup	178	22	490	4	1	---	---	---	130	105	5.3	90	.16	.17	3.9	0
268	Figs, dried, large, 2 by 1 in. 1 fig	21	23	60	1	Trace	---	---	---	15	26	.6	20	.02	.02	.1	0
269	Fruit cocktail, canned, in heavy sirup. 1 cup	256	80	195	1	Trace	---	---	---	50	23	1.0	360	.05	.03	1.3	5

[5] Measure and weight apply to entire vegetable or fruit including parts not usually eaten.

[7] Year-round average. Samples marketed from November through May, average 20 milligrams per 200-gram tomato; from June through October, around 52 milligrams.

[8] This is the amount from the fruit. Additional ascorbic acid may be added by the manufacturer. Refer to the label for this information.

[9] Value for varieties with orange-colored flesh; value for varieties with green flesh would be about 540 I.U.

[10] Value listed is based on products with label stating 30 milligrams per 6 fl. oz. serving.

Table of Food Composition (continued)

[Dashes in the columns for nutrients show that no suitable value could be found although there is reason to believe that a measurable amount of the nutrient may be present]

	Food, approximate measure, and weight (in grams)	Water	Food energy	Protein	Fat	Fatty acids — Saturated (total)	Fatty acids — Unsaturated Oleic	Fatty acids — Unsaturated Linoleic	Carbohydrate	Calcium	Iron	Vitamin A value	Thiamin	Riboflavin	Niacin	Ascorbic acid
		Percent	kCalories	Grams	Grams	Grams	Grams	Grams	Grams	Milligrams	Milligrams	International units	Milligrams	Milligrams	Milligrams	Milligrams
	FRUITS AND FRUIT PRODUCTS—Con.															
	Grapefruit:															
270	Raw, medium, 3¾-in. diam.⁵ White — ½ grapefruit.	89	45	1	Trace				12	19	0.5	10	0.05	0.02	0.2	44
271	Pink or red — ½ grapefruit.	89	50	1	Trace				13	20	0.5	540	0.05	0.02	0.2	44
272	Canned, sirup pack — 1 cup	81	180	2	Trace				45	33	.8	30	.08	.05	.5	76
	Grapefruit juice:															
273	Fresh — 1 cup	90	95	1	Trace				23	22	.5	(¹¹)	.09	.04	.4	92
	Canned, white:															
274	Unsweetened — 1 cup	89	100	1	Trace				24	20	1.0	20	.07	.04	.4	84
275	Sweetened — 1 cup	86	130	1	Trace				32	20	1.0	20	.07	.04	.4	78
	Frozen, concentrate, unsweetened:															
276	Undiluted, can, 6 fluid ounces. — 1 can	62	300	4	1				72	70	.8	60	.29	.12	1.4	286
277	Diluted with 3 parts water, by volume. — 1 cup	89	100	1	Trace				24	25	.2	20	.10	.04	.5	96
278	Dehydrated crystals — 4 oz.	1	410	6	1				102	100	1.2	80	.40	.20	2.0	396
279	Prepared with water — 1 cup (1 pound yields about 1 gallon).	90	100	1	Trace				24	22	.2	20	.10	.05	.5	91
	Grapes, raw:⁵															
280	American type (slip skin). — 1 cup	82	65	1	1				15	15	.4	100	.05	.03	.2	3
281	European type (adherent skin). — 1 cup	81	95	1	Trace				25	17	.6	140	.07	.04	.4	6
	Grapejuice:															
282	Canned or bottled — 1 cup	83	165	1	Trace				42	28	.8	---	.10	.05	.5	Trace
	Frozen concentrate, sweetened:															
283	Undiluted, can, 6 fluid ounces. — 1 can	53	395	1	Trace				100	22	.9	40	.13	.22	1.5	(¹²)

(Grams weights, reading the food column: 270 = 241; 271 = 241; 272 = 254; 273 = 246; 274 = 247; 275 = 250; 276 = 207; 277 = 247; 278 = 113; 279 = 247; 280 = 153; 281 = 160; 282 = 253; 283 = 216.)

No.	Food, approximate measure	Measure	Grams	Water (%)	Food energy (Cal.)	Protein (g)	Fat (g)	Saturated fatty acids	Oleic	Linoleic	Carbohydrate (g)	Calcium (mg)	Iron (mg)	Vitamin A (I.U.)	Thiamine (mg)	Riboflavin (mg)	Niacin (mg)	Ascorbic acid (mg)
284	Diluted with 3 parts water, by volume.	1 cup	250	86	135	1	Trace	—	—	—	33	8	.3	10	.05	.08	.5	(12)
285	Grapejuice drink, canned.	1 cup	250	86	135	Trace	Trace	—	—	—	35	8	.3	10	.03	.03	.3	(12)
286	Lemons, raw, 2⅛-in. diam., size 165.⁵ Used for juice.	1 lemon	110	90	20	1	Trace	—	—	—	6	19	.4	—	.03	.01	.1	39
287	Lemon juice, raw.	1 cup	244	91	60	1	Trace	—	—	—	20	17	.5	50	.07	.02	.2	112
288	Lemonade concentrate: Frozen, 6 fl. oz. per can.	1 can	219	48	430	Trace	Trace	—	—	—	112	9	.4	40	.04	.07	.7	66
289	Diluted with 4⅓ parts water, by volume.	1 cup	248	88	110	Trace	Trace	—	—	—	28	2	Trace	Trace	Trace	.02	.2	17
290	Lime juice: Fresh.	1 cup	246	90	65	1	Trace	—	—	—	22	22	.5	20	.05	.02	.2	79
291	Canned, unsweetened.	1 cup	246	90	65	1	Trace	—	—	—	22	22	.5	20	.05	.02	.2	52
292	Limeade concentrate, frozen: Undiluted, can, 6 fluid ounces.	1 can	218	50	410	Trace	Trace	—	—	—	108	11	.2	Trace	.02	.02	.2	26
293	Diluted with 4⅓ parts water, by volume.	1 cup	247	90	100	Trace	Trace	—	—	—	27	2	Trace	Trace	Trace	Trace	Trace	5
294	Oranges, raw, 2⅝-in. diam., all commercial varieties.⁵	1 orange	180	86	65	1	Trace	—	—	—	16	54	.5	260	.13	.05	.5	66
295	Orange juice, fresh, all varieties.	1 cup	248	88	110	2	1	—	—	—	26	27	.5	500	.22	.07	1.0	124
296	Canned, unsweetened.	1 cup	249	87	120	2	Trace	—	—	—	28	25	1.0	500	.17	.05	.7	100
297	Frozen concentrate:⁵ Undiluted, can, 6 fluid ounces.	1 can	213	55	360	5	Trace	—	—	—	87	75	.9	1,620	.68	.11	2.8	360
298	Diluted with 3 parts water, by volume.	1 cup	249	87	120	2	Trace	—	—	—	29	25	.2	550	.22	.02	1.0	120
299	Dehydrated crystals.	4 oz.	113	1	430	6	2	—	—	—	100	95	1.9	1,900	.76	.24	3.3	408
300	Prepared with water (1 pound yields about 1 gallon).	1 cup	248	88	115	2	1	—	—	—	27	25	.5	500	.20	.07	1.0	109
301	Orange-apricot juice drink.	1 cup	249	87	125	1	Trace	—	—	—	32	12	.2	1,440	.05	.02	.5	¹⁰ 40

⁵ Measure and weight apply to entire vegetable or fruit including parts not usually eaten.

¹⁰ Value listed is based on product with label stating 30 milligrams per 6 fl. oz. serving.

¹¹ For white-fleshed varieties value is about 20 I.U. per cup; for red-fleshed varieties, 1,080 I.U. per cup.

¹² Present only if added by the manufacturer. Refer to the label for this information.

Table of Food Composition (continued)

[Dashes in the columns for nutrients show that no suitable value could be found although there is reason to believe that a measurable amount of the nutrient may be present]

	Food, approximate measure, and weight (in grams)	Water	Food energy	Protein	Fat	Fatty acids Saturated (total)	Fatty acids Unsaturated Oleic	Fatty acids Unsaturated Linoleic	Carbo-hy-drate	Calcium	Iron	Vita-min A value	Thia-min	Ribo-flavin	Niacin	Ascor-bic acid
		Per-cent	kCalo-ries	Grams	Grams	Grams	Grams	Grams	Grams	Milli-grams	Milli-grams	Inter-national units	Milli-grams	Milli-grams	Milli-grams	Milli-grams
	FRUITS AND FRUIT PRODUCTS—Con.															
	Orange and grapefruit juice:															
	Frozen concentrate:															
302	Undiluted, can, 6 fluid ounces. 1 can — 210	59	330	4	1				78	61	0.8	800	0.48	0.06	2.3	302
303	Diluted with 3 parts water, by volume. 1 cup — 248	88	110	1	Trace				26	20	.2	270	.16	.02	.8	102
304	Papayas, raw, ½-inch cubes. 1 cup — 182	89	70	1	Trace				18	36	.5	3,190	.07	.08	.5	102
	Peaches:															
	Raw:															
305	Whole, medium, 2-inch diameter, about 4 per pound.[5] 1 peach — 114	89	35	1	Trace				10	9	.5	[13]1,320	.02	.05	1.0	7
306	Sliced. 1 cup — 168	89	65	1	Trace				16	15	.8	[13]2,230	.03	.08	1.6	12
	Canned, yellow-fleshed, solids and liquid:															
	Sirup pack, heavy:															
307	Halves or slices. 1 cup — 257	79	200	1	Trace				52	10	.8	1,100	.02	.06	1.4	7
308	Water pack. 1 cup — 245	91	75	1	Trace				20	10	.7	1,100	.02	.06	1.4	7
309	Dried, uncooked. 1 cup — 160	25	420	5	1				109	77	9.6	6,240	.02	.31	8.5	28
310	Cooked, unsweetened, 10–12 halves and juice. 1 cup — 270	77	220	3	1				58	41	5.1	3,290	.01	.15	4.2	6
	Frozen:															
311	Carton, 12 ounces, not thawed. 1 carton — 340	76	300	1	Trace				77	14	1.7	2,210	.03	.14	2.4	[14]135
	Pears:															
312	Raw, 3 by 2½-inch diameter.[5] 1 pear — 182	83	100	1	1				25	13	.5	30	.04	.07	.2	7
	Canned, solids and liquid:															
	Sirup pack, heavy:															
313	Halves or slices. 1 cup — 255	80	195	1	1				50	13	.5	Trace	.03	.05	.3	4

Item	Food	Measure	Grams	Water (%)	Food energy (Cal)	Protein (g)	Fat (g)	Saturated	Oleic	Linoleic	Carbohydrate (g)	Calcium (mg)	Iron (mg)	Vitamin A (I.U.)	Thiamine (mg)	Riboflavin (mg)	Niacin (mg)	Ascorbic acid (mg)
314	Pineapple: Raw, diced	1 cup	140	85	75	1	Trace				19	24	.7	100	.12	.04	.3	24
	Canned, heavy sirup pack, solids and liquid:																	
315	Crushed	1 cup	260	80	195	1	Trace				50	29	.8	120	.20	.06	.5	17
316	Sliced, slices and juice	2 small or 1 large	122	80	90	Trace	Trace				24	13	.4	50	.09	.03	.2	8
317	Pineapple juice, canned	1 cup	249	86	135	1	Trace				34	37	.7	120	.12	.04	.5	[8]22
	Plums, all except prunes:																	
318	Raw, 2-inch diameter, 1 plum about 2 ounces.[5]	1 plum	60	87	25	Trace	Trace				7	7	.3	140	.02	.02	.3	3
319	Canned, sirup pack (Italian prunes): Plums (with pits) and juice.[5]	1 cup	256	77	205	1	Trace				53	22	2.2	2,970	.05	.05	.9	4
	Prunes, dried, "softenized", medium:																	
320	Uncooked [5]	4 prunes	32	28	70	1	Trace				18	14	1.1	440	.02	.04	.4	1
321	Cooked, unsweetened, 17-18 prunes and 1/3 cup liquid.[5]	1 cup	270	66	295	2	1				78	60	4.5	1,860	.08	.18	1.7	2
322	Prune juice, canned or bottled.	1 cup	256	80	200	1	Trace				49	36	10.5	-----	.03	.03	1.0	[8]5
	Raisins, seedless:																	
323	Packaged, 1/2 oz. or 1 1/2 tbsp. per pkg.	1 pkg	14	18	40	Trace	Trace				11	9	.5	Trace	.02	.01	.1	Trace
324	Cup, pressed down	1 cup	165	18	480	4	Trace				128	102	5.8	30	.18	.13	.8	2
	Raspberries, red:																	
325	Raw	1 cup	123	84	70	1	1				17	27	1.1	160	.04	.11	1.1	31
326	Frozen, 10-ounce carton, not thawed.	1 carton	284	74	275	2	1				70	37	1.7	200	.06	.17	1.7	59
327	Rhubarb, cooked, sugar added.	1 cup	272	63	385	1	Trace				98	212	1.6	220	.06	.15	.7	17
	Strawberries:																	
328	Raw, capped	1 cup	149	90	55	1	1				13	31	1.5	90	.04	.10	1.0	88
329	Frozen, 10-ounce carton, not thawed.	1 carton	284	71	310	1	1				79	40	2.0	90	.06	.17	1.5	150
330	Tangerines, raw, medium, 2 3/8-in. diam., size 176.[5]	1 tangerine	116	87	40	1	Trace				10	34	.3	360	.05	.02	.1	27
331	Tangerine juice, canned, sweetened.	1 cup	249	87	125	1	1				30	45	.5	1,050	.15	.05	.2	55
332	Watermelon, raw, wedge, 4 by 8 inches (1/16 of 10 by 16-inch melon, about 2 pounds with rind).[5]	1 wedge	925	93	115	2	1				27	30	2.1	2,510	.13	.13	.7	30

[5] Measure and weight apply to entire vegetable or fruit including parts not usually eaten.

[8] This is the amount from the fruit. Additional ascorbic acid may be added by the manufacturer. Refer to the label for this information.

[13] Based on yellow-fleshed varieties; for white-fleshed varieties value is about 50 I.U. per 114-gram peach and 80 I.U. per cup of sliced peaches.

[14] This value includes ascorbic acid added by manufacturer.

Table of Food Composition (continued)

[Dashes in the columns for nutrients show that no suitable value could be found although there is reason to believe that a measurable amount of the nutrient may be present]

	Food, approximate measure, and weight	(in grams)	Water	Food energy	Protein	Fat	Fatty acids			Carbohydrate	Calcium	Iron	Vitamin A value	Thiamin	Riboflavin	Niacin	Ascorbic acid
							Saturated (total)	Unsaturated Oleic	Linoleic								
		Grams	Percent	kCalories	Grams	Grams	Grams	Grams	Grams	Grams	Milligrams	Milligrams	International units	Milligrams	Milligrams	Milligrams	Milligrams
	GRAIN PRODUCTS																
	Bagel, 3-in. diam.:																
333	Egg	1 bagel	55	32	165	6	2	—	—	—	28	9	1.2	30	0.14	0.10	1.2	0
334	Water	1 bagel	55	29	165	6	2	—	—	—	30	8	1.2	0	.15	.11	1.4	0
335	Barley, pearled, light, uncooked.	1 cup	200	11	700	16	2	Trace	1	1	158	32	4.0	0	.24	.10	6.2	0
336	Biscuits, baking powder from home recipe with enriched flour, 2-in. diam.	1 biscuit	28	27	105	2	5	1	2	1	13	34	.4	Trace	.06	.06	.1	Trace
337	Biscuits, baking powder from mix, 2-in. diam.	1 biscuit	28	28	90	2	3	1	1	1	15	19	.6	Trace	.08	.07	.6	Trace
338	Bran flakes (40% bran), added thiamin and iron.	1 cup	35	3	105	4	1	—	—	—	28	25	12.3	0	.14	.06	2.2	0
339	Bran flakes with raisins, added thiamin and iron.	1 cup	50	7	145	4	1	—	—	—	40	28	13.5	Trace	.16	.07	2.7	0
	Breads:																	
340	Boston brown bread, slice 3 by ¾ in.	1 slice	48	45	100	3	1	—	—	—	22	43	.9	0	.05	.03	.6	0
	Cracked-wheat bread:																	
341	Loaf, 1 lb.	1 loaf	454	35	1,190	40	10	2	5	2	236	399	5.0	Trace	.53	.41	5.9	Trace
342	Slice, 18 slices per loaf.	1 slice	25	35	65	2	1	—	—	—	13	22	.3	Trace	.03	.02	.3	Trace
	French or vienna bread:																	
343	Enriched, 1 lb. loaf.	1 loaf	454	31	1,315	41	14	3	8	2	251	195	10.0	Trace	1.27	1.00	11.3	Trace
344	Unenriched, 1 lb. loaf.	1 loaf	454	31	1,315	41	14	3	8	2	251	195	3.2	Trace	.36	.36	3.6	Trace
	Italian bread:																	
345	Enriched, 1 lb. loaf.	1 loaf	454	32	1,250	41	4	Trace	1	2	256	77	10.0	0	1.32	.91	11.8	0
346	Unenriched, 1 lb. loaf.	1 loaf	454	32	1,250	41	4	Trace	1	2	256	77	3.2	0	.41	.27	3.6	0
	Raisin bread:																	
347	Loaf, 1 lb.	1 loaf	454	35	1,190	30	13	3	8	2	243	322	5.9	Trace	.23	.41	3.2	Trace

No.	Food	Measure	Weight (g)	Water (%)	Food energy (Cal.)	Protein (g)	Fat (g)	Saturated (g)	Oleic (g)	Linoleic (g)	Carbohydrate (g)	Calcium (mg)	Iron (mg)	Vitamin A (I.U.)	Thiamin (mg)	Riboflavin (mg)	Niacin (mg)	Ascorbic acid (mg)
348	Slice, 18 slices per loaf.	1 slice	25	35	65	2	1	---	---	---	13	18	.3	Trace	.01	.02	.2	Trace
	Rye bread:																	
	American, light (⅓ rye, ⅔ wheat):																	
349	Loaf, 1 lb.	1 loaf	454	36	1,100	41	5	---	---	---	236	340	7.3	0	.82	.32	6.4	0
350	Slice, 18 slices per loaf.	1 slice	25	36	60	2	Trace	---	---	---	13	19	.4	0	.05	.02	.4	0
351	Pumpernickel, loaf, 1 lb.	1 loaf	454	34	1,115	41	5	---	---	---	241	381	10.9	0	1.04	.64	5.4	0
	White bread, enriched: [15]																	
	Soft-crumb type:																	
352	Loaf, 1 lb.	1 loaf	454	36	1,225	39	15	3	8	2	229	381	11.3	Trace	1.13	.95	10.9	Trace
353	Slice, 18 slices per loaf.	1 slice	25	36	70	2	1	---	---	---	13	21	.6	Trace	.06	.05	.6	Trace
354	Slice, toasted.	1 slice	22	25	70	2	1	---	---	---	13	21	.6	Trace	.05	.05	.6	Trace
355	Slice, 22 slices per loaf.	1 slice	20	36	55	2	1	---	---	---	10	17	.5	Trace	.05	.04	.5	Trace
356	Slice, toasted.	1 slice	17	25	55	2	1	---	---	---	10	17	.5	Trace	.05	.04	.5	Trace
357	Loaf, 1½ lbs.	1 loaf	680	36	1,835	59	22	5	12	3	343	571	17.0	Trace	1.70	1.43	16.3	Trace
358	Slice, 24 slices per loaf.	1 slice	28	36	75	2	1	---	---	---	14	24	.7	Trace	.07	.06	.7	Trace
359	Slice, toasted.	1 slice	24	25	75	2	1	---	---	---	14	24	.7	Trace	.07	.06	.7	Trace
360	Slice, 28 slices per loaf.	1 slice	24	36	65	2	1	---	---	---	12	20	.6	Trace	.06	.05	.6	Trace
361	Slice, toasted.	1 slice	21	25	65	2	1	---	---	---	12	20	.6	Trace	.06	.05	.6	Trace
	Firm-crumb type:																	
362	Loaf, 1 lb.	1 loaf	454	35	1,245	41	17	4	10	2	228	435	11.3	Trace	1.22	.91	10.9	Trace
363	Slice, 20 slices per loaf.	1 slice	23	35	65	2	1	---	---	---	12	22	.6	Trace	.06	.05	.6	Trace
364	Slice, toasted.	1 slice	20	24	65	2	1	---	---	---	12	22	.6	Trace	.06	.05	.6	Trace
365	Loaf, 2 lbs.	1 loaf	907	35	2,495	82	34	8	20	4	455	871	22.7	Trace	2.45	1.81	21.8	Trace
366	Slice, 34 slices per loaf.	1 slice	27	35	75	2	1	---	---	---	14	26	.7	Trace	.07	.05	.6	Trace
367	Slice, toasted.	1 slice	23	35	75	2	1	---	---	---	14	26	.7	Trace	.07	.05	.6	Trace
	Whole-wheat bread, soft-crumb type:																	
368	Loaf, 1 lb.	1 loaf	454	36	1,095	41	12	2	6	2	224	381	13.6	Trace	1.36	.45	12.7	Trace
369	Slice, 16 slices per loaf.	1 slice	28	36	65	3	1	---	---	---	14	24	.8	Trace	.09	.03	.8	Trace
370	Slice, toasted.	1 slice	24	24	65	3	1	---	---	---	14	24	.8	Trace	.09	.03	.8	Trace

[15] Values for iron, thiamin, riboflavin, and niacin per pound of unenriched white bread would be as follows:

	Iron Milligrams	Thiamin Milligrams	Riboflavin Milligrams	Niacin Milligrams
Soft crumb	3.2	.31	.39	5.0
Firm crumb	3.2	.32	.59	4.1

Table of Food Composition (continued)

[Dashes in the columns for nutrients show that no suitable value could be found although there is reason to believe that a measurable amount of the nutrient may be present]

	Food, approximate measure, and weight (in grams)		Water	Food energy	Protein	Fat	Fatty acids			Carbohydrate	Calcium	Iron	Vitamin A value	Thiamin	Riboflavin	Niacin	Ascorbic acid
							Saturated (total)	Unsaturated									
								Oleic	Linoleic								
		Grams	Percent	kCalories	Grams	Grams	Grams	Grams	Grams	Grams	Milligrams	Milligrams	International units	Milligrams	Milligrams	Milligrams	Milligrams
	GRAIN PRODUCTS—Continued																
	Bread—Continued																
	Whole-wheat bread, firm-crumb type:																
371	Loaf, 1 lb.	454	36	1,100	48	14	3	6	3	216	449	13.6	Trace	1.18	0.54	12.7	Trace
372	Slice, 18 slices per loaf.	25	36	60	3	1	-	-	-	12	25	.8	Trace	.06	.03	.7	Trace
373	Slice, toasted	21	24	60	3	1	-	-	-	12	25	.8	Trace	.06	.03	.7	Trace
374	Breadcrumbs, dry, grated. 1 cup	100	6	390	13	5	1	2	1	73	122	3.6	Trace	.22	.30	3.5	Trace
375	Buckwheat flour, light, sifted. 1 cup	98	12	340	6	1	-	-	-	78	11	1.0	0	.08	.04	.4	0
376	Bulgur, canned, seasoned 1 cup	135	56	245	8	4	-	-	-	44	27	1.9	0	.08	.05	4.1	0
	Cakes made from cake mixes:																
	Angelfood:																
377	Whole cake 1 cake	635	34	1,645	36	1	-	-	-	377	603	1.9	0	.03	.70	.6	0
378	Piece, 1/12 of 10-in. diam. cake. 1 piece	53	34	135	3	Trace	-	-	-	32	50	.2	0	Trace	.06	.1	0
	Cupcakes, small, 2½ in. diam.:																
379	Without icing 1 cupcake	25	26	90	1	3	1	1	1	14	40	.1	40	.01	.03	.1	Trace
380	With chocolate icing 1 cupcake	36	22	130	2	5	2	2	1	21	47	.3	60	.01	.04	.1	Trace
	Devil's food, 2-layer, with chocolate icing:																
381	Whole cake 1 cake	1,107	24	3,755	49	136	54	58	16	645	653	8.9	1,660	.33	.89	3.3	1
382	Piece, ¹⁄₁₆ of 9-in. diam. cake. 1 piece	69	24	235	3	9	3	4	1	40	41	.6	100	.02	.06	.2	Trace
383	Cupcake, small, 2½ in. diam. 1 cupcake	35	24	120	2	4	1	2	Trace	20	21	.3	50	.01	.03	.1	Trace
	Gingerbread:																
384	Whole cake 1 cake	570	37	1,575	18	39	10	19	9	291	513	9.1	Trace	.17	.51	4.6	2
385	Piece, ⅑ of 8-in. square cake. 1 piece	63	37	175	2	4	1	2	1	32	57	1.0	Trace	.02	.06	.5	Trace
	White, 2-layer, with chocolate icing:																
386	Whole cake 1 cake	1,140	21	4,000	45	122	45	54	17	716	1,129	5.7	680	.23	.91	2.3	2

No.	Food	Measure	Grams															
387	Piece, 1/16 of 9-in. diam. cake.	1 piece	71	21	250	3	8	3	3	1	45	70	.4	40	.01	.06	.1	Trace
388	**Cakes made from home recipes:**[16] Boston cream pie; piece 1/12 of 8-in. diam.	1 piece	69	35	210	4	6	2	3	1	34	46	.3	140	.02	.08	.1	Trace
	Fruitcake, dark, made with enriched flour:																	
389	Loaf, 1-lb.	1 loaf	454	18	1,720	22	69	15	37	13	271	327	11.8	540	.59	.64	3.6	2
390	Slice, 1/30 of 8-in. loaf.	1 slice	15	18	55	1	2	Trace	1	Trace	9	11	.4	20	.02	.02	.1	Trace
	Plain sheet cake: Without icing:																	
391	Whole cake.	1 cake	777	25	2,830	35	108	30	52	21	434	497	3.1	1,320	.16	.70	1.6	2
392	Piece, 1/9 of 9-in. square cake.	1 piece	86	25	315	4	12	3	6	2	48	55	.3	150	.02	.08	.2	Trace
393	With boiled white icing, piece, 1/9 of 9-in. square cake.	1 piece	114	23	400	4	12	3	6	2	71	56	.3	150	.02	.08	.2	Trace
	Pound:																	
394	Loaf, 8½ by 3½ by 3in.	1 loaf	514	17	2,430	29	152	34	68	17	242	108	4.1	1,440	.15	.46	1.0	0
395	Slice, ½-in. thick.	1 slice	30	17	140	2	9	2	4	1	14	6	.2	80	.01	.03	.1	0
	Sponge:																	
396	Whole cake.	1 cake	790	32	2,345	60	45	14	20	4	427	237	9.5	3,560	.40	1.11	1.6	Trace
397	Piece, 1/12 of 10-in. diam. cake.	1 piece	66	32	195	5	4	1	2	Trace	36	20	.8	300	.03	.09	.1	Trace
	Yellow, 2-layer, without icing:																	
398	Whole cake.	1 cake	870	24	3,160	39	111	31	53	22	506	618	3.5	1,310	.17	.70	1.7	2
399	Piece, 1/16 of 9-in. diam. cake.	1 piece	54	24	200	2	7	2	3	1	32	39	.2	80	.01	.04	.1	Trace
	Yellow, 2-layer, with chocolate icing:																	
400	Whole cake.	1 cake	1,203	21	4,390	51	156	55	69	23	727	818	7.2	1,920	.24	.96	2.4	Trace
401	Piece, 1/16 of 9-in. diam. cake.	1 piece	75	21	275	3	10	3	4	1	45	51	.5	120	.02	.06	.2	Trace
	Cake icings. See Sugars, Sweets.																	
	Cookies: Brownies with nuts:																	
402	Made from home recipe with enriched flour.	1 brownie	20	10	95	1	6	1	3	1	10	8	.4	40	.04	.02	.1	Trace
403	Made from mix.	1 brownie	20	11	85	1	4	1	2	1	13	9	.4	20	.03	.02	.1	Trace

[16] Unenriched cake flour used unless otherwise specified.

Table of Food Composition (continued)

[Dashes in the columns for nutrients show that no suitable value could be found although there is reason to believe that a measurable amount of the nutrient may be present]

	Food, approximate measure, and weight (in grams)		Water	Food energy	Protein	Fat	Fatty acids Saturated (total)	Fatty acids Unsaturated Oleic	Fatty acids Unsaturated Linoleic	Carbohydrate	Calcium	Iron	Vitamin A value	Thiamin	Riboflavin	Niacin	Ascorbic acid
		Grams	Percent	kCalories	Grams	Grams	Grams	Grams	Grams	Grams	Milligrams	Milligrams	International units	Milligrams	Milligrams	Milligrams	Milligrams
	GRAIN PRODUCTS—Continued																
	Cookies—Continued																
	Chocolate chip:																
404	Made from home recipe with enriched flour. 1 cookie	10	3	50	1	3	1	1	1	6	4	0.2	10	0.01	0.01	0.1	Trace
405	Commercial 1 cookie	10	3	50	1	2	1	1	Trace	7	4	.2	10	Trace	Trace	Trace	Trace
406	Fig bars, commercial 1 cookie	14	14	50	1	1				11	11	.2	20	Trace	.01	.1	Trace
407	Sandwich, chocolate or vanilla, commercial. 1 cookie	10	2	50	1	2	1	1	Trace	7	2	.1	0	Trace	Trace	.1	0
	Corn flakes, added nutrients:																
408	Plain 1 cup	25	4	100	2	Trace				21	4	.4	0	.11	.02	.5	0
409	Sugar-covered 1 cup	40	2	155	2	Trace				36	5	.4	0	.16	.02	.8	0
	Corn (hominy) grits, degermed, cooked:																
410	Enriched 1 cup	245	87	125	3	Trace				27	2	.7	[17]150	.10	.07	1.0	0
411	Unenriched 1 cup	245	87	125	3	Trace				27	2	.2	[17]150	.05	.02	.5	0
	Cornmeal:																
412	Whole-ground, unbolted, dry. 1 cup	122	12	435	11	5	1	2	2	90	24	2.9	620	.46	.13	2.4	0
413	Bolted (nearly whole-grain) dry. 1 cup	122	12	440	11	4	Trace	1	2	91	21	2.2	590	.37	.10	2.3	0
	Degermed, enriched:																
414	Dry form 1 cup	138	12	500	11	2				108	8	4.0	[17]610	.61	.36	4.8	0
415	Cooked 1 cup	240	88	120	3	1				26	2	1.0	[17]140	.14	.10	1.2	0
	Degermed, unenriched:																
416	Dry form 1 cup	138	12	500	11	2				108	8	1.5	[17]610	.19	.07	1.4	0
417	Cooked 1 cup	240	88	120	3	1				26	2	.5	[17]140	.03	.02	.2	0
418	Corn muffins, made with enriched degermed cornmeal and enriched flour; muffin 2⅜-in. diam. 1 muffin	40	33	125	3	4	2	2	Trace	19	42	.7	[17]120	.08	.09	.6	Trace

No.	Food	Measure	Grams	Water (%)	Food energy	Protein (g)	Fat (g)	Saturated (g)	Oleic (g)	Linoleic (g)	Carbohydrate (g)	Calcium (mg)	Iron (mg)	Vitamin A (IU)	Thiamin (mg)	Riboflavin (mg)	Niacin (mg)	Ascorbic acid (mg)
419	Corn muffins, made with mix, egg, and milk; muffin 2⅜-in. diam.	1 muffin	40	30	130	3	4	1	2	1	20	96	.6	100	.07	.08	.6	Trace
420	Corn, puffed, presweetened, added nutrients.	1 cup	30	2	115	1	Trace	—	—	—	27	3	.5	0	.13	.05	.6	0
421	Corn, shredded, added nutrients.	1 cup	25	3	100	2	Trace	—	—	—	22	1	.6	0	.11	.05	.5	0
	Crackers:																	
422	Graham, 2½-in. square	4 crackers	28	6	110	2	3	—	1	—	21	11	.4	0	.01	.06	.4	0
423	Saltines	4 crackers	11	4	50	1	1	—	1	—	8	2	.1	0	Trace	Trace	.1	0
424	Danish pastry, plain (without fruit or nuts): Packaged ring, 12 ounces.	1 ring	240	22	1,435	25	80	24	37	15	155	170	3.1	1,050	.24	.51	2.7	Trace
425	Round piece, approx. 4¼-in. diam. by 1 in.	1 pastry	65	22	275	5	15	5	7	3	30	33	.6	200	.05	.10	.5	Trace
426	Ounce	1 oz.	28	22	120	2	7	2	3	1	13	14	.3	90	.02	.04	.2	Trace
427	Doughnuts, cake type	1 doughnut	32	24	125	1	6	1	4	Trace	16	13	[18].4	30	[18].05	[18].05	[18].4	Trace
428	Farina, quick-cooking, enriched, cooked.	1 cup	245	89	105	3	Trace	—	—	—	22	147	[19].7	0	[19].12	[19].07	[19]1.0	0
	Macaroni, cooked: Enriched:																	
429	Cooked, firm stage (undergoes additional cooking in a food mixture).	1 cup	130	64	190	6	1	—	—	—	39	14	[19]1.4	0	[19].23	[19].14	[19]1.8	0
430	Cooked until tender	1 cup	140	72	155	5	1	—	—	—	32	8	[19]1.3	0	[19].20	[19].11	[19]1.5	0
	Unenriched:																	
431	Cooked, firm stage (undergoes additional cooking in a food mixture).	1 cup	130	64	190	6	1	—	—	—	39	14	.7	0	.03	.03	.5	0
432	Cooked until tender	1 cup	140	72	155	5	1	—	—	—	32	11	.6	0	.01	.01	.4	0
433	Macaroni (enriched) and cheese, baked.	1 cup	200	58	430	17	22	10	9	2	40	362	1.8	860	.20	.40	1.8	Trace
434	Canned	1 cup	240	80	230	9	10	4	3	1	26	199	1.0	260	.12	.24	1.0	Trace
435	Muffins, with enriched white flour; muffin, 3-inch diam.	1 muffin	40	38	120	3	4	1	2	1	17	42	.6	40	.07	.09	.6	Trace
	Noodles (egg noodles), cooked:																	
436	Enriched	1 cup	160	70	200	7	2	1	1	Trace	37	16	[19]1.4	110	[19].22	[19].13	[19]1.9	0
437	Unenriched	1 cup	160	70	200	7	2	1	1	Trace	37	16	1.0	110	.05	.03	.6	0

[17] This value is based on product made from yellow varieties of corn; white varieties contain only a trace.

[18] Based on product made with enriched flour. With unenriched flour, approximate values per doughnut are: Iron, 0.2 milligram; thiamin, 0.01 milligram; riboflavin, 0.03 milligram; niacin, 0.2 milligram.

[19] Iron, thiamin, riboflavin, and niacin are based on the minimum levels of enrichment specified in standards of identity promulgated under the Federal Food, Drug, and Cosmetic Act.

Table of Food Composition (continued)

[Dashes in the columns for nutrients show that no suitable value could be found although there is reason to believe that a measurable amount of the nutrient may be present]

	Food, approximate measure, and weight (in grams)	Water	Food energy	Protein	Fat	Fatty acids Saturated (total)	Fatty acids Unsaturated Oleic	Fatty acids Unsaturated Linoleic	Carbohydrate	Calcium	Iron	Vitamin A value	Thiamin	Riboflavin	Niacin	Ascorbic acid
		Percent	kCalories	Grams	Grams	Grams	Grams	Grams	Grams	Milligrams	Milligrams	International units	Milligrams	Milligrams	Milligrams	Milligrams
	GRAIN PRODUCTS—Continued															
438	Oats (with or without corn) puffed, added nutrients. 1 cup — 25 Grams	3	100	3	1	---	---	---	19	44	1.2	0	0.24	0.04	0.5	0
439	Oatmeal or rolled oats, cooked. 1 cup — 240	87	130	5	2	---	---	1	23	22	1.4	0	.19	.05	.2	0
	Pancakes, 4-inch diam.:															
440	Wheat, enriched flour (home recipe). 1 cake — 27	50	60	2	2	Trace	1	Trace	9	27	.4	30	.05	.06	.4	Trace
441	Buckwheat (made from mix with egg and milk). 1 cake — 27	58	55	2	2	1	1	Trace	6	59	.4	60	.03	.04	.2	Trace
442	Plain or buttermilk (made from mix with egg and milk). 1 cake — 27	51	60	2	2	1	1	Trace	9	58	.3	70	.04	.06	.2	Trace
	Pie (piecrust made with unenriched flour): Sector, 4-in., 1/7 of 9-in. diam. pie:															
443	Apple (2-crust). 1 sector — 135	48	350	3	15	4	7	3	51	11	.4	40	.03	.03	.5	1
444	Butterscotch (1-crust). 1 sector — 130	45	350	6	14	5	6	2	50	98	1.2	340	.04	.13	.3	Trace
445	Cherry (2-crust). 1 sector — 135	47	350	4	15	4	7	3	52	19	.4	590	.03	.03	.7	Trace
446	Custard (1-crust). 1 sector — 130	58	285	8	14	5	6	2	30	125	.8	300	.07	.21	.4	0
447	Lemon meringue (1-crust). 1 sector — 120	47	305	4	12	4	6	2	45	17	.6	200	.04	.10	.2	4
448	Mince (2-crust). 1 sector — 135	43	365	3	16	4	8	3	56	38	1.4	Trace	.09	.05	.5	1
449	Pecan (1-crust). 1 sector — 118	20	490	6	27	4	16	5	60	55	3.3	190	.19	.08	.4	Trace
450	Pineapple chiffon (1-crust). 1 sector — 93	41	265	6	11	3	5	2	36	22	.8	320	.04	.08	.4	1
451	Pumpkin (1-crust). 1 sector — 130	59	275	5	15	5	6	2	32	66	.7	3,210	.04	.13	.7	Trace
	Piecrust, baked shell for pie made with:															
452	Enriched flour. 1 shell — 180	15	900	11	60	16	28	12	79	25	3.1	0	.36	.25	3.2	0
453	Unenriched flour. 1 shell — 180	15	900	11	60	16	28	12	79	25	.9	0	.05	.05	.9	0

No.	Food	Measure	Grams	Water (%)	Food energy (cal)	Protein (g)	Fat (g)	Saturated (g)	Oleic (g)	Linoleic (g)	Carbohydrate (g)	Calcium (mg)	Iron (mg)	Vitamin A (I.U.)	Thiamin (mg)	Riboflavin (mg)	Niacin (mg)	Ascorbic acid (mg)
	Piecrust mix including stick form:																	
454	Package, 10-oz., for double crust.	1 pkg	284	9	1,480	20	93	23	46	21	141	131	1.4	0	.11	.11	2.0	0
455	Pizza (cheese) 5½-in. sector; ⅛ of 14-in. diam. pie.	1 sector	75	45	185	7	6	2	3	Trace	27	107	.7	290	.04	.12	.7	4
	Popcorn, popped:																	
456	Plain, large kernel	1 cup	6	4	25	1	Trace				5	1	.2		—	.01	.1	0
457	With oil and salt	1 cup	9	3	40	1	2		Trace	1	5	1	.2		—	.01	.2	0
458	Sugar coated	1 cup	35	4	135	2	1				30	2	.5		—	.02	.4	0
	Pretzels:																	
459	Dutch, twisted	1 pretzel	16	5	60	2	1				12	4	.2	0	Trace	Trace	.1	0
460	Thin, twisted	1 pretzel	6	5	25	1	Trace				5	1	.1	0	Trace	Trace	Trace	0
461	Stick, small, 2¼ inches	10 sticks	3	5	10	Trace	Trace				2	1	Trace	0	Trace	Trace	Trace	0
462	Stick, regular, 3⅛ inches	5 sticks	3	5	10	Trace	Trace				2	1	Trace	0	Trace	Trace	Trace	0
	Rice, white: Enriched:																	
463	Raw	1 cup	185	12	670	12	1				149	44	[20]5.4	0	[20].81	[20].06	[20]6.5	0
464	Cooked	1 cup	205	73	225	4	Trace				50	21	[20]1.8	0	[20].23	[20].02	[20]2.1	0
465	Instant, ready-to-serve.	1 cup	165	73	180	4	Trace				40	5	[20]1.3	0	[20].21	[20] —	[20]1.7	0
466	Unenriched, cooked	1 cup	205	73	225	4	Trace				50	21	.4	0	.04	.02	.8	0
467	Parboiled, cooked	1 cup	175	73	185	4	Trace				41	33	[20]1.4	0	[20].19	[20] —	[20]2.1	0
468	Rice, puffed, added nutrients.	1 cup	15	4	60	1	Trace				13	3	.3	0	.07	.01	.7	0
	Rolls, enriched: Cloverleaf or pan:																	
469	Home recipe	1 roll	35	26	120	3	3	1	1	Trace	20	16	.7	30	.09	.09	.8	Trace
470	Commercial	1 roll	28	31	85	2	2	Trace	1	Trace	15	21	.5	Trace	.08	.05	.6	Trace
471	Frankfurter or hamburger.	1 roll	40	31	120	3	2	1	1	Trace	21	30	.8	Trace	.11	.07	.9	Trace
472	Hard, round or rectangular.	1 roll	50	25	155	5	2	Trace	1	Trace	30	24	1.2	Trace	.13	.12	1.4	Trace
473	Rye wafers, whole-grain, 1⅞ by 3½ inches.	2 wafers	13	6	45	2	Trace				10	7	.5	0	.04	.03	.2	0
474	Spaghetti, cooked, tender stage, enriched.	1 cup	140	72	155	5	1				32	11	[19]1.3	0	[19].20	[19].11	[19]1.5	0

[19] Iron, thiamin, riboflavin, and niacin are based on the minimum levels of enrichment specified in standards of identity promulgated under the Federal Food, Drug, and Cosmetic Act.

[20] Iron, thiamin, and niacin are based on the minimum levels of enrichment specified in standards of identity promulgated under the Federal Food, Drug, and Cosmetic Act. Riboflavin is based on unenriched rice. When the minimum level of enrichment for riboflavin specified in the standards of identity becomes effective the value will be 0.12 milligram per cup of parboiled rice and of white rice.

Table of Food Composition (continued)

[Dashes in the columns for nutrients show that no suitable value could be found although there is reason to believe that a measurable amount of the nutrient may be present]

	Food, approximate measure, and weight (in grams)		Water	Food energy	Protein	Fat	Fatty acids			Carbohydrate	Calcium	Iron	Vitamin A value	Thiamin	Riboflavin	Niacin	Ascorbic acid
							Saturated (total)	Unsaturated Oleic	Unsaturated Linoleic								
		Grams	Percent	kCalories	Grams	Grams	Grams	Grams	Grams	Grams	Milligrams	Milligrams	International units	Milligrams	Milligrams	Milligrams	Milligrams
	GRAIN PRODUCTS—Continued																
	Spaghetti with meat balls, and tomato sauce:																
475	Home recipe, 1 cup	248	70	330	19	12	4	6	1	39	124	3.7	1,590	0.25	0.30	4.0	22
476	Canned, 1 cup	250	78	260	12	10	2	3	4	28	53	3.3	1,000	.15	.18	2.3	5
	Spaghetti in tomato sauce with cheese:																
477	Home recipe, 1 cup	250	77	260	9	9	2	5	1	37	80	2.3	1,080	.25	.18	2.3	13
478	Canned, 1 cup	250	80	190	6	2	1	1	1	38	40	2.8	930	.35	.28	4.5	10
479	Waffles, with enriched flour, 7-in. diam., 1 waffle	75	41	210	7	7	2	4	1	28	85	1.3	250	.13	.19	1.0	Trace
480	Waffles, made from mix, enriched, egg and milk added, 7-in. diam., 1 waffle	75	42	205	7	8	3	3	1	27	179	1.0	170	.11	.17	.7	Trace
481	Wheat, puffed, added nutrients, 1 cup	15	3	55	2	Trace	-----	-----	-----	12	4	.6	0	.08	.03	1.2	0
482	Wheat, shredded, plain, 1 biscuit	25	7	90	2	1	-----	-----	-----	20	11	.9	0	.06	.03	1.1	0
483	Wheat flakes, added nutrients, 1 cup	30	4	105	3	Trace	-----	-----	-----	24	12	1.3	0	.19	.04	1.5	0
	Wheat flours:																
484	Whole-wheat, from hard wheats, stirred, 1 cup	120	12	400	16	2	Trace	1	1	85	49	4.0	0	.66	.14	5.2	0
	All-purpose or family flour, enriched:																
485	Sifted, 1 cup	115	12	420	12	1	-----	-----	-----	88	18	[19] 3.3	0	[19] .51	[19] .30	[19] 4.0	0
486	Unsifted, 1 cup	125	12	455	13	1	-----	-----	-----	95	20	[19] 3.6	0	[19] .55	[19] .33	[19] 4.4	0
487	Self-rising, enriched, 1 cup	125	12	440	12	1	-----	-----	-----	93	331	[19] 3.6	0	[19] .55	[19] .33	[19] 4.4	0
488	Cake or pastry flour, sifted, 1 cup	96	12	350	7	1	-----	-----	-----	76	16	.5	0	.03	.03	.7	0
	FATS, OILS																
	Butter:																
	Regular, 4 sticks per pound:																
489	Stick, ½ cup	113	16	810	1	92	51	30	3	1	23	0	[12] 3,750				0

Item No.	Food, approximate measure, and weight	Measure	Grams	Water (%)	Food energy (cal.)	Protein (g)	Fat (g)	Saturated (total) (g)	Oleic (g)	Linoleic (g)	Carbohydrate (g)	Calcium (mg)	Iron (mg)	Vitamin A (I.U.)	Thiamin (mg)	Riboflavin (mg)	Niacin (mg)	Ascorbic acid (mg)
490	Tablespoon (approx. ⅛ stick).	1 tbsp	14	16	100	Trace	12	6	4	Trace	Trace	3	0	[21]470	—	—	—	0
491	Pat (1-in. sq. ⅓-in. high; 90 per lb.).	1 pat	5	16	35	Trace	4	2	1	Trace	Trace	1	0	[21]170	—	—	—	0
	Whipped, 6 sticks or 2, 8-oz. containers per pound:																	
492	Stick.	½ cup	76	16	540	1	61	34	20	2	Trace	15	0	[22]2,500	—	—	—	0
493	Tablespoon (approx. ⅛ stick).	1 tbsp	9	16	65	Trace	8	4	3	Trace	Trace	2	0	[21]310	—	—	—	0
494	Pat (1¼-in. sq. ⅓-in. high; 120 per lb.).	1 pat	4	16	25	Trace	3	2	1	Trace	Trace	1	0	[21]130	—	—	—	0
	Fats, cooking:																	
495	Lard.	1 cup	205	0	1,850	0	205	78	94	20	0	0	0	0	0	0	0	0
496	Lard.	1 tbsp	13	0	115	0	13	5	6	1	0	0	0	0	0	0	0	0
497	Vegetable fats.	1 cup	200	0	1,770	0	200	50	100	44	0	0	0	—	0	0	0	0
498	Vegetable fats.	1 tbsp	13	0	110	0	13	3	6	3	0	0	0	—	0	0	0	0
	Margarine:																	
	Regular, 4 sticks per pound:																	
499	Stick.	½ cup	113	16	815	1	92	17	46	25	1	23	0	[23]3,750	—	—	—	0
500	Tablespoon (approx. ⅛ stick).	1 tbsp	14	16	100	Trace	12	2	6	3	Trace	3	0	[22]470	—	—	—	0
501	Pat (1-in. sq. ⅓-in. high; 90 per lb.).	1 pat	5	16	35	Trace	4	1	2	1	Trace	1	0	[22]170	—	—	—	0
	Whipped, 6 sticks per pound:																	
502	Stick.	½ cup	76	16	545	1	61	11	31	17	Trace	15	0	[22]2,500	—	—	—	0
	Soft, 2 8-oz. tubs per pound:																	
503	Tub.	1 tub	227	16	1,635	1	184	34	68	68	1	45	0	[27]7,500	—	—	—	0
504	Tablespoon.	1 tbsp	14	16	100	Trace	11	2	4	4	Trace	3	0	[22]470	—	—	—	0
	Oils, salad or cooking:																	
505	Corn.	1 cup	220	0	1,945	0	220	22	62	117	0	0	0	0	0	0	0	0
506	Corn.	1 tbsp	14	0	125	0	14	1	4	7	0	0	0	0	0	0	0	0
507	Cottonseed.	1 cup	220	0	1,945	0	220	55	46	110	0	0	0	0	0	0	0	0
508	Cottonseed.	1 tbsp	14	0	125	0	14	4	3	7	0	0	0	0	0	0	0	0
509	Olive.	1 cup	220	0	1,945	0	220	24	167	15	0	0	0	0	0	0	0	0
510	Olive.	1 tbsp	14	0	125	0	14	2	11	1	0	0	0	0	0	0	0	0
511	Peanut.	1 cup	220	0	1,945	0	220	40	103	64	0	0	0	0	0	0	0	0
512	Peanut.	1 tbsp	14	0	125	0	14	3	7	4	0	0	0	0	0	0	0	0
513	Safflower.	1 cup	220	0	1,945	0	220	18	37	165	0	0	0	0	0	0	0	0
514	Safflower.	1 tbsp	14	0	125	0	14	1	2	10	0	0	0	0	0	0	0	0
515	Soybean.	1 cup	220	0	1,945	0	220	33	44	114	0	0	0	0	0	0	0	0
516	Soybean.	1 tbsp	14	0	125	0	14	2	3	7	0	0	0	0	0	0	0	0

[19] Iron, thiamin, riboflavin, and niacin are based on the minimum levels of enrichment specified in standards of identity promulgated under the Federal Food, Drug, and Cosmetic Act.

[21] Year-round average.

[22] Based on the average vitamin A content of fortified margarine. Federal specifications for fortified margarine require a minimum of 15,000 I.U. of vitamin A per pound.

Table of Food Composition (continued)

[Dashes in the columns for nutrients show that no suitable value could be found although there is reason to believe that a measurable amount of the nutrient may be present]

	Food, approximate measure, and weight (in grams)	Water	Food energy	Protein	Fat	Fatty acids — Saturated (total)	Fatty acids — Unsaturated — Oleic	Fatty acids — Unsaturated — Linoleic	Carbohydrate	Calcium	Iron	Vitamin A value	Thiamin	Riboflavin	Niacin	Ascorbic acid
	Grams	*Percent*	*kCalories*	*Grams*	*Grams*	*Grams*	*Grams*	*Grams*	*Grams*	*Milligrams*	*Milligrams*	*International units*	*Milligrams*	*Milligrams*	*Milligrams*	*Milligrams*
	FATS, OILS—Continued															
	Salad dressings:															
517	Blue cheese --- 1 tbsp --- 15	32	75	1	8	2	2	4	1	12	Trace	30	Trace	0.02	Trace	Trace
	Commercial, mayonnaise type:															
518	Regular --- 1 tbsp --- 15	41	65	Trace	6	1	1	3	2	2	Trace	30	Trace	Trace	Trace	---
519	Special dietary, low-calorie. 1 tbsp --- 16	81	20	Trace	2	Trace	Trace	1	1	3	Trace	40	Trace	Trace	Trace	---
	French:															
520	Regular --- 1 tbsp --- 16	39	65	Trace	6	1	1	3	3	2	.1	---	---	---	---	---
521	Special dietary, low-fat with artificial sweeteners. 1 tbsp --- 15	95	Trace	Trace	Trace	---	---	---	Trace	2	.1	---	---	---	---	---
522	Home cooked, boiled. 1 tbsp --- 16	68	25	1	2	1	1	Trace	2	14	.1	80	.01	.03	Trace	Trace
523	Mayonnaise --- 1 tbsp --- 14	15	100	Trace	11	2	2	6	Trace	3	.1	40	Trace	.01	Trace	Trace
524	Thousand island --- 1 tbsp --- 16	32	80	Trace	8	1	2	4	3	2	.1	50	Trace	Trace	Trace	Trace
	SUGARS, SWEETS															
	Cake icings:															
525	Chocolate made with milk and table fat. 1 cup --- 275	14	1,035	9	38	21	14	1	185	165	3.3	580	.06	.28	.6	1
526	Coconut (with boiled icing). 1 cup --- 166	15	605	3	13	11	1	Trace	124	10	.8	0	.02	.07	.3	0
527	Creamy fudge from mix with water only. 1 cup --- 245	15	830	7	16	5	8	3	183	96	2.7	Trace	.05	.20	.7	Trace
528	White, boiled --- 1 cup --- 94	18	300	1	0	---	---	---	76	2	Trace	0	Trace	.03	Trace	0
	Candy:															
529	Caramels, plain or chocolate. 1 oz --- 28	8	115	1	3	2	1	Trace	22	42	.4	Trace	.01	.05	.1	Trace
530	Chocolate, milk, plain --- 1 oz --- 28	1	145	2	9	5	3	Trace	16	65	.3	80	.02	.10	.1	Trace
531	Chocolate-coated peanuts. 1 oz --- 28	1	160	5	12	3	6	2	11	33	.4	Trace	.10	.05	2.1	Trace

Item	Food, approximate measure	Grams	Water (%)	Food energy (cal)	Protein (g)	Fat (g)	Saturated (g)	Unsaturated Oleic (g)	Unsaturated Linoleic (g)	Carbohydrate (g)	Calcium (mg)	Iron (mg)	Vitamin A (I.U.)	Thiamine (mg)	Riboflavin (mg)	Niacin (mg)	Ascorbic acid (mg)
532	Fondant; mints, uncoated; candy corn. — 1 oz.	28	8	105	Trace	1	—	—	—	25	4	.3	0	Trace	Trace	Trace	0
533	Fudge, plain — 1 oz.	28	8	115	1	4	2	1	Trace	21	22	.3	Trace	.01	.03	.1	Trace
534	Gum drops — 1 oz.	28	12	100	Trace	Trace	—	—	—	25	2	.1	0	0	Trace	Trace	0
535	Hard — 1 oz.	28	1	110	0	Trace	—	—	—	28	6	.5	0	0	0	0	0
536	Marshmallows — 1 oz.	28	17	90	1	Trace	—	—	—	23	5	.5	0	0	Trace	Trace	0
	Chocolate-flavored sirup or topping:																
537	Thin type — 1 fl. oz.	38	32	90	1	1	Trace	Trace	Trace	24	6	.6	Trace	.01	.03	.2	0
538	Fudge type — 1 fl. oz.	38	25	125	2	5	2	2	Trace	20	48	.5	60	.02	.08	.2	Trace
	Chocolate-flavored beverage powder (approx. 4 heaping teaspoons per oz.):																
539	With nonfat dry milk — 1 oz.	28	2	100	5	1	Trace	Trace	Trace	20	167	.5	10	.04	.21	.2	1
540	Without nonfat dry milk — 1 oz.	28	1	100	1	1	Trace	Trace	Trace	25	9	.6	0	.01	.03	.1	0
541	Honey, strained or extracted — 1 tbsp.	21	17	65	Trace	0	—	—	—	17	1	.1	0	Trace	.01	.1	Trace
542	Jams and preserves — 1 tbsp.	20	29	55	Trace	Trace	—	—	—	14	4	.2	Trace	Trace	.01	Trace	Trace
543	Jellies — 1 tbsp.	18	29	50	Trace	Trace	—	—	—	13	4	.3	Trace	Trace	.01	Trace	1
	Molasses, cane:																
544	Light (first extraction) — 1 tbsp.	20	24	50	—	—	—	—	—	13	33	.9	—	.01	.01	Trace	—
545	Blackstrap (third extraction) — 1 tbsp.	20	24	45	—	—	—	—	—	11	137	3.2	—	.02	.04	.4	—
	Sirups:																
546	Sorghum — 1 tbsp.	21	23	55	—	—	—	—	—	14	35	2.6	—	—	.02	Trace	0
547	Table blends, chiefly corn, light and dark. — 1 tbsp.	21	24	60	—	—	—	—	—	15	9	.8	—	—	0	0	0
	Sugars:																
548	Brown, firm packed — 1 cup	220	2	820	2	0	—	—	—	212	187	7.5	0	.02	.07	.4	0
	White:																
549	Granulated — 1 cup	200	Trace	770	0	0	—	—	—	199	0	.2	0	0	0	0	0
550	— 1 tbsp.	11	Trace	40	0	0	—	—	—	11	0	Trace	0	0	0	0	0
551	Powdered, stirred before measuring. — 1 cup	120	Trace	460	0	0	—	—	—	119	0	.1	0	0	0	0	0
	MISCELLANEOUS ITEMS																
552	Barbecue sauce — 1 cup	250	81	230	4	17	2	5	9	20	53	2.0	900	.03	.03	.8	13
	Beverages, alcoholic:																
553	Beer — 12 fl. oz.	360	92	150	1	0	—	—	—	14	18	Trace	—	.01	.11	2.2	—
	Gin, rum, vodka, whiskey:																
554	80-proof — 1½ fl. oz. jigger.	42	67	100	—	—	—	—	—	Trace	—	—	—	—	—	—	—
555	86-proof — 1½ fl. oz. jigger.	42	64	105	—	—	—	—	—	Trace	—	—	—	—	—	—	—
556	90-proof — 1½ fl. oz. jigger.	42	62	110	—	—	—	—	—	Trace	—	—	—	—	—	—	—

Table of Food Composition (continued)

[Dashes in the columns for nutrients show that no suitable value could be found although there is reason to believe that a measurable amount of the nutrient may be present]

MISCELLANEOUS ITEMS—Continued

	Food, approximate measure, and weight	Weight (Grams)	Water (Percent)	Food energy (kCalories)	Protein (Grams)	Fat (Grams)	Fatty acids Saturated (total) (Grams)	Unsaturated Oleic (Grams)	Unsaturated Linoleic (Grams)	Carbohydrate (Grams)	Calcium (Milligrams)	Iron (Milligrams)	Vitamin A value (International units)	Thiamin (Milligrams)	Riboflavin (Milligrams)	Niacin (Milligrams)	Ascorbic acid (Milligrams)
	Beverages, alcoholic—Continued																
	Gin, rum, vodka, whiskey—Con.																
557	94-proof 1½ fl. oz. jigger.	42	60	115	Trace	0	---			Trace							
558	100-proof 1½ fl. oz. jigger.	42	58	125	Trace	0	---			Trace							
	Wines:																
559	Dessert 3½ fl. oz. glass.	103	77	140	Trace	0	---			8	8	---	---	.01	.02	.2	---
560	Table 3½ fl. oz. glass.	102	86	85	Trace	0	---			4	9	.4	---	Trace	.01	.1	---
	Beverages, carbonated, sweetened, nonalcoholic:																
561	Carbonated water 12 fl. oz.	366	92	115	0	0	---			29	---	---	0	0	0	0	0
562	Cola type 12 fl. oz.	369	90	145	0	0	---			37	---	---	0	0	0	0	0
563	Fruit-flavored sodas and Tom Collins mixes. 12 fl. oz.	372	88	170	0	0	---			45	---	---	0	0	0	0	0
564	Ginger ale 12 fl. oz.	366	92	115	0	0	---			29	·	---	0	0	0	0	0
565	Root beer 12 fl. oz.	370	90	150	0	0	---			39	---	---	---	---	---	---	---
566	Bouillon cubes, approx. ½ in. 1 cube	4	4	5	1	Trace				Trace							
	Chocolate:																
567	Bitter or baking 1 oz.	28	2	145	3	15	8	6	Trace	8	22	1.9	20	.01	.07	.4	0
568	Semi-sweet, small pieces. 1 cup	170	1	860	7	61	34	22	1	97	51	4.4	30	.02	.14	.9	0
	Gelatin:																
569	Plain, dry powder in envelope. 1 envelope	7	13	25	6	Trace				0							
570	Dessert powder, 3-oz. package. 1 pkg.	85	2	315	8	0				75							
571	Gelatin dessert, prepared with water. 1 cup	240	84	140	4	0				34							

No.	Food and description	Measure	Grams	Water (%)	Food energy (cal.)	Protein (g)	Fat (g)	Saturated (total) (g)	Oleic (g)	Linoleic (g)	Carbohydrate (g)	Calcium (mg)	Iron (mg)	Vitamin A (I.U.)	Thiamin (mg)	Riboflavin (mg)	Niacin (mg)	Ascorbic acid (mg)
572	Olives, pickled: Green	4 medium or 3 extra large or 2 giant	16	78	15	Trace	2	Trace	2	Trace	Trace	8	.2	40	—	—	—	—
573	Ripe: Mission	3 small or 2 large	10	73	15	Trace	2	Trace	2	Trace	Trace	9	.1	10	Trace	Trace	Trace	—
574	Pickles, cucumber: Dill, medium, whole, 3¾ in. long, 1¼ in. diam.	1 pickle	65	93	10	1	Trace	—	—	—	1	17	.7	70	Trace	.01	Trace	4
575	Fresh, sliced, 1½ in. diam., ¼ in. thick.	2 slices	15	79	10	Trace	Trace	—	—	—	3	5	.3	20	Trace	Trace	Trace	1
576	Sweet, gherkin, small, whole, approx. 2½ in. long, ¾ in. diam.	1 pickle	15	61	20	Trace	Trace	—	—	—	6	2	.2	10	Trace	Trace	Trace	1
577	Relish, finely chopped, sweet.	1 tbsp.	15	63	20	Trace	Trace	—	—	—	5	3	.1	—	—	—	—	1
	Popcorn. See Grain Products.																	
578	Popsicle, 3 fl. oz. size	1 popsicle	95	80	70	0	0	0	0	0	18	0	Trace	0	0	0	0	0
	Pudding, home recipe with starch base:																	
579	Chocolate	1 cup	260	66	385	8	12	7	4	Trace	67	250	1.3	390	.05	.36	.3	1
580	Vanilla (blanc mange)	1 cup	255	76	285	9	10	5	3	Trace	41	298	Trace	410	.08	.41	.3	2
581	Pudding mix, dry form, 4-oz. package.	1 pkg.	113	2	410	3	2	1	1	Trace	103	23	1.8	Trace	.02	.08	.5	0
582	Sherbet	1 cup	193	67	260	2	2	—	—	—	59	31	Trace	120	.02	.06	Trace	4
	Soups: Canned, condensed, ready-to-serve: Prepared with an equal volume of milk:																	
583	Cream of chicken	1 cup	245	85	180	7	10	3	3	3	15	172	.5	610	.05	.27	.7	2
584	Cream of mushroom	1 cup	245	83	215	7	14	4	4	5	16	191	.5	250	.05	.34	.7	1
	Prepared with an equal volume of water:																	
585	Tomato	1 cup	250	84	175	7	7	3	2	1	23	168	.8	1,200	.10	.25	1.3	15
586	Bean with pork	1 cup	250	84	170	8	6	1	2	2	22	63	2.3	650	.13	.08	1.0	3
587	Beef broth, bouillon consomme.	1 cup	240	96	30	5	0	—	—	—	3	Trace	.5	Trace	Trace	.02	1.2	—
588	Beef noodle	1 cup	240	93	70	4	3	1	1	1	7	7	1.0	50	.05	.07	1.0	Trace
589	Clam chowder, Manhattan type (with tomatoes, without milk).	1 cup	245	92	80	2	3	—	—	—	12	34	1.0	880	.02	.02	1.0	Trace
590	Cream of chicken	1 cup	240	92	95	3	6	1	2	3	8	24	.5	410	.02	.05	.5	Trace
591	Cream of mushroom	1 cup	240	90	135	2	10	1	3	5	10	41	.5	70	.02	.12	.7	Trace
592	Minestrone	1 cup	245	90	105	5	3	—	—	—	14	37	1.0	2,350	.07	.05	1.0	—

Table of Food Composition (continued)

[Dashes in the columns for nutrients show that no suitable value could be found although there is reason to believe that a measurable amount of the nutrient may be present]

	Food, approximate measure, and weight (in grams)	Water	Food energy	Protein	Fat	Fatty acids Saturated (total)	Fatty acids Unsaturated Oleic	Fatty acids Unsaturated Linoleic	Carbohydrate	Calcium	Iron	Vitamin A value	Thiamin	Riboflavin	Niacin	Ascorbic acid
		Percent	kCalories	Grams	Grams	Grams	Grams	Grams	Grams	Milligrams	Milligrams	International units	Milligrams	Milligrams	Milligrams	Milligrams
	MISCELLANEOUS ITEMS—Continued Soups—Continued Canned, condensed, ready-to-serve—Con. Prepared with an equal volume of water—Con.															
593	Split pea — 1 cup — 245 Grams	85	145	9	3	1	2	Trace	21	29	1.5	440	0.25	0.15	1.5	1
594	Tomato — 1 cup — 245	90	90	2	3	Trace	1	1	16	15	.7	1,000	.05	.05	1.2	12
595	Vegetable beef — 1 cup — 245	92	80	5	2	---	---	---	10	12	.7	2,700	.05	.05	1.0	---
596	Vegetarian — 1 cup — 245	92	80	2	2				13	20	1.0	2,940	.05	.05	1.0	---
	Dehydrated, dry form:															
597	Chicken noodle (2-oz. package) — 1 pkg — 57	6	220	8	6	2	3	1	33	34	1.4	190	.30	.15	2.4	3
598	Onion mix (1½-oz. package) — 1 pkg — 43	3	150	6	5	1	2	1	23	42	.6	30	.05	.03	.3	6
599	Tomato vegetable with noodles (2½ oz. pkg.) — 1 pkg — 71	4	245	6	6	2	3	1	45	33	1.4	1,700	.21	.13	1.8	18
	Frozen, condensed: Clam chowder, New England type (with milk, without tomatoes):															
600	Prepared with equal volume of milk — 1 cup — 245	83	210	9	12	---	---	---	16	240	1.0	250	.07	.29	.5	Trace
601	Prepared with equal volume of water — 1 cup — 240	89	130	4	8	---	---	---	11	91	1.0	50	.05	.10	.5	---
	Cream of potato:															
602	Prepared with equal volume of milk — 1 cup — 245	83	185	8	10	5	3	Trace	18	208	1.0	590	.10	.27	.5	Trace
603	Prepared with equal volume of water — 1 cup — 240	90	105	3	5	3	2	Trace	12	58	1.0	410	.05	.05	.5	---

No.	Food	Measure	Grams	Water (%)	Food energy (Calories)	Protein (g)	Fat (g)	Fatty acids, Saturated (total)	Fatty acids, Unsaturated Oleic	Fatty acids, Unsaturated Linoleic	Carbohydrate (g)	Calcium (mg)	Iron (mg)	Vitamin A (I.U.)	Thiamin (mg)	Riboflavin (mg)	Niacin (mg)	Ascorbic acid (mg)
604	Cream of shrimp: Prepared with equal volume of milk.	1 cup	245	82	245	9	16	---	---	---	15	189	.5	290	.07	.27	.5	Trace
605	Prepared with equal volume of water.	1 cup	240	88	160	5	12	---	---	---	8	38	.5	120	.05	.05	.5	---
606	Oyster stew: Prepared with equal volume of milk.	1 cup	240	83	200	10	12	---	---	---	14	305	1.4	410	.12	.41	.5	Trace
607	Prepared with equal volume of water.	1 cup	240	90	120	6	8	---	---	---	8	158	1.4	240	.07	.19	.5	---
608	Tapioca, dry, quick-cooking.	1 cup	152	13	535	1	Trace	---	---	---	131	15	.6	0	0	0	0	0
609	Tapioca desserts: Apple.	1 cup	250	70	295	1	Trace	---	---	---	74	8	.5	30	Trace	Trace	Trace	Trace
610	Cream pudding.	1 cup	165	72	220	8	8	4	3	Trace	28	173	.7	480	.07	.30	.2	2
611	Tartar sauce.	1 tbsp	14	34	75	Trace	8	1	4	1	1	3	.1	30	Trace	Trace	Trace	Trace
612	Vinegar.	1 tbsp	15	94	Trace	Trace	0	---	---	---	1	1	.1	---	---	---	---	---
613	White sauce, medium.	1 cup	250	73	405	10	31	16	10	1	22	288	.5	1,150	.10	.43	.5	2
614	Yeast: Baker's, dry, active.	1 pkg.	7	5	20	3	Trace	---	---	---	3	3	1.1	Trace	.16	.38	2.6	Trace
615	Brewer's, dry.	1 tbsp.	8	5	25	3	Trace	---	---	---	3	17	1.4	Trace	1.25	.34	3.0	Trace

Yoghurt. See Milk, Cheese, Cream, Imitation Cream.

APPENDIX II

Fast Foods

The following table is reprinted from a publication by Ross Laboratories.[1] We appreciate their permission, and that of the authors, to use this information.

Notes

1. Table 1 from E. A. Young, E. H. Brennan, and G. L. Irving, Update: Nutritional analysis of fast foods, *Dietetic Currents, Ross Timesaver* Vol. 21, No. 3, May–June 1981.

Table 1. Nutritional Analyses of Fast Foods (Dashes indicate no data available. X = less than 2% RDA; tr = trace)

	Weight (g)	Energy (cal)	Protein (g)	Carbohydrate (g)	Fat (g)	Cholesterol (mg)	Vitamin A (IU)	Thiamin (mg)	Riboflavin (mg)	Niacin (mg)	Vitamin C (mg)	Calcium (mg)	Iron (mg)	Sodium (mg)
ARBY'S®														
Roast beef	140	350	22	32	15	45	X	0.30	0.34	5	X	80	3.6	880
Beef and cheese	168	450	27	36	22	55	X	0.38	0.43	6	X	200	4.5	1220
Super roast beef	263	620	30	61	28	85	X	0.53	0.43	7	X	100	5.4	1420
Junior roast beef	74	220	12	21	9	35	X	0.15	0.17	3	X	40	1.8	530
Ham and cheese	154	380	23	33	17	60	X	0.75	0.34	5	X	200	2.7	1350
Turkey deluxe	236	510	28	46	24	70	X	0.45	0.34	8	X	80	2.7	1220
Club sandwich	252	560	30	43	30	100	X	0.68	0.43	7	X	200	3.6	1610

Source: Consumer Affairs, Arby's, Inc., Atlanta, Georgia. Nutritional analysis by Technological Resources, Camden, New Jersey.

	Weight (g)	Energy (cal)	Protein (g)	Carbohydrate (g)	Fat (g)	Cholesterol (mg)	Vitamin A (IU)	Thiamin (mg)	Riboflavin (mg)	Niacin (mg)	Vitamin C (mg)	Calcium (mg)	Iron (mg)	Sodium (mg)
BURGER CHEF®														
Hamburger	91	244	11	29	9	27	114	0.17	0.16	2.7	1.2	45	2.0	—
Cheeseburger	104	290	14	29	13	39	267	0.18	0.21	2.8	1.2	132	2.2	—
Double cheeseburger	145	420	24	30	22	77	431	0.20	0.32	4.4	1.2	223	3.2	—
Fish filet	179	547	21	46	31	43	400	0.23	0.22	2.7	1.0	145	2.2	—
Super Shef® sandwich	252	563	29	44	30	105	754	0.31	0.40	6.0	9.3	205	4.5	—
Big Shef® sandwich	186	569	23	38	36	81	279	0.26	0.31	4.7	1.0	152	3.6	—
TOP Shef® sandwich	138	661	41	36	38	134	273	0.35	0.47	8.1	0	194	5.4	—
Funmeal® feast	—	545	15	55	30	27	123	0.25	0.21	4.6	12.8	61	2.8	—
Rancher® platter[a]	316	640	32	33	42	106	1750[a]	0.29	0.38	8.6	23.5	66	5.3	—
Mariner® platter[a]	373	734	29	78	34	35	2069[a]	0.34	0.23	5.2	23.5	63	3.3	—
French fries, small	68	250	2	20	19	0	0	0.07	0.04	1.7	11.5	9	0.7	—
French fries, large	85	351	3	28	26	0	0	0.10	0.06	2.4	16.2	13	0.9	—
Vanilla shake (12 oz)	336	380	13	60	10	40	387	0.10	0.66	0.5	0	497	0.3	—
Chocolate shake (12 oz)	336	403	10	72	9	36	292	0.16	0.76	0.4	0	449	1.1	—
Hot chocolate	—	198	8	23	8	30	288	0.93	0.39	0.3	2.1	271	0.7	—

[a] Includes salad. Source: Burger Chef Systems, Inc., Indianapolis, Indiana. Nutritional analysis from *Handbook No. 8.* Washington: US Dept of Agriculture.

	Weight (g)	Energy (cal)	Protein (g)	Carbo-hydrate (g)	Fat (g)	Cholesterol (mg)	Vitamin A (IU)	Thiamin (mg)	Riboflavin (mg)	Niacin (mg)	Vitamin C (mg)	Calcium (mg)	Iron (mg)	Sodium (mg)
CHURCH'S FRIED CHICKEN®														
White chicken portion	100	327	21	10	23	—	160	0.10	0.18	7.2	0.7	94	1.0	498
Dark chicken portion	100	305	22	7	21	—	140	0.10	0.27	5.3	1.0	15	1.3	475

Source: Church's Fried Chicken, San Antonio, Texas. Nutritional analysis by Medallion Laboratories, Minneapolis, Minnesota.

	Weight (g)	Energy (cal)	Protein (g)	Carbo-hydrate (g)	Fat (g)	Cholesterol (mg)	Vitamin A (IU)	Thiamin (mg)	Riboflavin (mg)	Niacin (mg)	Vitamin C (mg)	Calcium (mg)	Iron (mg)	Sodium (mg)
DAIRY QUEEN®														
Frozen dessert	113	180	5	27	6	20	100	0.09	0.17	X	X	150	X	—
DQ cone, small	71	110	3	18	3	10	100	0.03	0.14	X	X	100	X	—
DQ cone, regular	142	230	6	35	7	20	300	0.09	0.26	X	X	200	X	—
DQ cone, large	213	340	10	52	10	30	400	0.15	0.43	X	X	300	X	—
DQ dip cone, small	78	150	3	20	7	10	100	0.03	0.17	X	X	100	X	—
DQ dip cone, small	156	300	7	40	13	20	300	0.09	0.34	X	X	200	0.4	—
DQ dip cone, regular	234	450	10	58	20	30	400	0.12	0.51	X	X	300	0.4	—
DQ dip cone, large	106	170	4	30	4	15	100	0.03	0.17	X	X	100	0.7	—
DQ sundae, small	177	290	6	51	7	20	300	0.06	0.26	X	X	200	1.1	—
DQ sundae, regular	248	400	9	71	9	30	400	0.09	0.43	X	X	300	1.8	—
DQ sundae, large	241	340	10	51	11	30	400	0.06	0.34	0.4	2.4	300	1.8	—
DQ malt, small	418	600	15	89	20	50	750	0.12	0.60	0.8	3.6	500	3.6	—
DQ malt, regular	588	840	22	125	28	70	750	0.15	0.85	1.2	6	600	5.4	—
DQ malt, large	397	330	6	59	8	20	100	0.12	0.17	X	X	200	X	—
DQ float	383	540	10	91	15	30	750	0.60	0.60	0.8	18	350	1.8	—
DQ banana split	284	460	10	81	11	30	400	0.12	0.43	0.4	X	300	1.8	—
DQ parfait	397	520	11	89	13	35	200	0.15	0.34	X	X	300	X	—
DQ freeze	411	500	10	87	12	35	200	0.15	0.34	X	X	300	X	—
Mr. Misty® freeze	404	440	6	85	8	20	100	0.12	0.17	X	X	200	X	—
Mr. Misty® float	85	240	4	22	15	10	100	0.06	0.17	X	X	100	0.4	—
''Dilly''® bar	60	140	3	24	4	10	100	0.03	0.14	0.4	X	60	0.4	—
DQ sandwich	89	70	0	17	0	0	X	X	X	X	X	X	X	—
Mr Misty Kiss®	113	330	15	24	19	—	—	—	0.18	3.3	—	168	1.6	939
Brazier® cheese dog	128	330	13	25	20	—	—	0.15	0.23	3.9	11.0	86	2.0	939
Brazier® chili dog	99	273	11	23	15	—	—	0.12	0.15	2.6	11.0	75	1.5	868

Table 1. Nutritional Analyses of Fast Foods (*continued*)

	Weight (g)	Energy (cal)	Protein (g)	Carbo-hydrate (g)	Fat (g)	Cholesterol (mg)	Vitamin A (IU)	Thiamin (mg)	Riboflavin (mg)	Niacin (mg)	Vitamin C (mg)	Calcium (mg)	Iron (mg)	Sodium (mg)
DAIRY QUEEN® (*continued*)														
Fish sandwich	170	400	20	41	17	—	tr	0.15	0.26	3.0	tr	60	1.1	—
Fish sandwich with cheese	177	440	24	39	21	—	100	0.15	0.26	3.0	tr	150	0.4	—
Super Brazier® dog	182	518	20	41	30	—	tr	0.42	0.44	7.0	14.0	158	4.3	1552
Super Brazier® dog with cheese	203	593	26	43	36	—	—	0.43	0.48	8.1	14.0	297	4.4	1986
Super Brazier® chili dog	210	555	23	42	33	—	—	0.42	0.48	8.8	18.0	158	4.0	1640
Brazier® fries, small	71	200	2	25	10	—	tr	0.06	tr	0.8	3.6	tr	0.4	—
Brazier® fries, large	113	320	3	40	16	—	tr	0.09	0.03	1.2	4.8	tr	0.4	—
Brazier® onion rings	85	300	6	33	17	—	tr	0.09	tr	0.4	2.4	20	0.4	—

Source: International Dairy Queen, Inc., Minneapolis, Minnesota. Nutritional analysis by Raltech Scientific Services, Inc. (formerly WARF), Madison, Wisconsin. (Nutritional analysis not applicable in the state of Texas.)

	Weight (g)	Energy (cal)	Protein (g)	Carbo-hydrate (g)	Fat (g)	Cholesterol (mg)	Vitamin A (IU)	Thiamin (mg)	Riboflavin (mg)	Niacin (mg)	Vitamin C (mg)	Calcium (mg)	Iron (mg)	Sodium (mg)
JACK IN THE BOX®														
Hamburger	97	263	13	29	11	26	49	0.27	0.18	5.6	1.1	82	2.3	566
Cheeseburger	109	310	16	28	15	32	338	0.27	0.21	5.4	<1.1	172	2.6	877
Jumbo Jack® hamburger	246	551	28	45	29	80	246	0.47	0.34	11.6	3.7	134	4.5	1134
Jumbo Jack® hamburger with cheese	272	628	32	45	35	110	734	0.52	0.38	11.3	4.9	273	4.6	1666
Regular taco	83	189	8	15	11	22	356	0.07	0.08	1.8	<0.9	116	1.2	460
Super taco	146	285	12	20	17	37	599	0.10	0.12	2.8	1.6	196	1.9	968
Moby Jack® sandwich	141	455	17	38	26	56	240	0.30	0.21	4.5	1.4	167	1.7	837
Breakfast Jack® sandwich	121	301	18	28	13	182	442	0.41	0.47	5.1	3.4	177	2.5	1037
French fries	80	270	3	31	15	13	—	0.12	0.02	1.9	3.7	19	0.7	128
Onion rings	85	351	5	32	23	24	—	0.24	0.12	3.1	<1.2	26	1.4	318
Apple turnover	119	411	4	45	24	17	—	0.23	0.12	2.5	<1.2	11	1.4	352
Vanilla shake[a]	317	317	10	57	6	26	—	0.16	0.38	0.5	<3.2	349	0.2	229

JACK IN THE BOX® (continued)

	Weight (g)	Energy (cal)	Protein (g)	Carbo-hydrate (g)	Fat (g)	Cholesterol (mg)	Vitamin A (IU)	Thiamin (mg)	Riboflavin (mg)	Niacin (mg)	Vitamin C (mg)	Calcium (mg)	Iron (mg)	Sodium (mg)
Strawberry shake[a]	328	323	11	55	7	26	—	0.16	0.46	0.6	<3.3	371	0.6	241
Chocolate shake[a]	322	325	11	55	7	26	—	0.16	0.64	0.6	<3.2	348	0.7	270
Vanilla shake	314	342	10	54	9	36	440	0.16	0.47	0.5	3.5	349	0.4	263
Strawberry shake	328	380	11	63	10	33	426	0.16	0.62	0.5	<3.3	351	0.3	268
Chocolate shake	317	365	11	59	10	35	380	0.16	0.60	0.6	<3.2	350	1.2	294
Ham and cheese omelette	174	425	21	32	23	355	766	0.45	0.70	3.0	<1.7	260	4.0	975
Double cheese omelette	166	423	19	30	25	370	797	0.33	0.68	2.5	1.7	276	3.6	899
Ranchero style omelette	196	414	20	33	23	343	853	0.33	0.74	2.6	<2.0	278	3.8	1098
French toast	180	537	15	54	29	115	522	0.56	0.30	4.4	9.2	119	3.0	1130
Pancakes	232	626	16	79	27	87	488	0.63	0.44	4.6	<26.2	105	2.8	1670
Scrambled eggs	267	719	26	55	44	259	694	0.69	0.56	5.2	<12.8	257	5.0	1110

[a] Special formula for shakes sold in California, Arizona, Texas, and Washington. Source: Jack-in-the-Box, Foodmaker, Inc., San Diego, California. Nutritional analysis by Raltech Scientific Services, Inc. (formerly WARF), Madison, Wisconsin.

KENTUCKY FRIED CHICKEN®

	Weight (g)	Energy (cal)	Protein (g)	Carbo-hydrate (g)	Fat (g)	Cholesterol (mg)	Vitamin A (IU)	Thiamin (mg)	Riboflavin (mg)	Niacin (mg)	Vitamin C (mg)	Calcium (mg)	Iron (mg)	Sodium (mg)
Original Recipe® dinner[a]														
Wing and rib	322	603	30	48	32	133	25.5	0.22	0.19	10.0	36.6	—	—	—
Wing and thigh	341	661	33	48	38	172	25.5	0.24	0.27	8.4	36.6	—	—	—
Drum and thigh	346	643	35	46	35	180	25.5	0.25	0.32	8.5	36.6	—	—	—
Extra crispy dinner[a]														
Wing and rib	349	755	33	60	43	132	25.5	0.31	0.29	10.4	36.6	—	—	—
Wing and thigh	371	812	36	58	48	176	25.5	0.31	0.35	10.3	36.6	—	—	—
Drum and thigh	376	765	38	55	44	183	25.5	0.32	0.38	10.4	36.6	—	—	—
Mashed potatoes	85	64	2	12	1	0	<18	<0.01	0.02	0.8	4.9	—	—	—
Gravy	14	23	0	1	2	0	<3	0.00	0.01	0.1	<0.2	—	—	—
Cole slaw	91	122	1	13	8	7	—	—	—	—	—	—	—	—
Rolls	21	61	2	11	1	1	<5	0.10	0.04	1.0	0.3	—	—	—
Corn (5.5-inch ear)	135	169	5	31	3	X	162	0.12	0.07	1.2	2.6	—	—	—

[a] Includes two pieces of chicken, mashed potato and gravy, coleslaw, and roll. Source: Kentucky Fried Chicken, Inc., Louisville, Kentucky. Nutritional analysis by Raltech Scientific Services, Inc. (formerly WARF), Madison, Wisconsin.

Table 1. Nutritional Analyses of Fast Foods *(continued)*

	Weight (g)	Energy (cal)	Protein (g)	Carbo-hydrate (g)	Fat (g)	Cholesterol (mg)	Vitamin A (IU)	Thiamin (mg)	Riboflavin (mg)	Niacin (mg)	Vitamin C (mg)	Calcium (mg)	Iron (mg)	Sodium (mg)
LONG JOHN SILVER'S®														
Fish with batter (2 pc)	136	366	22	21	22	—	—	—	—	—	—	—	—	—
Fish with batter (3 pc)	207	549	32	32	32	—	—	—	—	—	—	—	—	—
Treasure Chest®	143	506	30	32	33	—	—	—	—	—	—	—	—	—
Chicken Planks® (4 pc)	166	457	27	35	23	—	—	—	—	—	—	—	—	—
Peg Legs® with batter (5 pc)	125	350	22	26	28	—	—	—	—	—	—	—	—	—
Ocean Scallop (6 pc)	120	283	11	30	13	—	—	—	—	—	—	—	—	—
Shrimp with batter (6 pc)	88	268	8	30	13	—	—	—	—	—	—	—	—	—
Breaded oysters (6 pc)	156	441	13	53	19	—	—	—	—	—	—	—	—	—
Breaded clams	142	617	18	61	34	—	—	—	—	—	—	—	—	—
Fish sandwich	193	337	22	49	31	—	—	—	—	—	—	—	—	—
French Fryes	85	288	4	33	16	—	—	—	—	—	—	—	—	—
Cole slaw	113	138	1	16	8	—	—	—	—	—	—	—	—	—
Corn on the cob (1 ear)	150	176	5	29	4	—	—	—	—	—	—	—	—	—
Hushpuppies (3)	45	153	3	20	7	—	—	—	—	—	—	—	—	—
Clam chowder (8 oz)	170	107	5	15	3	—	—	—	—	—	—	—	—	—

Source: Long John Silver's Food Shoppes, Lexington, Kentucky. Nutritional analysis by L. V. Packett, PhD, Department of Nutrition and Food Science, University of Kentucky.

	Weight (g)	Energy (cal)	Protein (g)	Carbo-hydrate (g)	Fat (g)	Cholesterol (mg)	Vitamin A (IU)	Thiamin (mg)	Riboflavin (mg)	Niacin (mg)	Vitamin C (mg)	Calcium (mg)	Iron (mg)	Sodium (mg)
McDONALD'S®														
Egg McMuffin®	138	327	19	31	15	229	97	0.47	0.44	3.8	<1.4	226	2.9	885
English muffin, buttered	63	186	5	30	5	13	164	0.28	0.49	2.6	0.8	117	1.5	318
Hotcakes with butter and syrup	214	500	8	94	10	47	257	0.26	0.36	2.3	4.7	103	2.2	1070
Sausage (pork)	53	206	9	tr	19	43	<32	0.27	0.11	2.1	0.5	16	0.8	615
Scrambled eggs	98	180	13	3	13	349	652	0.08	0.47	0.2	1.2	61	2.5	205
Hashbrown potatoes	55	125	2	14	7	7	<14	0.06	<0.01	0.8	4.1	5	0.4	325
Big Mac®	204	563	26	41	33	86	530	0.39	0.37	6.5	2.2	157	4.0	1010
Cheeseburger	115	307	15	30	14	37	345	0.25	0.23	3.8	1.6	132	2.4	767
Hamburger	102	255	12	30	10	25	82	0.25	0.18	4.0	1.7	51	2.3	520

McDONALDS® (continued)

	Weight (g)	Energy (cal)	Protein (g)	Carbo-hydrate (g)	Fat (g)	Cholesterol (mg)	Vitamin A (IU)	Thiamin (mg)	Riboflavin (mg)	Niacin (mg)	Vitamin C (mg)	Calcium (mg)	Iron (mg)	Sodium (mg)
Quarter Pounder®	166	424	24	33	22	67	133	0.32	0.28	6.5	<1.7	63	4.1	735
Quarter Pounder® with cheese	194	524	30	32	31	96	660	0.31	0.37	7.4	2.7	219	4.3	1236
Filet-O-Fish®	139	432	14	37	25	47	42	0.26	0.20	2.6	<1.4	93	1.7	781
Regular fries	68	220	3	26	12	9	<17	0.12	0.02	2.3	12.5	9	0.6	109
Apple pie	85	253	2	29	14	12	<34	0.02	0.02	0.2	<0.8	14	0.6	398
Cherry pie	88	260	2	32	14	13	114	0.03	0.02	0.4	<0.8	12	0.6	427
McDonaldland® cookies	67	308	4	49	11	10	<27	0.23	0.23	2.9	0.9	12	1.5	358
Chocolate shake	291	383	10	66	9	30	349	0.12	0.44	0.5	<2.9	320	0.8	300
Strawberry shake	290	362	9	62	9	32	377	0.12	0.44	0.4	4.1	322	0.2	207
Vanilla shake	291	352	9	60	8	31	349	0.12	0.70	0.3	3.2	329	0.2	201
Hot fudge sundae	164	310	7	46	11	18	230	0.07	0.31	1.1	2.5	215	0.6	175
Caramel sundae	165	328	7	53	10	26	279	0.07	0.31	1.0	3.6	200	0.2	195
Strawberry sundae	164	289	7	46	9	20	230	0.07	0.30	1.0	2.8	174	0.4	96

Source: McDonald's Corporation, Oak Brook, Illinois. Nutritional analysis by Raltech Scientific Services, Inc. (formerly WARF), Madison, Wisconsin.

TACO BELL®

	Weight (g)	Energy (cal)	Protein (g)	Carbo-hydrate (g)	Fat (g)	Cholesterol (mg)	Vitamin A (IU)	Thiamin (mg)	Riboflavin (mg)	Niacin (mg)	Vitamin C (mg)	Calcium (mg)	Iron (mg)	Sodium (mg)
Bean burrito	166	343	11	48	12	—	1657	0.37	0.22	2.2	15.2	98	2.8	272
Beef burrito	184	466	30	37	21	—	1675	0.30	0.39	7.0	15.2	83	4.6	327
Beefy tostada	184	291	19	21	15	—	3450	0.16	0.27	3.3	12.7	208	3.4	138
Bellbeefer®	123	221	15	23	7	—	2961	0.15	0.20	3.7	10.0	40	2.6	231
Bellbeefer® with cheese	137	278	19	23	12	—	3146	0.16	0.27	3.7	10.0	147	2.7	330
Burrito Supreme®	225	457	21	43	22	—	3462	0.33	0.35	4.7	16.0	121	3.8	367
Combination burrito	175	404	21	43	16	—	1666	0.34	0.31	4.6	15.2	91	3.7	300
Enchirito®	207	454	25	42	21	—	1178	0.31	0.37	4.7	9.5	259	3.8	1175
Pintos 'n cheese	158	168	11	21	5	—	3123	0.26	0.16	0.9	9.3	150	2.3	102
Taco	83	186	15	14	8	—	120	0.09	0.16	2.9	0.2	120	2.5	79
Tostada	138	179	9	25	6	—	3152	0.18	0.15	0.8	9.7	191	2.3	101

Sources: (1) *Menu Item Portions* (San Antonio, Texas: Taco Bell Co., July 1976); (2) Adams, C. F., *Nutritive value of American foods in common units*, in *Handbook No. 456* (Washington, D.C.: USDA Agricultural Research Service, November 1975); (3) Church, E. F., Church, H. N., eds. *Food Values of Portions Commonly Used*, 12th ed. (Philadelphia: J. B. Lippincott Co., 1975); (4) Valley Baptist Medical Center. Food Service Department, *Descriptions of Mexican-American Foods* (Fort Atkinson, Wisconsin: NASCO).

Table 1. Nutritional Analyses of Fast Foods (continued)

	Weight (g)	Energy (cal)	Protein (g)	Carbo-hydrate (g)	Fat (g)	Cholesterol (mg)	Vitamin A (IU)	Thiamin (mg)	Riboflavin (mg)	Niacin (mg)	Vitamin C (mg)	Calcium (mg)	Iron (mg)	Sodium (mg)
WENDY'S®														
Single hamburger	200	470	26	34	26	70	94	0.24	0.36	5.8	0.6	84	5.3	774
Double hamburger	285	670	44	34	40	125	128	0.43	0.54	10.6	1.5	138	8.2	980
Triple hamburger	360	850	65	33	51	205	220	0.47	0.68	14.7	2.0	104	10.7	1217
Single with cheese	240	580	33	34	34	90	221	0.38	0.43	6.3	0.7	228	5.4	1085
Double with cheese	325	800	50	41	48	155	439	0.49	0.75	11.4	2.3	177	10.2	1414
Triple with cheese	400	1040	72	35	68	225	472	0.80	0.84	15.1	3.4	371	10.9	1848
Chili	250	230	19	21	8	25	1188	0.22	0.25	3.4	2.9	83	4.4	1065
French fries	120	330	5	41	16	5	40	0.14	0.07	3.0	6.4	16	1.2	112
Frosty	250	390	9	54	16	45	355	0.20	0.60	X	0.7	270	0.9	247

Source: Wendy's International, Inc., Dublin, Ohio. Nutritional analysis by Medallion Laboratories, Minneapolis, Minnesota.

PIZZA HUT®a serving size: 2 slices of medium (13") pizza / 4 servings per pizza

	Weight (g)	Energy (cal)	Protein (g)	Carbo-hydrate (g)	Fat (g)	Cholesterol (mg)	Vitamin A (IU)	Thiamin (mg)	Riboflavin (mg)	Niacin (mg)	Vitamin C (mg)	Calcium (mg)	Iron (mg)	Sodium (mg)
THIN 'N CRISPY®														
Standard cheese	—	340	19	42	11	22	600	0.45	0.51	4	X	500	3.6	900
Superstyle cheese	—	410	26	45	14	30	750	0.53	0.60	4	X	800	3.6	1100
Standard pepperoni	—	370	19	42	15	27	700	0.45	0.43	4	X	400	3.2	1000
Superstyle pepperoni	—	430	23	43	19	34	800	0.60	0.43	5	X	550	3.6	1200
Standard pork with mushrooms	—	380	21	44	14	35	750	0.53	0.51	6	X	120	4.5	1200
Superstyle pork with mushrooms	—	450	26	46	19	40	750	0.60	0.60	6	1.2	150	6.3	1400
Supreme	—	400	21	44	17	13	750	0.68	0.51	6	2.4	400	4.5	1200
Super supreme	—	520	30	46	26	44	1100	1.05	0.68	8	3.6	550	5.4	1500
THICK 'N CHEWY®														
Standard cheese	—	390	24	53	10	18	800	0.75	1.19	8	X	600	4.5	800
Superstyle cheese	—	450	31	54	14	21	1000	0.83	0.68	8	1.2	950	4.5	1000
Standard pepperoni	—	450	25	52	16	21	1500	0.83	0.68	5	X	500	4.5	900
Superstyle pepperoni	—	490	27	52	20	24	1000	0.83	0.68	6	1.2	500	3.6	1200
Standard pork with mushrooms	—	430	27	53	14	21	1000	0.90	0.60	11	2.4	400	5.4	1000

	Weight (g)	Energy (cal)	Protein (g)	Carbo- hydrate (g)	Fat (g)	Cholesterol (mg)	Vitamin A (IU)	Thiamin (mg)	Riboflavin (mg)	Niacin (mg)	Vitamin C (mg)	Calcium (mg)	Iron (mg)	Sodium (mg)
PIZZA HUT® (continued)														
Superstyle pork														
with mushrooms	—	500	30	54	18	21	1000	0.90	0.68	12	2.4	550	6.3	1200
Supreme	—	480	29	52	18	24	1000	0.90	0.77	10	3.6	550	5.4	1000
Super supreme	—	590	34	55	26	38	1000	1.20	0.94	12	3.6	550	6.3	1400

a ''PIZZA HUT, THIN 'N CRISPY, and THICK 'N CHEWY are all registered trademarks of Pizza Hut, Inc., and are being used with permission.'' Source: Pizza Hut, Inc., Wichita, Kansas. Nutritional analysis determined in 1979 by Raltech Scientific Services, Inc. (formerly WARF), Madison, Wisconsin.

	Weight (g)	Energy (cal)	Protein (g)	Carbo- hydrate (g)	Fat (g)	Cholesterol (mg)	Vitamin A (IU)	Thiamin (mg)	Riboflavin (mg)	Niacin (mg)	Vitamin C (mg)	Calcium (mg)	Iron (mg)	Sodium (mg)
BEVERAGES														
Coffee[a]	180	2	tr	tr	tr	—	0	0	tr	0.5	0	4	0.2	2
Tea[a]	180	2	tr	—	tr	—	0	0	0.04	0.1	1	5	0.2	—
Orange juice	183	82	1	20	tr	—	366	0.17	0.02	0.6	82.4	17	0.2	2
Chocolate milk	250	213	9	28	9	—	330	0.08	0.40	0.3	3.0	278	0.5	118
Skim milk	245	88	9	13	tr	—	10	0.09	0.44	0.2	2.0	296	0.1	127
Whole milk	244	159	9	12	9	27	342	0.07	0.41	0.2	2.4	188	tr	122
Coca-Cola®	246	96	0	24	0	—	—	—	—	—	—	—	—	20[b]
Fanta® ginger ale	244	84	0	21	0	—	—	—	—	—	—	—	—	30[b]
Fanta® grape	247	114	0	29	0	—	—	—	—	—	—	—	—	21[b]
Fanta® orange	248	117	0	30	0	—	—	—	—	—	—	—	—	21[b]
Fanta® root beer	246	103	0	27	0	—	—	—	—	—	—	—	—	23[b]
Mr. Pibb®	245	95	0	25	0	—	—	—	—	—	—	—	—	23[b]
Mr. Pibb® without sugar	236	1	0	tr	0	—	—	—	—	—	—	—	—	37[b]
Sprite®	245	95	0	24	0	—	—	—	—	—	—	—	—	42[b]
Sprite® without sugar	236	3	0	0	0	—	—	—	—	—	—	—	—	42[b]
Tab®	236	tr	0	tr	0	—	—	—	—	—	—	—	—	30[b]
Fresca®	236	2	0	0	0	—	—	—	—	—	—	—	—	38

a 6-oz serving; all other data are for 8-oz serving.

b Value when bottling water with average sodium content (12 mg/8 oz) is used.

Sources: (1) Adams, C. F., Nutritive value of American foods in common units, in *Handbook No. 456* (Washington, D. C.: USDA Agricultural Research Service, November 1975); (2) The Coca-Cola Company, Atlanta, Georgia, January 1977; (3) *American Hospital Formulary Service* (Washington, D. C.: American Society of Hospital Pharmacists, March 1978) Section 28:20.

APPENDIX III

Food Units

gram = g. = 1/454 of a pound

milligram = mg. = 1/1000 of a gram

microgram = μg. = 1/1,000,000 of a gram

kilogram = kg. = 1000 grams = 2.2 pounds

100 cc = unit of volume about 4 ounces

1000 cc = slightly more than 1 quart

calorie = small calorie

Calorie = large calorie = 1000 small calories

1 ounce = 28.4 grams

100 grams = 3.5 ounces

IU = International Unit—designated for some vitamins based on an amount of different forms which has equivalent biological effects.

INDEX

†